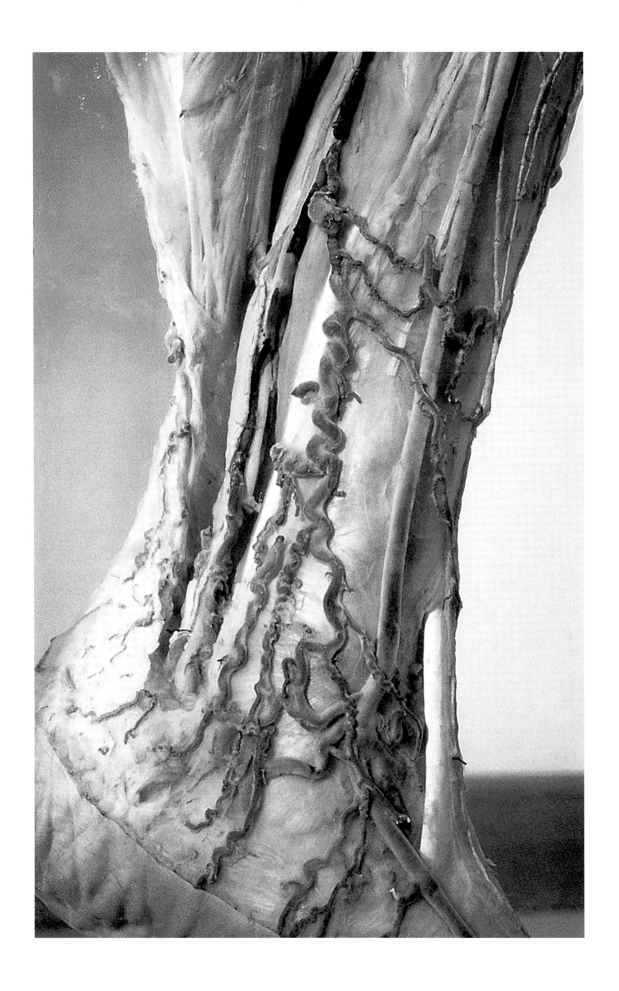

Leg Ulcers

Wounds cannot be healed without searching.
    Francis Bacon 1561–1626

It has been unpropitious to the improvement of the treatment of ulcers on the leg, that they have been universally admitted to be the most unmanageable cases which become the object of surgery; that they are cases in which the most eminent surgeons are too often known to fail in performing a cure; and therefore, bring no imputation of want of skill on those practitioners who happen to prove unsuccessful. This has led the younger part of the profession … to be too diffident of their own ability; to disparage success where so many have failed, and to follow a beaten track, in which so little advance has been made, that ulcers on the leg are not unjustly considered as the opprobrium of surgery.
    Sir Everard Home, *Practical Observations on the Treatment of Ulcers of the Leg*, London, Bulmer, 1801.

Leg Ulcers
Diagnosis and Management
Third edition

Edited by

David Negus MA DM MCh FRCS(Eng.)
Emeritus Consultant Surgeon, University Hospital,
Lewisham, London; and Honorary Senior Lecturer,
Guy's, King's and St Thomas' School of Medicine,
London, UK

Philip D. Coleridge Smith MA DM FRCS
Consultant Vascular Surgeon and Reader in Surgery,
UCL Medical School, The Middlesex Hospital,
London, UK

John J. Bergan MD FACS(Hon) FRCS(Eng.)
Professor of Surgery, University of California,
San Diego, California;
Scripps Memorial Hospital,
La Jolla; and Vein Institute of La Jolla,
California, USA

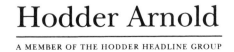

A MEMBER OF THE HODDER HEADLINE GROUP

First published in Great Britain in 2005 by
Hodder Education, a member of the Hodder Headline Group,
338 Euston Road, London NW1 3BH

http://www.hoddereducation.com

Distributed in the United States of America by
Oxford University Press Inc.,
198 Madison Avenue, New York, NY10016
Oxford is a registered trademark of Oxford University Press

Whilst the advice and information in this book are believed to be true and
accurate at the date of going to press, neither the author[s] nor the publisher
can accept any legal responsibility or liability for any errors or omissions
that may be made. In particular, (but without limiting the generality of the
preceding disclaimer) every effort has been made to check drug dosages;
however it is still possible that errors have been missed. Furthermore,
dosage schedules are constantly being revised and new side-effects
recognized. For these reasons the reader is strongly urged to consult the
drug companies' printed instructions before administering any of the drugs
recommended in this book.

British Library Cataloguing in Publication Data
A catalogue record for this book is available from the British Library

Library of Congress Cataloging-in-Publication Data
A catalog record for this book is available from the Library of Congress

ISBN-10   0 340 81013 0
ISBN-13   978 0 340 81013 2

1 2 3 4 5 6 7 8 9 10

Commissioning Editor: Sarah Burrows
Project Editor: Naomi Wilkinson
Production Controller: Joanna Walker
Cover Design: Georgina Hewitt
Index: Lisa Footitt

Typeset in 10/12 Minion by Charon Tec Pvt. Ltd, Chennai
www.charontec.com
Printed and bound in the UK by CPI Bath

What do you think about this book? Or any other Hodder Arnold
title? Please visit our website at www.hoddereducation.com

Contents

Contributors

John J. Bergan MD FACS Hon. FRCS (Eng.)
Professor of Surgery,
University of California, San Diego;
Scripps Memorial Hospital, La Jolla; and
Vein Institute of La Jolla,
California, USA

David C. Berridge DM FRCS (Ed., Eng.)
Consultant Vascular Surgeon,
St James's University Hospital,
Leeds, UK

Jayne Chambers
Melbourne Vascular Ultrasound,
Epworth Hospital,
Melbourne, Australia

Amy Clough
Melbourne Vascular Ultrasound,
Epworth Hospital,
Melbourne, Australia

Philip D. Coleridge Smith DM FRCS
Consultant Vascular Surgeon and Reader in Surgery,
UCL Medical School,
The Middlesex Hospital,
London, UK

Bo Eklof MD PhD
Clinical Professor Emeritus,
University of Lund,
Helsingborg,
Sweden

Peter J. Franks
Professor of Health Sciences,
Centre for Research & Implementation of Clinical Practice,
Faculty of Health & Human Sciences,
Thames Valley University,
London, UK

Robert Gardiner BPharm MRPharmS
STD Pharmaceutical Products Ltd,
Hereford, UK

Peter Gloviczki MD
Professor of Surgery, Mayo Clinic College of Medicine
Chair, Division of Vascular Surgery; and
Director, Gonda Vascular Center,
Mayo Clinic and Mayo Foundation,
Rochester, MN, USA

Manju Kalra MBBS
Assistant Professor of Surgery,
Mayo Clinic College of Medicine,
Rochester, MN, USA

Robert L. Kistner MD
Straub Clinic & Hospital,
Honolulu, HI, USA

Fedor Lurie MD PhD
Straub Foundations,
Honolulu, HI, USA

S. J. Machin
Professor of Haematology,
Haemostasis Research Unit,
University College Hospital London,
Middlesex Hospital,
London, UK

M. Mathias
Research Fellow,
Haemostasis Research Unit,
University College Hospital London,
Middlesex Hospital,
London, UK

Christine J. Moffatt
Professor of Nursing,
Centre for Research & Implementation of Clinical Practice,
Faculty of Health & Human Sciences,
Thames Valley University,
London, UK

Kenneth Myers
Melbourne Vascular Ultrasound,
Epworth Hospital and Monash Medical Centre,
Melbourne, Australia

Peter Neglén MD PhD
Vascular Surgeon,
River Oaks Hospital,
Jackson, Mississippi, USA

David Negus MA DM MCh FRCS
Membre d'Honeur, Société Française de Phlebologie
Emeritus Consultant Surgeon,
University Hospital, Lewisham; and
Honorary Senior Lecturer,
Guy's, King's and St Thomas' School of Medicine,
London, UK

Hugo Partsch MD
Professor of Dermatology,
Emeritus Head of the Dermatological Department of
the Wilhelminenspital,
Vienna, Austria

Luigi Pascarella MD
Fellow, Whitaker Institute of Biomedical Engineering,
Department of Bioengineering,
Jacobs School of Engineering,
University of California, San Diego,
La Jolla, CA, USA

Michelle Rodeh
Melbourne Vascular Ultrasound,
Epworth Hospital,
Melbourne, Australia

S. S. Rose MB Chj.B Hons FRCS (Hons)
Consultant Vascular Surgeon (Retired),
University Hospital of South Manchester,
Manchester, UK

Geert W. Schmid Schönbein PhD
Professor, Whitaker Institute of Biomedical Engineering,
Department of Bioengineering,
Jacobs School of Engineering,
University of California, San Diego,
La Jolla, CA, USA

Philipp A. Stalder MD
Specialist Registrar in Vascular Surgery,
St James's University Hospital,
Leeds, UK

Peter R. Taylor MA MB MChir FRCS
Department of Vascular Surgery,
St Thomas' Hospital,
London, UK

Huw Walters
Department of Radiology,
King's College Hospital,
London, UK

Foreword

In the field of phlebology, the most expensive complication of it all is the catastrophe of venous ulceration; it is expensive in terms of whichever parameter is considered: economic, time, effort and, not least, quality of life. Progress in the understanding of the fundamentals of this dreaded complication, the outcome of uncontrolled venous hypertension, and the strict assessment of methods and results, have led to rational scientific management. The important consideration nowadays is not so much how to heal a venous ulcer but how to prevent its recurrence. This has become the challenge, bearing in mind that for various reasons, the underlying venous hypertension often cannot be corrected surgically and treatment has to rely upon acceptable and effective external methods of control. The role of pharmacological treatment is still being established.

It is a compliment to David Negus and confirmation of the quality, relevance and success of his previous editions that the publishers have asked him to produce a new edition of *Leg Ulcers*.

As the co-editors state in the preface to this third edition of the book: 'the manifold advances ... have demanded that this become a multi-authored text'. David Negus, single editor of the previous editions, and his two wisely-chosen co-editors, Philip Coleridge Smith and John Bergan, are to be warmly congratulated on having responded to the demand for a third edition in this way, and to have produced a text of such quality on all aspects of venous ulceration.

With its reasonable size, numerous and relevant illustrations, and clear and uniform style, this book is easy reading. How pleasant and appropriate it is to be greeted in the very first illustration by such a splendid and imposing photograph of Virchow, father-figure of venous pathology!

Most chapters have been rewritten or updated and the new venous anatomical nomenclature has been adopted. Completely new chapters have been added on venous thrombosis, microcirculation, functional tests, compression therapy, skin grafting, recent advances in the surgery of superficial venous insufficiency, sclerotherapy and echosclerotherapy, surgery of the perforating veins, treatment of venous obstruction and recurrent ulceration together with new texts on pharmacology and topical agents – all written by experts, and thus highly relevant and informative.

This new edition is intended to be a text of reference for the initiated rather than a basic textbook on the subject and in this it is entirely successful. It will surely become compulsory reading for all those concerned with the management of chronic venous disorders.

Georges Jantet
Past President, Union Internationale de Phlébologie
Past President, Venous Forum of the Royal Society
of Medicine, London, UK

Preface

In ancient times, treatment of leg ulcers was an important part of surgical practice. Witness the lasting contributions of Ambroise Paré. Even into the middle of the twentieth century, leg ulcers were an important part of surgical research and patient care. As modern vascular surgery dawned, important observations on causation of leg ulcer in Boston by Linton and in London by Cockett stirred surgical imagination. The subsequent introduction of safe, reliable anesthesia, safe blood transfusions, the development of antibiotics and the perfection of anticoagulation allowed surgeons to enter the no-man's land of arterial repair. Vascular operations were no longer restricted to varicose vein surgery, sympathectomy and amputation. Direct surgery of atherosclerosis, total excision of aneurysms with confidence in subsequent arterial reconstruction attracted a new generation of young and aggressive surgeons.

Interest in varicose veins languished just as belief in the powers of sympathectomy vanished. The heavy workload of arterial reconstructive surgery in an ever-aging population left vascular surgeons little time for the treatment of leg ulcers. Diagnosis became largely relegated to dermatologists and treatment to nurses.

Just as surgical interest in leg ulcers waned, new tools of patient investigation emerged. Physiological investigation developed beyond non-specific venous pressure determination to precise delineation of venous abnormalities in the ulcerated limb. Ultrasound imaging was introduced and has now largely replaced phlebography. Other imaging methods became available and the new instrumentation confirmed that leg ulcers were not exclusively in the province of the post-phlebitic limb but that many were caused by easily repairable superficial venous incompetence, as had been originally observed by John Homans of Boston in 1916.

Some surgical interest in venous abnormalities persisted during the last half of the twentieth century. At the turn of the century, the place of valve repair became defined more clearly,

the limitations of the bypass principle became recognized, and the reopening of occluded venous segments using interventional radiological techniques showed promise. Investigations into the molecular biology of venous insufficiency and valve destruction and the causes of venous-related dermatitis, lipodermatosclerosis and skin breakdown hinted at pharmacological manipulation to ease the burdens of the chronic, intractable and recurrent venous ulcer.

As these many venous-related events transpired, this volume passed through infancy and adolescence marked by the first and second editions. Now, this third edition shows the promise of maturity, fortified with new information, new tools and the need for expert and efficient care. Many of the individuals who contributed to the last quarter century's advances in venous diagnosis and new methods of venous care of have now contributed to this new volume. The manifold advances in all aspects of venous investigations and patient care have demanded that this become a multi-authored text.

This book is therefore no longer 'a practical guide to management' but a collection of expert contributions and the subtitle 'diagnosis and management' seems more appropriate. A gratifying number of distinguished specialist authors, from many countries, accepted our invitation and have together created a work of which they can be proud. We are most grateful to each and to all of them.

Without the patience and efficiency of the staff of Hodder Arnold, it is doubtful if our task would have been completed and we are most grateful for their help.

The international authorship of this volume reflects the widespread growth of interest in the treatment of leg ulcers. This growth has been much helped by the Union Internationale de Phlébologie, whose conferences are increasingly well attended, and we are honored that Dr Georges Jantet, immediate past president, has provided the foreword.

The Editors

Sources of illustrations

Permission to reproduce illustrations from the following authors, publishers and institutions in Chapters 1, 3, 8 and 25 is gratefully acknowledged.

Figure 1.2: The Wellcome Institute Library, London.

Plate 3.1: The late Harold Dodd Ch.M., FRCS.

Frontispiece, Figures 3.2, 3.6: The Wellcome Museum of Anatomy, by kind permission of The President and Council of the Royal College of Surgeons of England.

Plates 8.3, 8.4, 8.5, 13.1: Mark Tyrrell Ph.D., FRCS, Vascular Surgeon, Kent and Sussex Hospital, Tunbridge Wells, Kent, UK.

Figure 25.2: Segar Design, Nottingham, UK.

Historical background

DAVID NEGUS

VENOUS DISORDERS

The first written reference to veins is probably in the Ebers papyrus, written 1550 BC, which notes certain 'serpentine windings' thought to be varicose veins. The oldest known illustration is a votive tablet in Athens dated the fourth century BC, showing the medial side of a massive leg with what appears to be a varicose vein.[1]

The first known mention of leg ulcers is by Hippocrates (460–377 BC)[2], who noted the association between varicose veins and ulceration, and recommended that patients with ulcers in the leg should avoid standing. He introduced 'puncturing and bandaging' for the treatment of leg ulcers and associated varicose veins, and advocated that superficial varices should not be incised, as ulcers often resulted from this.

A Roman physician, Aurelius Cornelius Celsus (25 BC–50 AD)[3] advised the use of plasters and linen bandages in the treatment of ulcers and also treated varicose veins by avulsion and cauterization. These procedures were also described by the later Roman physicians Claudius Galen (130–200 AD)[4] and Aetios of Amida (502–574 AD)[5].

During the Dark Ages, those with unsightly and ulcerated legs were denied even simple remedies. Haly, son of Abbas (d. 994),[6] believed that bandaging varicose legs would reintroduce 'black bile' into the circulation and lead to madness. In the tenth century,[7] Avicenna believed that to cure an ulcer was to prevent the efflux of dangerous humors and this widely-held belief persisted until the eighteenth century, when it was expounded by Le Dran in France in 1731[8] and by Heister (but only in elderly patients) in 1739.[9]

However, as early as the sixteenth century there were some surgeons who believed in healing leg ulcers and who recognized the need to control local venous hypertension in order to do so. Ambroise Paré (1510–1590) is well recognized for his work in improving the treatment of war injuries. His contributions to the healing of leg ulcers are equally important.[10] After being taken prisoner at the siege of Hesdin in 1553, he was summoned to attend Lord Vaudeville, Governor of Graveline, who had suffered from a chronic leg ulcer for 6 or 7 years. After debriding the ulcer and excising the indurated edge, Paré applied a dressing soaked in plantain juice and bandaged the leg from foot to knee. His account continues '… and do not forget to put a little compress on the varicose vein to prevent the reflux of liquid to the said ulcer'. He advised bed rest as recommended by Hippocrates and the dressings were changed once daily (and not more frequently, as had been done previously). The ulcer was almost completely healed 2 weeks later.

During the seventeenth century, the humoral theory gradually began to lose ground and a new confidence was exhibited in the treatment of leg ulcers. Richard Wiseman described a laced stocking in 1676[11] and its use was later recommended by Benjamin Bell (1779).[12] Wiseman made another significant contribution: he described the formation of a blood coagulum and stated that this was due to stagnation 'by reason of dependence of the part or some other pressure on the vessel'. He mentions pregnancy and riding horses as contributory causes.

John Hunter (1775)[13] described the association of thrombosis and phlebitis, both in man after venesection and in horses which had been bled by their ostlers. His specimens illustrate venous and perivenous inflammation, although the prevalence of infection at that time makes it likely this was bacterial in origin rather than an aseptic thrombophlebitis. He also showed interest in leg ulcers and wrote: 'The sores of poor people are often in a bad condition from bad living and are often healed by rest in a horizontal position, fresh provisions and warmth in hospitals, and the change is generally very speedy.'

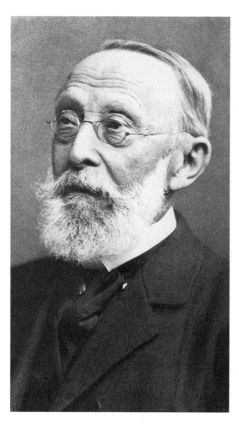

Figure 1.1 *Rudolph Virchow, 1821–1902, Professor of Pathological Anatomy, University of Würzburg, Germany.*

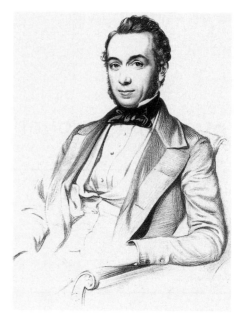

Figure 1.2 *John Gay, 1812(13)–1885, surgeon, The Royal Northern Hospital, London. (From the original lithograph of 1853 by TH Maguire in the Wellcome Institute Library, London.)*

The next century saw significant advances in knowledge of the processes involved in thrombosis. Hewson described a 'coagulable lymph' in 1772[14] and phlebitis and periphlebitic inflammation were described by Carl Rokitansky in 1852.[15] In 1860, Rudolph Virchow (Fig. 1.1)[16] described the association between thrombosis in the legs and emboli in the lungs, and in subsequent publications he introduced the term 'fibrinogen' and also his famous triad of the causes of thrombosis (stasis, endothelial damage and changes in coagulability). Von Strauch observed venous thrombosis following surgical operation in 1894[17] and this relationship was studied by Cordiér in 1905,[18] who found a 2 percent incidence of phlebitis following abdominal and pelvic operations in a study of 232 cases.

During the eighteenth century it began to be realized that leg ulcers were not necessarily accompanied by visible varicose veins. Many eighteenth-century writers, including Bell (1779),[12] Baynton (1797)[19] and Whately (1799),[20] make no reference to varicose veins as a cause of ulceration, although Benjamin Brodie (1846)[21] still held to the varicose theory of ulceration. Baynton introduced paste bandaging and Brodie also used plaster and bandages to heal ulcers and recognized that some dressings caused sensitivity reactions.

In 1868 John Gay (Fig. 1.2) described the calf and ankle perforating veins,[22] which had previously been illustrated by von Loder, a Russian anatomist, in 1803.[23] Gay also recorded the fact that ulcers could occur in the absence of varicose veins if there had been post-thrombotic damage to the deep veins, and introduced the term 'venous ulcer'. He described clot formation and post-thrombotic recanalization. His observations were fully supported by those of Spender (1868), who worked separately and reached the same conclusions from his own work.[24] Gay was also the first to describe compression of the left common iliac vein as it passes beneath the right common iliac artery, and also correctly described the subfascial course of the proximal short saphenous vein in the upper one-third of the calf which, until recently, has been incorrectly described in most anatomical textbooks.

Gay's work seems to have been overlooked by early twentieth-century writers until, in 1916, John Homans (Fig. 1.3)[25] introduced the title 'post-phlebitic syndrome'. Homans divided ulcers into those associated with varicose veins of the leg, easily cured by removal of these veins, and post-phlebitic ulcers, 'rapid in development, always intractable to palliative treatment, generally incurable by the removal of varicose veins alone and must be excised to be cured'. Homans described valve destruction by the organization of thrombus. Later, in 1928,[26] he found that nearly all severe post-phlebitic cases had at some time had a 'milk leg' or iliofemoral venous thrombosis.

In 1927, Franklin[27] published an historical survey of the discovery of valves in veins and this stimulated interest in venous physiology and pathology. In his monograph published in 1931, Turner Warwick[28] reviewed the history of the subject and described the 'bleed back' test which is still used at operation to test the competence of valves in the perforating veins. In 1937, Edwards and Edwards[29] showed that venous thrombosis destroyed valves but was frequently followed by recanalization. Also in 1937 the use of heparin was first described by Murray *et al.*[30]

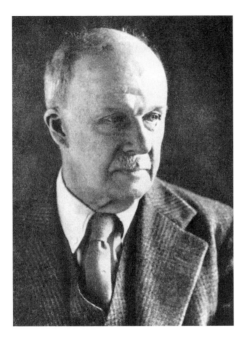

Figure 1.3 *John Homans, 1877–1954, Clinical Professor of Surgery, Harvard University Medical School, USA.*

In 1930 Crafoord[31] described the use of heparin in the treatment of postoperative deep vein thrombosis, and in 1941 Crafoord and Jorpes[32] used heparin as a prophylactic drug in the prevention of deep vein thrombosis. In 1950 the use of low doses of heparin for the prevention of deep vein thrombosis was suggested by De Takats,[33] and further advances in this method of prophylaxis have been much assisted by advances in phlebography and by the introduction of the isotope-labelled fibrinogen uptake method of detecting deep vein thrombosis. De Takats' work has been continued in numerous studies, of which the largest was the International Multicentre Trial (1974).[34]

Clinical phlebography was described by Dos Santos in 1938,[35] based on Ratschow's introduction of water-soluble X-ray contrast material in 1930.[36] Dos Santos's technique was subsequently used by Gunnar Bauer in Sweden in 1940[37] to study the effect of anticoagulation on deep vein thrombosis, and in 1942[38] he undertook an important phlebographic study of the post-thrombotic syndrome. The development, in 1984,[39] of low osmolality, non-ionic contrast media, which are virtually non-thrombogenic, has much improved the safety and applicability of phlebography.

In 1960 Hobbs and Davis[40] described the detection of venous thrombi with radioisotopes and this was subsequently validated by comparison with phlebography in clinical studies by Flanc *et al.*[41] and Negus *et al.*[42] in 1968. Phlebography and the ^{125}I-fibrinogen uptake technique stimulated a flood of research into the prevention of deep vein thrombosis. This technique allowed the development of much of our present knowledge of factors responsible for venous thrombosis. The development of duplex ultrasonography has superseded this technique, which is now no longer in use.

The ligation of incompetent perforating veins had been practiced by some surgeons since Gay's description in 1868, but many must have been discouraged from treating venous ulcers in this way by the difficulty of dissection and finding the offending veins in indurated subcutaneous tissue affected by lipodermatosclerosis. A significant advance was made by Linton of Boston in 1938,[43] who described the subfascial ligation of incompetent perforating veins. In 1953, Cockett and Elgin Jones[44] undertook careful cadaver dissections to obtain precise information on the sites of the calf and ankle perforating veins. They introduced the phrase 'ankle blow-out syndrome'. A modification of Linton's operation was introduced in 1964 by Harold Dodd,[45] who showed that improved skin healing could be obtained by placing the incision for subfascial ligation posteromedially rather than through medial liposclerotic skin. These authors stimulated a wave of interest in perforating vein ligation in the treatment of venous ulceration, and between 1961 and 1971 a number of carefully conducted follow-up studies of this operation were reported. Taking these together, over 1000 patients were followed up for between 5 and 9 years, with a success rate of around 90 percent.[46–51] However, in the subsequent 10 years, disappointing results in patients with deep venous incompetence as well as perforating vein incompetence led to a widespread reluctance to undertake perforating vein ligation,[52–57] and many surgeons advised against any attempt at surgical treatment for these patients, relying on elastic compression hosiery alone. In an attempt to reduce the morbidity of operations to ligate perforating veins, subfascial endoscopic perforator vein surgery (SEPS) has been introduced. This has been found greatly to reduce the morbidity of perforating vein ligation since the leg incision is made remote from the liposclerotic skin.[58] Debate continues over the role of this operation and in which patients it should be used.[59]

In 1954, Warren and Thayer[60] described the use of the saphenous vein for bypassing a post-thrombotic occlusion of the superficial femoral vein and this operation was further developed by Husni in 1970.[61] Iliac vein occlusion was first similarly treated by femorofemoral bypass by Palma *et al.* in 1958,[62,63] and these operations have been followed by a number of other ingenious procedures to improve venous function.

At the same time as these advances in diagnosis and treatment, physiological tests of venous function have been developed and are now invaluable in the investigation of the post-thrombotic syndrome and other venous disorders. Venous pressure in the dorsal veins of the foot was first measured by Beecher *et al.* in 1936[64] and has since been used by many workers.[65–69] Early measurements were made using a saline manometer; the subsequent introduction of the more sophisticated pressure transducer has allowed precise analysis of pressure changes.[70]

The introduction of the ultrasonic Doppler-shift velocity meter by Satomura and Kanecko in 1960[71] was the first of the new non-invasive measurement techniques. Venous disorders can now be investigated by a variety of non-invasive methods which provide an accurate evaluation of venous function without any patient discomfort. The most useful is the colour-coded Duplex scanner which is now used almost universally in the investigation and management of venous disorders in the lower limb.

ISCHEMIC ULCERATION

As many leg ulcers are now ischemic in origin, this account would be incomplete without including the more important milestones in the investigation and treatment of arterial disease. Arteriography was first described by Brooks in 1924[72] and was followed by Reynaldo Dos Santos's introduction of translumbar aortography in 1929.[73] The evaluation of occlusive arterial disease by Doppler ultrasound was introduced by Strandness and his colleagues in 1966,[74] and this is now an essential investigation in distinguishing between ischemic and venous ulceration. More recently, computed tomography (CT) scanning and magnetic resonance imaging (MRI) have also become available for the investigation of arterial disease. Now that direct arterial surgery is widely available for the treatment of peripheral arterial disease, it is often forgotten that, until the introduction of heparin in 1937, direct arterial surgery was not possible, and lumbar sympathectomy was the only available option. In 1913, Leriche[75] described the effect of peri-arterial sympathectomy in increasing peripheral blood flow and this was followed in 1924 by Hunter and Royles' introduction of lumbar sympathectomy in the treatment of Raynaud's disease.[75] Surgical lumbar sympathectomy has now been largely superseded by paravertebral injection of the lumbar sympathetic ganglia, first described by Labat in 1924.[75]

The introduction of heparin in 1937 encouraged further attempts at direct arterial surgery and embolectomy was frequently performed. While working with Leriche, J. Cid Dos Santos removed some atheromatous intima while performing an embolectomy. In spite of this 'mistake', the artery remained patent.[76] Dos Santos[77] and Leriche were encouraged by this success to remove atherosclerotic intima from chronically occluded arteries, the operation of thromboendarterectomy. In the 1950s and 1960s, the long endarterectomy became the standard procedure for atherosclerotic arterial occlusions. An additional technical advance was Edwards' introduction of the patch graft to widen the artery and maintain full flow.[78]

Following Kunlin's introduction of the reversed saphenous vein graft in 1951,[79] endarterectomy was gradually superseded by this operation. Occlusions of the aorta and iliac arteries were initially treated by arterial homografts, with generally poor results, and when synthetic grafts such as crimped Dacron (Terylene) became available,[80] homograft transplantation was abandoned. A number of other synthetic grafts were developed, of which the expanded polytetrafluoroethylene (PTFE)[81] Gortex graft remains the most popular. Short occlusive lesions can now be treated by balloon angioplasty (percutaneous transluminal angioplasty, PTA), which was developed by Gruntzig in 1974,[82] and this technique is often successful in treating ischemic ulceration or relieving rest pain and impending gangrene in elderly patients considered unfit for direct arterial surgery.

In addition to these technical advances, there have been some encouraging developments in the drug treatment of peripheral vascular disease, particularly the introduction of the vasoactive prostaglandins.

REFERENCES

1. Majno G. *The Healing Hand: Man and Wound in the Ancient World.* Cambridge: Harvard University Press, 1975; 90.
2. Hippocrates. De ulceribus and de carnibus. In: Adams F, ed. *The Genuine Works of Hippocrates.* London: Sydenham Society, 1849.
3. Celsus A. C. *Medicine (in Eight Books)* (translated by James Grieve; revised by George Futvoye). London: Renshaw, 1838.
4. Galen C. *Ad scripti libri*, Venice, Vincentium Valgressium, 1562 p. 34, quoted by Anning ST. In: Dodd H, Cockett FB, eds. *The Pathology and Surgery of the Veins of the Lower Limb.* Edinburgh: Churchill Livingstone, 1976; 4.
5. Aetios of Amida, Ricci JV (translator). *Cornarius* (publ. 1542). Philadelphia: Blakeston, 1950.
6. Haly filius Abbas, Michaele of Capella (translator – from Arabic into Latin) (1523). Quoted by Anning ST. In: Dodd H, Cockett FB, eds. *The Pathology and Surgery of the Veins of the Lower Limb*, 2nd edn. Edinburgh: Churchill Livingstone, 1976.
7. Avicenna. *De ulceribus, Liber IV.* Quoted by Underwood M. In: *A Treatise on Ulcers of the Legs*, London: Matthews, 1783.
8. Le Dran HF. *Observations de Chirurgie*, Vol. 1. Paris: Osmont, 1731.
9. Heister L. *A General System of Surgery* (author's preface: Helmstaadt, 1739). London: Whiston, Innys, Davis, Clarke, Mansby, Cox, Whiston, 1748.
10. Ouvry PA, Laruelle PE, Ouvry PAG. La Traitment d'un Ulcere Variqueux par Ambroise Paré. *Phlebologie* 2001; **3**: 323–6.
11. Wiseman R. *Several Chirurgical Treatises.* London: Wilthoe and Knapton, 1676.
12. Bell B. *Treatise on the Theory and Management of Ulcers etc.* Edinburgh: C Elliot, 1779.
13. Hunter J. Observation on the inflammation of the internal coats of veins (1775). In: Palmer JI, ed. *The Works of John Hunter.* London: Longman, Rees, Orme, Green and Longman, 1837; 581–6.
14. Hewson W. *Experimental Enquiries. Part I. An Enquiry into the Properties of Blood.* London: Cadell, 1772.
15. Rokitansky C, Gay GE (translator). *A Manual of Pathological Anatomy.* London: Sydenham Society, 1852; 336.
16. Virchow R. *Cellular Pathology as Based upon Physiological and Pathological Histology.* London: Churchill, 1860.
17. Von Strauch N. Über Venenthrombose der Unteren Extremitäten nach Köliotomien bei Beckenhochlagerung und Äthernarkose. *Zentralbl Gynäkol* 1894; **18**: 304–6.
18. Cordiér AN. Phlebitis following abdominal and pelvic operations. *J Am Med Assoc* 1905; **45**: 1792–6.
19. Baynton T. *Descriptive Account of New Method of Treating Old Ulcers of the Legs.* Bristol: Biggs, 1797.
20. Whately T. *Practical Observations on the Cure of Wounds and Ulcers of the Legs Without Rest.* London: Cadell and Davies, 1799.

21. Brodie B. *Lectures Illustrative of Various Subjects in Pathology and Surgery*. London: Longmans, 1846; 158.

22. Gay J. On varicose disease of the lower extremities and its allied disorders. *Lettsomian Lectures of 1867*. London: Churchill, 1868.

23. Von Loder JC. *Anatomische Tafeln*. Weimar: Landes Industrien Comptoir 1803.

24. Spender JK. *A Manual of the Pathology and Treatment of Ulcers and Cutaneous Diseases of the Lower Limbs*, London: Churchill, 1868.

25. Homans J. The operative treatment of varicose veins and ulcers, based on a classification of these lesions. *Surg Gynecol Obstet* 1916; **22**: 143–58.

26. Homans J. Thrombophlebitis of the lower extremities. *Ann Surg* 1928; **87**: 641–51.

27. Franklin KJ. The valves in veins. An historical survey. *Proc R Soc Med* (Section of History of Medicine) 1927; **21**: 1–33.

28. Warwick WT. *The Rational Treatment of Varicose Veins and Varicocele*, London: Faber, 1931.

29. Edwards FA, Edwards JE. The effect of thrombophlebitis on the venous valves. *Surg Gynecol Obstet* 1937; **65**: 310–20.

30. Murray DWG, Jaques LB, Perrett TS, Best CH. Heparin and the thrombosis of veins following injury. *Surgery* 1937; **ii**: 163–87.

31. Crafoord C. Heparin and post-operative thrombosis. *Acta Chir Scand* 1939; **82**: 319–35.

32. Crafoord C, Jorpes E. Heparin as a prophylactic against thrombosis. *J Am Med Assoc* 1941; **116**: 2831–5.

33. De Takats G. Anticoagulant therapy in surgery. *J Am Med Assoc* 1950; **142**: 527–34.

34. International Multicentre Trial. Heparin versus dextran in the prevention of deep vein thrombosis. *Lancet* 1974; **ii**: 118–20.

35. Dos Santos JC. La phlebographie directe. Conception, technique, premiers resultats. *J Int Chir* 1938; **3**: 625–69.

36. Ratschow M. Euroselektan in der Vasographie. Unter spezieller Berucksichtigung der Varikographie. *Fortsch Rontgenstr* 1930; **42**: 37.

37. Bauer G. A venographic study of thromboembolic patients. *Acta Chir Scand* 1940; **84**: suppl. 61.

38. Bauer G. A roentgenological and clinical study of the sequels of thrombosis. *Acta Chir Scand* 1942; **86**: suppl. 74.

39. Lea Thomas M, Biggs GM. Low osmolality contrast media for phlebography. *Int Angiol* 1984; **3**: 73–6.

40. Hobbs JT, Davis JWL. Detection of venous thrombosis with ^{131}I-labelled fibrinogen in the rabbit. *Lancet* 1960; **ii**: 134–5.

41. Flanc C, Kakkar VV, Clark MB. The detection of venous thrombosis of the legs using ^{125}I-labelled fibrinogen. *Br J Surg* 1968; **55**: 742–7.

42. Negus D, Pinto DJ, Le Quesne LP, Brown N, Chapman H. ^{125}I-labelled fibrinogen in the diagnosis of deep vein thrombosis and its correlation with phlebography. *Br J Surg* 1968; **55**: 835–9.

43. Linton RR. The communicating veins of the lower leg and the operative technique for their ligation. *Ann Surg* 1938; **107**: 582–93.

44. Cockett FB, Elgin Jones DE. The ankle blow-out syndrome. A new approach to the venous ulcer problem. *Lancet* 1953; **i**: 17–23.

45. Dodd H. The diagnosis and ligation of incompetent perforating veins. *Ann R Coll Surg Engl* 1964; **34**: 186–96.

46. Burnley JJ, Krausers Trasser ES. Chronic venous insufficiency of the lower extremities. *Surgery* 1961; **49**: 48–58.

47. Hansson LO. Venous ulcers of the lower limb. *Acta Chir Scand* 1964; **128**: 269–77.

48. Bertelsen S, Gammelgaard A. Surgical treatment of post-thrombotic leg ulcers. *J Cardiovasc Surg* 1965; **6**: 452–5.

49. Silver D, Gleysteen JJ, Rhodes GR *et al.* Surgical treatment of the refractory post-thrombotic ulcers. *Arch Surg* 1971; **103**: 554–60.

50. Field P, Van Boxall P. The role of the Linton flap procedure on the management of stasis dermatitis and ulceration in the lower limbs. *Surgery* 1971; **70**: 920–6.

51. Arnoldi IC, Haeger K. Ulcus cruris venosum – crux medicorum? *Läkartidningen* 1967; **64**: 2149–57.

52. Recek EA. critical appraisal of the role of ankle perforators for the genesis of venous ulcers in the lower legs. *J Cardiovasc Surg* 1971; **12**: 45–9.

53. Burnand KG, Lea Thomas M, O'Donnell E *et al.* Relation between post-phlebitic changes in the deep veins and results of surgical treatment of venous ulcers. *Lancet* 1976; **i**: 936–8.

54. Kiely PE. Surgery should be avoided in patients with deep vein incompetence and without superficial varices. Personal communication, 1982.

55. Strandness DE, Thiele DL. *Selected Topics in Venous Disorders*. New York: Futura, 1981.

56. Lumley JSP. Surgical treatment of varicose veins. In: Marston A, ed. *Contemporary Operative Surgery*. London: Northwood Books, 1979.

57. Browse NL, Burnand KG. The causes of venous ulceration. *Lancet* 1982; **ii**: 243–5.

58. Sybrandy JE, van Gent WB, Pierik EG, Wittens CH. Endoscopic versus open subfascial division of incompetent perforating veins in the treatment of venous leg ulceration: long-term follow-up. *J Vasc Surg* 2001; **33**: 1028–32.

59. Kalra M, Gloviczki P. Surgical treatment of venous ulcers: role of subfascial endoscopic perforator vein ligation. *Surg Clin North Am* 2003; **83**: 671–705.

60. Warren R, Thayer T. Transplantation of the saphenous vein for post-phlebitic stasis. *Surgery* 1954; **35**: 867–76.

61. Husni EA. *In situ* saphenopopliteal bypass graft for incompetence of the femoral and popliteal veins. *Surg Gynecol Obstet* 1970; **130**: 279–84.

62. Palma EC, Ricci F, De Campo F. Tratamiento de los trastornos post flebiticos mediante anastomosis venosa safenofemoral contro-lateral. *Bull Soc Surg Uruguay* 1958; **29**: 135.

63. Palma EC, Esperon R. Vein transplants and grafts in the surgical treatment of the post-phlebitic syndrome. *J Cardiovasc Surg* 1960; **1**: 94–107.

64. Beecher HK, Field ME, Krogh L. The effect of walking on the venous pressure at the ankle. *Scand Arch Physiol* 1936; **73**: 133.

65. Warren R, White EA, Beecher CD. Venous pressures in the saphenous system in normal, varicose and post-phlebitic extremities. *Surgery* 1949; **26**: 435–45.

66. Pollack AA, Wood EH. Venous pressure in the saphenous vein of the ankle in man during exercise and changes in posture. *J Appl Physiol* 1949; **1**: 649–62.

67. De Camp PT, Schramel RJ, Roy CJ *et al.* Ambulatory venous pressure determinations in post-phlebitic and related syndromes. *Surgery* 1951; **29**: 44–70.

68. Höjensgard JC, Sturup H. Static and dynamic pressures in superficial and deep veins of the lower extremities in man. *Acta Physiol Scand* 1953; **27**: 49–67.

69. Arnoldi CCE, Greitz T, Linderholme H. Variations in cross-sectional area and pressure in the veins of the normal human leg during rhythmical muscular exercise. *Acta Chir Scand* 1966; **132**: 507–52.

70. Nicolaides AN, Hoare M, Miles CR *et al.* Value of ambulatory venous pressures in the assessment of venous insufficiency. *Vasc Diagn Ther* 1982; **3**: 41.

71. Satomura S, Kanecko Z Ultrasonic blood rheograph. *Proceedings of the Third International Conference on Medical Electronics*. London: The Institute of Electrical Engineers, 1960; 254–8.

72. Brooks B. Intraarterial injection of sodium iodide. *J Am Med Assoc* 1924; **82**: 1016.

73. Dos Santos R, Lamas AC, Pereira-Caldas J. L'arteriographie des membres, de l'aorta et de ses branches abdominales. *Bull Soc Nat Chir* 1929; **55**: 587.

74. Strandness DE Jr, McCutcheon EP, Rushmer RF. Application of a transcutaneous Doppler flowmeter in evaluation of occlusive arterial disease. *Surg Gynecol Obstet* 1966; **122**: 1039.

75. White JC, Smethwick RH. *The Autonomic Nervous System.* London: Macmillan, 1944.

76. Dos Santos JC. From embolectomy to endarterectomy or the fall of a myth. *J Cardiovasc Surg* 1976; **17**: 113–28.

77. dos Santos JC. Sur la desobstruction des thromboses arterielles anciennes. *Mem Acad Chir* 1947; **73**: 409–11.

78. Edwards WS. Composite reconstruction of the femoral artery with saphenous vein after endarterectomy. *Surg Gynecol Obstet* 1960; **111**: 651–3.

79. Kunlin J. Le traitement de l'ischemie arthritique par la greffe veineuse longue. *Rev Chir (Paris)* 1951; **70**: 206–35.

80. Crawford ES, De Bakey ME, Cooley DA, Morris JC Jnr. Use of crimped knitted Dacron grafts in patients with occlusive disease of the aorta and of the iliac, femoral and popliteal arteries. In: Wesolowska SA, Dennis C, eds. *Fundamentals of Vascular Grafting.* New York: McGraw Hill, 1963; 356–66.

81. Soyer T, Lempinen M, Cooper P *et al.* A new venous prosthesis. *Surgery* 1972; **72**: 864–72.

82. Gruntzig A, Hopff H. Perkutane rekanalisationn chronischer arterieller Verschlusse mit einem neuen Dilatationskatheter. Modifikation der Dotter-technik. *Dtsch Med Wschr* 1974; **99**: 2502–5.

2

Epidemiology – the extent of the problem

PHILIP D. COLERIDGE SMITH

INTRODUCTION

Venous disease in the lower limb is a common finding but usually causes only limited morbidity in the majority of patients. However, a proportion of patients develop skin changes and leg ulceration leading to discomfort, pain and the need for frequent treatment and dressing changes. This imposes a substantial financial burden on health care systems. The more severe symptoms of venous disease result in considerable morbidity in Western societies.

The prevalence of venous diseases has been studied in a modest number of epidemiological surveys. The findings in these studies vary considerably both in the overall prevalence of venous disease and in the variation between male and female patients. This is partly due to the way in which populations were selected. In many studies, an easily accessible population was found, such as the group of chemical factory workers studied by Widmer.[1] He made no attempt to assess a cross-section of all of society but instead investigated a group of people who could easily be studied. Consequently, his cohort was drawn from only one section of society. This limitation has been addressed in subsequent surveys, such as the Edinburgh Vein Study.[2]

A further limitation of some publications in this field are the types of venous disease which were included and the definitions of venous disease that have been employed. In some studies, patients with minor varices such as telangiectases and reticular varices have been excluded from assessment. In others they have been included. Our developing understanding of venous disease has resulted in a series of changes of definition and description of venous valvular incompetence. In the earlier studies, these were based principally on clinical examination, or on photography in the case of Widmer's study. He recognized three classes of varicose vein and that patients with skin changes of any type reflected a more severe stage of venous disease. He referred to such patients as having 'chronic venous insufficiency'. His classification is shown in Box 2.1.

Widmer's classification was used for several years but has largely been superseded by a classification which was originally instigated by an *ad hoc* Committee on Reporting Standards of the Joint Council of the Society for Vascular Surgery and the North American Chapter of the International Society for Cardiovascular Surgery. A group of experts agreed on a method of classification of venous disease and this was published in

---

Box 2.1   Widmer's classification of venous disease[1]

Varicose veins

1 'Hyphenwebs' (telangiectases, spiders): intradermal veinectasias
2 Reticular varicose veins: dilated, tortuous subcutaneous veins, not belonging to the main trunk or its major branches
3 Trunk varicosities: dilated, tortuous trunks of the long (greater) or short (lesser) saphenous veins and their first- or second-order branches

Chronic venous insufficiency

Grade I   Dilated subcutaneous veins at the ankle, 'Corona phlebectatica'
Grade II   Hyperpigmented or depigmented areas, with or without 'Corona phlebectatica'
Grade III Active or healed ulcer

Box 2.2 A system of classification of venous disease suggested by Porter *et al.*[3]

Class 0 Asymptomatic CVI

Class 1 Mild CVI with signs and symptoms including mild to moderate ankle swelling, mild discomfort (e.g. sensation of leg heaviness or painful varicosities), and local or generalized dilatation of subcutaneous veins. In this clinical class, CVI is usually limited to involvement of the superficial veins only

Class 2 Moderate CVI, including skin hyperpigmentation in the gaiter area, moderate brawny edema, and subcutaneous fibrosis, which may be either limited in extent or involve the whole malleolar and pretibial area, but with no ulceration. There is usually prominent local or regional dilation of the subcutaneous veins

Class 3 Severe CVI. Chronic distal leg pain associated with ulcerative or pre-ulcerative skin changes, eczematoid changes, and/or severe edema. This category is usually associated with extensive involvement of the deep venous system with widespread loss of venous valvular function and/or chronic deep vein obstruction

---

Box 2.3 The CEAP classification

Class 0 No visible or palpable signs of venous disease
Class 1 Telangiectases or reticular veins
Class 2 Varicose veins
Class 3 Edema
Class 4 Skin changes ascribed to venous disease, e.g. pigmentation, venous eczema, lipodermatosclerosis
Class 5 Skin changes as defined above with healed ulceration
Class 6 Skin changes as defined above with active ulceration

1988.[3] This system of classification has been used to a moderate extent and is summarized in Box 2.2.

Although a number of refinements to Porter's classification have been proposed, it was recognized that this too had deficiencies and the American Venous Forum organized a consensus meeting during a congress in Hawaii in 1995 to better define a classification for venous disease. One of the problems that this was intended to overcome was the confusion that had arisen as the consequence of the term 'chronic venous insufficiency', which was understood in different ways by different people. A multi-axial system was proposed which took into account the clinical signs (C), aetiology (E), anatomic distribution (A) and pathophysiologic dysfunction (P). Thus the CEAP classification was born and is shown in Box 2.3.[4] A number of revisions to this have been published subsequently as our understanding of venous disease improves. Modern-day phlebologists regard this as a 'living classification' which may be revised as our knowledge improves. It may be used to define a patient group or to describe the clinical condition of one patient as his or her venous disease evolves over a period of time. This classification is described more completely in Chapter 6.

The CEAP classification is supplemented with mode of presentation: (A) for asymptomatic or (S) for symptomatic limb. Symptoms include aching pain, congestion, skin irritation, and muscle cramps as well as other complaints attributable to venous dysfunction. The etiological classification recognizes three categories of venous dysfunction: congenital (E_C),

primary, with undetermined cause (E_P), and secondary – post-thrombotic, post-traumatic, or other (E_S). The anatomic classification describes the anatomic extent of venous disease, i.e. in the superficial (A_S), deep (A_D) or perforating (A_P) veins. The site and extent of involvement of the superficial, deep, and perforating veins may be categorized using the anatomic segments. The pathophysiological classification includes reflux (P_R), obstruction (P_O) or both (P_{RO}), and allows for reporting of the location and anatomical extent of reflux and/or obstruction in greater detail by using the anatomic segments.

The CEAP classification requires the use of investigations such as duplex ultrasonography or phlebography in order to establish fully the extent of venous disease and its causes. This is a reflection of the increased use of such diagnostic methods which commenced in the mid-1980s as ultrasound imaging was introduced in the diagnosis of venous disease. Most of the early epidemiological studies relied on history-taking and clinical examination alone, or on photography in the case of Widmer's study. More recent publications, such as the Edinburgh Vein Study, have employed duplex ultrasonography to assess the extent of underlying venous disease.[2] This addition to epidemiological surveys has shown that in many cases venous valvular incompetence in deep or superficial veins may produce no symptom or clinical evidence of venous disease. This is best illustrated in the Bochum studies where a longitudinal investigation was performed in a group of schoolchildren starting with 10- to 12-year-olds.[5] Schultz-Ehrenburg *et al.* found that, of 14- to 16-year-olds, 12 percent had saphenous reflux but only 1.7 percent had trunk varices. In 18- to 20-year-olds he found that 20 percent had saphenous reflux but only 3.3 percent had trunk varices. The method of investigation used in this study was continuous-wave (CW) Doppler ultrasound. Longitudinal studies of this type add greatly to our knowledge of how venous disease evolves, but unfortunately these are rather few and far between.

PREVALENCE OF VARICOSE VEINS

The prevalence of varicose veins in published studies is shown in Table 2.1. This shows a very wide range of frequency of

Table 2.1 *Prevalence of varicose veins in adult males and females in epidemiological surveys*

Year	Country	Population	Definition used	(n)	Female (%)	Male (%)
1957	Denmark[6]	Hospital patients	All varicosities	293	49	–
1966	Wales[7]	Population sample	All varicosities	289	53	37
1967	Switzerland[8]	Chemical industry employees	All varicosities	4376	68	57
1969	Egypt[9]	Cotton mill workers	Excluding telangiectases	467	5.8	–
1969	England[9]	Cotton mill workers	Excluding telangiectases	504	31	–
1972	India (South)[10]	Railway sweepers	All varicosities	323	–	25
1972	India (North)[10]	Railway sweepers	All varicosities	354	–	6.8
1973	Switzerland[1]	Chemical industry employees	All varicosities	4529	55	56
1973	Switzerland[11]	Shop and factory employees	Excluding telangiectases	610	29	–
1973	United States[12]	Population sample	All varicosities	6389	26	13
1975	Cook Is. Pukapuka[13]	Selected population	All varicosities	377	4.0	2.1
1975	Cook Is. Rarotonga[13]	Selected population	All varicosities	417	15	16
1975	New Guinea[14]	Villagers	All varicosities	1457	0.1	5.1
1975	New Zealand (Maori)[15]	Selected population	All varicosities	721	44	33
1975	New Zealand (Euro)[15]	Selected population	All varicosities	356	38	20
1975	Tokelau Island[13]	Selected population	All varicosities	786	0.8	2.9
1977	Tanzania[16]	Outpatients	All varicosities	1000	5.0	6.1
1981	Israel[17]	Population sample	Excluding small varicosities	4888	29	10
1986	Brazil[18]	Health centre patients	Excluding telangiectases and reticular varices	1755	51	38
1988	Sicily[19]	Villagers	All varicosities	1122	46	19
1990	Japan[20]	Patients, hospital staff, elderly residents	All varicosities	541	45	–
1991	Czechoslovakia[21]	Shop employees	All varicosities	696	61	–
1994	Turkey[22]	General population	All varicosities	850	38	35
1995	Finland[23]	General population	Varicose veins	7217	25	6.8
1998	Italy[24]	General population	All varicosities	1319	35	17
1999	Scotland[2]	General population	Trunk varicosities	1566	32	40
2000	United States[25]	University employees	Trunk varicosities	600	33	17

venous disease which is a little difficult to understand at first sight. As I have pointed out, a range of definitions has been used in these series which, combined with different inclusion and exclusion criteria and different methods of selection of populations for study, probably accounts for the differences. The studies included populations of different types and ages. The results are not age-standardized.

In attempting to establish the prevalence of venous disease in Western populations, the data from the Tecumseh study in the USA,[12] Beaglehole *et al.*'s study from New Zealand,[13] a study from Israel[17] and the Edinburgh Vein Study[2] can be considered. General populations were investigated here and are probably representative of the overall picture. In these studies, the prevalence of varicose veins in women was 25–30 percent and in men 10–20 percent, although the Edinburgh Vein Study found that the prevalence in men was 40 percent. The last finding remains unusual amongst epidemiological studies since venous diseases were more common in men than in women. This study was rigorously conducted and involved clinical examination, photography and duplex ultrasonography.

A self-reported study is included in Table 2.1[23] and the findings from this investigation are similar to those obtained from studies which included clinical examination. However, it is well known that patients and their doctors may differ greatly in opinions concerning varicose veins!

Table 2.1 reveals an interesting difference between Westernized populations and those in primitive societies. In general, the data for Westernized countries in this table are fairly similar whether the population lives in Europe, the Middle East, Australasia, North or South America. However, the prevalence of varicose veins is far lower in the subjects studied in remote Pacific islands.[13,14] This could be attributable to a number of factors, including the way in which the studies were conducted. However, Beaglehole *et al.* conducted a similar study amongst the population of New Zealand comparing the native Maori (Polynesian) population with the immigrant European people.[15] Here he found a slightly higher incidence of varicose veins in the Maoris. This suggests that genetic differences do not account for the low prevalence observed in the remote Pacific islands but that the Western way of life enjoyed by the residents of New Zealand may include factors predisposing to the development of varicose veins.

Epidemiological studies tend to show an increasing prevalence of varicose veins with age. For example, in the Edinburgh Vein Study the incidence of varicose veins is 16 percent in the age range 25–34 years and 51 percent in the age range 55–64 years.[2] The Bochum studies, conducted in a cohort of schoolchildren, similarly showed a rising prevalence of venous disease, including reticular and truncal varices.[5] The rate of development of varicose veins was assessed in the Framingham

Table 2.2 *Venous status of parents of cases of varicose veins and controls*

	% Mothers		% Fathers	
	Cases (n = 67)	Controls (n = 67)	Cases (n = 67)	Controls (n = 67)
Varicose veins				
Great saphenous	46.3	26.9	38.8	14.9
Small saphenous	32.8	16.4	23.9	4.5
Non-saphenous	19.4	10.4	10.4	6.0
Telangiectasia	83.6	73.1	41.8	28.8
Varicose vein treatment				
Surgery	28.4	6.0	19.4	0.0
Sclerotherapy	44.8	19.4	21.9	3.0

Study.[26] A large group of middle-aged men and women living in the town of Framingham in the USA were followed up from 1948 and the development of new cases of varicose veins was identified over a 16-year period from 1966. The annual incidence was 2.6 percent in women and 1.9 percent in men. The incidence rate, from the age of 40 years, did not increase with age. It would appear that the increasing prevalence with age is due to the relatively constant development of new cases as people grow older.

In the Basle study, 660 subjects of average age 53 years were considered to be disease-free at baseline. When followed up after a period of 11 years, the annual incidence of 'mild' varicose veins was 8 percent and of 'pronounced' varicosities was 0.4 percent. The incidence rate was similar in men and women. At the end of the 11-year period, over 90 percent of the population had acquired varicosities, although these were mostly of the 'mild' category.[27]

Several studies suggest a strong inherited component for the risk of developing venous disease.[28,29] Some studies have relied on patients' recollection of varicose veins in their parents; however, in the study of Cornu-Thénard *et al.*, the investigators examined both patients and their parents in comparison with controls to obtain an objective view of the presence of venous disease.[30] The results from this investigation are summarized in Table 2.2.

The results of this study show a much higher prevalence of venous disease in the parents of patients compared with control subjects, confirming the role of genetic predisposition in venous disease.

SKIN CHANGES ASSOCIATED WITH VENOUS DISEASE

Very few studies have reported on skin changes associated with venous disease. The only studies where this has been done systematically are the Tecumseh study in the USA[12] and the Basle study in Switzerland.[27] Evidence of skin changes was

seen in 3.7 percent of women and 3.0 percent of men, and the prevalence increased markedly with age.[12] In women, 1.8 percent of those aged 30–39 years had skin changes compared with 20.7 percent of those over 70 years of age. In the Basle study (II), the prevalence of 'pronounced' skin changes (dilatation of subcutaneous veins, hyper- or hypo-pigmentation) was found to be 9.6 percent in women and 8.7 percent in men.[8] Mild skin changes in the form of a venous flare occurred in 15 percent of women and 10 percent of men. In the Basle study (III), a lower prevalence of skin changes (14 percent) was found.[1] The data of the Basle study are based on a very specific population rather than being a general study. These data show that skin changes are far less frequent than the associated varicose veins. During the 11-year follow-up of this study it was found that for subjects with mild varicose veins, 21 percent developed chronic venous insufficiency (CVI, skin changes according to Widmer's classification), whereas 50 percent of those with severe varicose veins developed CVI. Twenty percent of subjects with severe varicose veins developed venous ulceration compared with 0.8 percent of those with mild varicose veins.

VENOUS ULCERATION

Venous ulceration occurs in a small proportion of the population but those affected require considerable health care resources to manage this problem. A limited number of epidemiological surveys addressing the frequency of this disease have been published and are summarized in Table 2.3. Methodological problems may result in difficulty in interpretation of some of the data contained in these studies. Although the presence of a leg ulcer is easy to establish, it may be the result of a number of diseases, not just venous disease. In a recent study, patients with leg ulcers had venous disease, arterial disease, diabetes, lymphedema and rheumatoid disease.[31] In this study, patients had combined pathologies in 35 percent of cases.

These data show a wide variation in the overall prevalence of venous ulceration. However, the data reflect differing populations and most of the differences between the findings are probably attributable to the way in which populations were selected for study. The prevalence of leg ulceration is highly age-dependent,[31] with leg ulcers becoming far more frequent with advancing age. Any variation in the age range included in a study will also result in variation in the findings.

The overall prevalence of open venous ulceration from these studies in adults over the age of 18 years is about 0.3 percent. For every patient with an open ulcer there are probably three or four with healed venous ulcers.[41,42] This means that approximately 1 percent of the adult population is affected by ulceration, either open or healed. Table 2.3 shows that where the prevalence of leg ulcers has been reported separately in men and women, the crude prevalence of ulceration is greater in men than in women. However, due to the greater

Table 2.3 *Prevalence of venous ulcers in adult males and females in selected epidemiological surveys*

	Location	Survey method	n	Population	Type of ulcer	Prevalence of ulcer (%)		
						M	M + F	F
1973	Tecumseh, USA[12]	Examination	6389	General, 10 years+	Venous, active or healed	0.1		0.3
1978	Basle, Switzerland[1]	Examination	4529	Chemical workers, 25 years+	Chronic, active or healed	1.0		1.0
1985	Edinburgh, Scotland[32]	Postal	586	General, 15 years+	Chronic ? active		0.8	
1985	Lothian/Forth Valley, Scotland[33]	Health service	1 million	General, 20 years+	Chronic active		0.15	
1986	Harrow, England[34]	Health service	92 100	General, 40 years+	Chronic active		0.38	
1986	Ireland[35]	Postal	2012	General, all ages	Chronic active	1.0		2.1
1991	Perth, Australia[36]	Health service	238 000	General, ? ages	Chronic active		0.11	
1991	Skaraborg, Sweden[37]	Health service	270 800	General, all ages	Chronic active	0.22		0.39
1992	Malmo, Sweden[38]	Health service	232 908	General, all ages	Chronic ? active		0.12	
1992	Newcastle, England[39]	Health service	107 400	General, 45 years+	Chronic active		0.19	
1993	Gothenburg, Sweden[40]	Postal	5140	General, 65 years+	Chronic active	3.2		1.5
1996	Malmö, Skaraborg, Sweden[41]	Postal and examination	12 000	General, 50–89 years	Chronic active		0.63	
					Chronic, active or healed		1.8	
1996	Skövde, Sweden[42]	Postal	2785	Industrial workers, 30–65 years	Chronic active		0.6	
					Chronic, active or healed		1.6	

longevity of women, the populations studied will contain more women than men. In a recent study, age-corrected data show a similar prevalence of leg ulceration in men and women.[31] The prevalence of venous ulceration increases with age in both men and women in all the surveys reported in Table 2.3.[32,34,35,37,41,42] This probably reflects the fact that as venous disease continues to develop throughout life, more patients reach the point at which an ulcer develops. Those already affected by ulcers continue to suffer recurrent episodes between periods when treatment results in healing. In addition, in old age more limited mobility associated with degenerate diseases of joints and poorer healing probably contributes to the accumulation of ulceration in the most elderly patients. Widmer's Basle study showed that those patients with the more severe clinical presentations of varicose veins were the most likely to develop leg ulceration subsequently. The severity of impairment of venous physiology of the lower limb can be assessed by a number of investigations. Nicolaides *et al.*[43] investigated 220 patients with venous disease and measured the ambulatory foot vein pressure (AVP) to assess the severity of venous reflux. They found that in limbs with an AVP of less than 30 mmHg no ulceration was observed. Where the ankle pressure exceeded 90 mmHg, ulceration was invariable. A linear relationship between the risk of ulceration and the AVP was reported, although the confidence interval was not included. In practice, the exact risk of ulceration in any one patient is difficult to assess because of wide variation between patients in their susceptibility to ulceration in response to a particular AVP.

A further factor which is widely associated with venous ulceration is deep vein thrombosis (DVT). In a study reported from Western Australia, 17 percent of patients with chronic venous ulcers reported a history of DVT.[44] Follow-up of patients who had suffered an episode of deep vein thrombosis might be expected to reveal the extent of ulceration as a consequence of post-thrombotic syndrome. Follow-up of 61 patients for an average of 39 months revealed the development of three ulcers (5 percent); another small follow-up study for 25 months on 77 DVT patients identified five patients with ulcer (6 percent). In a larger study of 278 patients with unilateral DVT, 8 percent developed an ulcer over a 5-year period. There was also a relationship between the incidence of post-thrombotic syndrome and the extent of the original thrombosis.[45,46] A cohort of patients with venous disease has been investigated for the presence of thrombophilias, which have become much better understood in recent years.[47] Eighty-eight patients with chronic venous ulceration were investigated; 36 percent had a history or duplex ultrasound evidence of previous venous ulceration. The presence of inherited or acquired thrombophilias was sought by blood testing and 41 percent of this cohort were found to have a thrombophilia. This is much higher than would be expected in the overall population, which reflects an important mechanism in the development of ulceration in these patients. The presence of a thrombophilia was not predicted by a history of previous venous thrombosis in this cohort, confirming that the absence of a history of DVT is not reliable in excluding post-thrombotic damage to the lower limb veins.

Arterial disease is also increasingly prevalent in aging populations and commonly coexists with venous disease in patients with leg ulceration.[34,36] A recent study found that

Table 2.4 *Incidence of recurrence of ulcer after initial ulcer healing in selection of treatment trials*

Authors	Year	Treatment	Duration of follow-up (years)	Total recurrence (%)	Average annual recurrence (%)
Reiter[52]	1954	Skin grafting	2.5	71	28
Anning[53]	1956	Miscellaneous	5.5	59	11
Hansson [54]	1964	Surgery	5	15	3
Burnand et al.[55]	1976	Ligation perforators	5	55	11
Hansson et al.[56]	1987	Miscellaneous	3	44	15
Mayberry et al.[57]	1991	Compression therapy	5	29	6
Dinn and Henry[58]	1992	Sclerotherapy	5	30	6

arterial disease alone was responsible for 20 percent of ulcers being treated by a community leg ulcer service.[31]

Clinical course of venous leg ulceration

Venous ulceration tends to run a course of the healing process, taking a number of months to complete, followed at a later date by relapse to a further episode. In some patients healing is very protracted or never achieved. Usually half the patients attending a leg ulcer service achieve healing in about 4 months.[48] In the Lothian and Forth Valley Leg Ulcer Study in Scotland, 20 percent of ulcers had not healed after 2 years, and 8 percent had been open for 5 years. The longest duration was 62 years in an 85-year-old woman.[33] In this study, episodes of ulceration were reported for more than 10 years in 45 percent of patients and between 5 and 10 years in 21 percent. From these data we can say that approximately one-third of patients will only have had one episode and that at least one-third are likely to have had four or more episodes. The most important factors determining whether an ulcer will heal are its size and duration.[48–51] The recurrence of ulceration following healing is a common problem. The frequency of this in a number of studies is reported in Table 2.4.

A recent study has suggested a way in which recurrence of ulceration may be reduced.[59] An investigation was undertaken in 500 patients with open or recently healed leg ulcers. Those with superficial venous reflux alone or with mixed superficial and deep venous reflux were randomized to undergo compression treatment alone or in combination with superficial venous surgery. Surgical treatment consisted of stripping saphenous trunks and, in some cases, ligation of perforating veins. The healing rate was identical after 24 weeks in both groups (65 percent). The recurrence rate at 12 months was 12 percent in the compression and surgery group and 28 percent in the compression-only group. This study provides objective evidence of the value of obliterating incompetent superficial veins in patients with leg ulcers.

A detailed analysis of all aspects of chronic venous disease of the leg has been published by the VEINES International Task Force, which considers many aspects of the epidemiology, health economics, investigation and treatment of patients with this disease.[60]

CONCLUSIONS

Venous diseases in the lower limb are common and usually cause little morbidity. Only a limited number of epidemiological studies have been published and are referenced above. Varicose veins occur in 20–30 percent of the population in Westernized countries. Patients with more severe varicose veins are at increased risk of developing leg ulceration. About 1 percent of the total population will suffer from a leg ulcer. These patients are likely to experience healing of their ulcer if treated appropriately, but are at considerable risk of further episodes of ulceration. In patients with superficial venous reflux, surgical removal of incompetent saphenous trunks reduces the risk of recurrence.

Considerable international effort has resulted in the development of the CEAP classification, which is widely used in reporting data from clinical series and trials in venous disease. This classification allows comparison between the results obtained from different centres and should be included when reporting any clinical data in a publication.

REFERENCES

1. Widmer LK, ed. *Peripheral Venous Disorders – Prevalence and Socio-Medical Importance*. Bern: Hans Gruber, 1978.
2. Evans CJ, Fowkes FG, Ruckley CV, Lee AJ. Prevalence of varicose veins and chronic venous insufficiency in men and women in the general population: Edinburgh Vein Study. *J Epidemiol Community Health* 1999; **53**: 149–53.
3. Porter JP, Rutherford RB, Clagett GP, Raju S et al. Reporting standards in venous disease. *J Vasc Surg* 1988; **8**(2): 172–9.
4. Porter JM, Moneta GL. An International Consensus Committe on Chronic Venous Disease. Reporting standards in venous disease: An update. *J Vasc Surg* 1995; **21**: 635–45.
5. Schultz-Ehrenburg U, Weindorf N, Matthes U, Hirche H. An epidemiologic study of the pathogenesis of varices. The Bochum study I–III. *Phlebologie* 1992; **45**: 497–500.
6. Arnoldi CC. The aetiology of primary varicose veins. *Dan Med Bull* 1957; **4**: 102–7.
7. Weddell JM. Varicose veins pilot study, 1966. *Br J Prev Soc Medical* 1969; **23**: 179–86.

8. Da Silva A, Widmer LK, Martin H, Mall TH *et al*. Varicose veins and chronic venous insufficiency – prevalence and risk factors in 4376 subjects in the Basle Study II. *Vasa* 1974; **3**: 118–25.

9. Mekky S, Schilling RS F, Walford J. Varicose veins in women cotton workers. An epidemiological study in England and Egypt. *Br Med J* 1969; **2**: 591–5.

10. Malhotra SL. An epidemiological study of varicose veins in Indian railroad workers from the south and north of India, with special reference to the causation and prevention of varicose veins. *Int J Epidemiol* 1972; **1**: 117–83.

11. Guberan W, Widmer LK, Glaus L, Muller R *et al*. Causative factors of varicose veins: myths and facts. *Vasa* 1973; **2**: 115–20.

12. Coon WW, Willis PW, Keller JB. Venous thromboembolism and other venous disease in the Tecumseh community health study. *Circulation* 1973; **48**: 839–46.

13. Beaglehole R, Prior IAM, Salmond CE, Davidson F. Varicose veins in the South Pacific. *Int J Epidemiol* 1975; **4**: 295–9.

14. Stanhope JM. Varicose veins in a population of New Guinea. *Int J Epidemiol* 1975; **4**: 221–5.

15. Beaglehole R, Salmond CE, Prior IA. Varicose veins in New Zealand: prevalence and severity. *NZ Med J* 1976; **84**: 396–9.

16. Richardson JB, Dixon M. Varicose veins in tropical Africa. *Lancet* 1977; **i**: 791–2.

17. Abramson JH, Hopp C, Epstein LM. The epidemiology of varicose veins – a survey of Western Jerusalem. *J Epidemiol Community Health* 1981; **35**: 213–7.

18. Maffei FHA, Magaldi C, Pinho SZ, Lastoria S *et al*. Varicose veins and chronic venous insufficiency in Brazil: prevalence among 1755 inhabitants of a country town. *Int J Epidemiol* 1986; **15**: 210–7.

19. Novo S, Avellone G, Pinto A, Davi G *et al*. Prevalence of primitive varicose veins of the lower limbs in a randomized population sample of Western Sicily. *Int Angiol* 1988; **7**(2): 176–81.

20. Hirai M, Kenichi N, Nakayama R. Prevalence and risk factors of varicose veins in Japanese women. *Angiology* 1990; **41**: 228–32.

21. Stvrtinova V, Kolesar J, Wimmer G. Prevalence of varicose veins of the lower limbs in the women working at a department store. *Int Angiol* 1991; **10**(1): 2–5.

22. Komsuoglu B, Goldeli O, Kulan K *et al*. Prevalence and risk factors of varicose veins in an elderly population. *Gerontology* 1994; **40**: 25–31.

23. Sisto T, Reunanen A, Laurikka J *et al*. Prevalence and risk factors of varicose veins in lower extremities: mini-Finland health survey. *Eur J Surg* 1995; **161**: 405–14.

24. Canonico S, Gallo C, Paolisso G *et al*. Prevalence of varicose veins in an Italian elderly population. *Angiology* 1998; **49**: 129–35.

25. Langer RD, Criqui MH, Denenburg J, Fronek A. The prevalence of venous disease by gender and ethnicity in a balanced sample of four ethnic groups in southern California. *Phlebology* 2000; **15**: 99–105.

26. Brand FN, Dannenberg AL, Abbott RD, Kannel WB. The epidemiology of varicose veins: the Framingham study. *Am J Prev Med* 1988; **4**: 96–101.

27. Widmer LK, Holz D, Morselli B, Zbinden O *et al*. Progression of varicose veins in 11 years. Observations on 1441 working persons of the Basle Study. Unpublished paper. Basle: Angiology Division of University Department of Medicine, 1992.

28. Matousek V, Prerovsky I. A contribution to the problem of the inheritance of primary varicose veins. *Hum Hered* 1974; **24**: 225–35.

29. Hauge M, Gundersen J. Genetics of varicose veins of the lower extremities. *Hum Hered* 1969; **19**: 573–80.

30. Cornu-Thenard C, Boivin P, Baud J-M *et al*. Importance of the familial factor in varicose disease. *J Dermatol Surg Oncol* 1994; **20**: 313–26.

31. Moffatt CJ, Franks PJ, Doherty DC *et al*. Prevalence of leg ulceration in a London population. *QJM* 2004; **97**: 431–7.

32. Dale JJ, Callam MJ, Ruckley CV *et al*. Chronic ulcers of the leg: a study of prevalence in a Scottish community. *Health Bull* 1985; **41**: 310–4.

33. Callam MJ, Ruckley CV, Harper DR, Dale JJ. Chronic ulceration of the leg: extent of the problem and provision of care. *Br Med J* 1985; **290**: 1855–6.

34. Cornwall JV, Doré CJ, Lewis JD. Leg ulcers: epidemiology and aetiology. *Br J Surg* 1986; **73**: 693–6.

35. Henry M. Incidence of varicose ulcers in Ireland. *Ir Med J* 1986; **79**: 65–7.

36. Baker SR, Stacey MC, Singh G, Hoskin SE *et al*. Aetiology of chronic leg ulcers. *Eur J Vasc Surg* 1992; **6**: 245–51.

37. Nelzén O, Bergqvist D, Lindhagen A, Hallböök T. Chronic leg ulcers: an underestimated problem in primary health care among elderly patients. *J Epidemiol Community Health* 1991; **45**: 184–7.

38. Lindholm C, Bjellerup M, Christensen OB, Zederfeldt B. A demographic survey of leg and foot ulcer patients in a defined population. *Acta Derm Venereol* 1992; **72**: 227–30.

39. Lees TA, Lambert D. Prevalence of lower limb ulceration in an urban health district. *Br J Surg* 1992; **79**: 1032–4.

40. Andersson E, Hansson C, Swanbeck G. Leg and foot ulcer prevalence and investigation of the peripheral arterial and venous circulation in a randomised elderly population. An epidemiological survey and clinical investigation. *Acta Derm Venereol* 1993; **73**: 57–61.

41. Nelzen O, Bergqvist D, Lindhagen A. The prevalence of chronic lower-limb ulceration has been underestimated: results of a validated population questionnaire. *Br J Surg* 1996; **83**: 255–8.

42. Nelzen O, Bergqvist D, Fransson I, Lindhagen A. Prevalence and aetiology of leg ulcers in a defined population of industrial workers. *Phlebology* 1996; **11**: 50–4.

43. Nicolaides AN, Hussein MK, Szendro G *et al*. The relation of venous ulceration with ambulatory venous pressure measurements. *J Vasc Surg* 1993; **17**: 414–9.

44. Baker SR, Stacey MC, Jopp-McKay AG *et al*. Epidemiology of chronic venous ulcers. *Br J Surg* 1991; **78**: 864–7.

45. Strandness DE, Langlois Y, Cramer M *et al*. Long-term sequelae of acute venous thrombosis. *J Am Med Assoc* 1983; **250**: 1289–92.

46. Mudge M, Leinster SJ, Hughes LE. A prospective 10-year study of the post–thrombotic syndrome in a surgical population. *Ann R Coll Surg Engl* 1988; **70**: 249–52.

47. Mackenzie RK, Ludlam CA, Ruckley CV *et al*. The prevalence of thrombophilia in patients with chronic venous leg ulceration. *J Vasc Surg* 2002; **35**: 718–22.

48. Skene AI, Smith JM, Doré CJ, Charlett A *et al*. Venous leg ulcers: a prognostic index to predict time to healing. *Br Med J* 1992; **305**: 1119–21.

49. Colgan MP, Dormandy JA, Jones PW *et al*. Oxpentifylline treatment of venous ulcers of the leg. *Br Med J* 1990; **300**: 972–5.

50. Kikta MJ, Schuler JJ, Meyer JP *et al*. A prospective, randomized trial of Unna's boots versus hydroactive dressing in the treatment of venous statis ulcers. *J Vasc Surg* 1988; **7**: 478–86.

51. Franks P, Bosanquet N, Connolly M *et al*. Venous ulcers healing: effect of socioeconomic factors in London. *J Epidemiol Community Health* 1995; **49**: 385–8.

52. Reiter H. Ulcer cruris. Cure rate and stability after treatment by skin grafting according to Reverdin. *Acta Derm Venereol* 1954; **34**: 439–45.

53. Anning ST. Leg ulcers – the results of treatment. *Angiology* 1956; **112**: 135–44.

54. Hansson LO. Venous ulcers of the lower limbs. A follow-up study 5 years after surgical treatment. *Acta Chir Scand* 1964; **128**: 269–77.

55. Burnand K, Thomas ML, O'Donnell T, Browse NL. Relationship between postphlebitic changes in the deep veins and results of surgical treatment of venous ulcers. *Lancet* 1976; **i**: 936–8.

56. Hansson C, Andersson E, Swanbeck G. A follow-up study of leg and foot ulcer patients. *Acta Derm Venereol* 1987; **67**: 496–500.

57. Mayberry JC, Moneta GL, Taylor LM, Porter JM. Fifteen year results of ambulatory compression therapy for chronic venous ulcers. *Surgery* 1991; **109**: 575–81.

58. Dinn E, Henry M. Treatment of venous ulceration by injection sclerotherapy and compression hosiery: a 5 year study. *Phlebology* 1992; **7**: 23–6.

59. Barwell JR, Davies CE, Deacon J *et al*. Comparison of surgery and compression with compression alone in chronic venous ulceration (ESCHAR study): randomised controlled trial. *Lancet* 2004; **363**: 1854–9.

60. The Task Force on Chronic Venous Disorders of the Leg. The management of chronic venous disorders of the leg. *Phlebol* 1999; **14**(1): 1–126.

3

The blood vessels of the lower limb: applied anatomy

DAVID NEGUS, PHILIP D. COLERIDGE SMITH

The integrity of the skin of the lower limb depends on its microcirculation, and ulceration is the end result of microcirculatory failure. Those responsible for treating leg ulcers should therefore have a working knowledge of the lower limb circulation, a subject that is best considered under three headings: microcirculation, arteries and veins. Note, however, that the anatomy of the lower limb arteries is well described in anatomical textbooks and there is no need for repetition here.

MICROCIRCULATION

The dermal microcirculation consists of a network of arterioles, the rete subpapillae, or superficial plexus, from which capillaries loop into the dermal papillae and so approach the base of the epithelium, before passing back to a venous plexus which lies immediately below the rete subpapillae. This drains into a flat intermediate plexus in the middle of the reticular layer of the skin and this plexus further connects with a deep laminar venous plexus at the junction of the dermis and the superficial plexus. Arteriovenous anastomoses are common in the deeper layer of the dermis. Some (glomera) are surrounded by sphincter-like groups of smooth muscle and pursue a convoluted course.[1] Capillaries are tubes lined by a single layer of polygonal or lanceolate epithelial cells, and exchange of oxygen and other metabolites takes place through the wall of these cells and across the walls of venules and arterioles.

Blood flow in the microcirculation is altered by contraction and relaxation of smooth muscle in the arterioles and cutaneous veins, which affects both the total blood flow and its distribution by means of the precapillary sphincters and arteriovenous anastomoses. These alterations in arteriolar and venous tone are controlled by the sympathetic nervous system.[2] Leukocytes and platelets accumulate in the microcirculation during venous congestion, and their continued presence and subsequent activation are now considered responsible for some of the complications of chronic venous hypertension.[3]

THE VEINS OF THE LOWER LIMB

Histological features

The walls of veins are similar to those of arteries, being composed of three coats: an inner endothelium, a muscular media and an outer fibrous adventitia. However, they differ from arteries in a number of important details. The endothelium of the intima, secretes factor VIII, prostacyclins and fibrinolytic activator. Recurrent spontaneous thrombosis occurs in patients with inherited or acquired abnormalities in some of these mechanisms.[4] The media consists of collagen and elastin fibres and non-striated muscle fibres arranged circularly. The elastin fibres are in a smaller proportion than in arterial walls. The muscle fibres are most well developed in the superficial veins, and their contraction is controlled by postganglionic adrenergic sympathetic nerve fibres. By contrast, the media of the deep veins contains relatively little muscle and these veins act mainly as passive blood conduits. The adventitia consists of areolar tissue with longitudinal elastic fibres. In the largest veins, it is very much thicker than the tunica media and contains longitudinal muscle fibres.

Most veins contain bicuspid valves which direct flow proximally and from the superficial to the deep veins. Valves consist of collagen fibres covered by a thin layer of endothelium and are stronger than the vein wall.[5] Valves are most numerous in the deep veins of the calf and are fewer in the popliteal and femoral veins. The iliac veins are usually valveless.[6] The great saphenous vein contains between two and 13 valves,[7] and each direct calf perforating vein contains one valve.

ANATOMY

The venous drainage of the lower limb is divided into the superficial and deep systems, the drainage areas of which are separated by the deep fascia. Thus the superficial veins, the great and small saphenous veins and tributaries of the perforating veins drain the skin and subcutaneous fat (the so-called superficial fascia), and the deep veins are responsible for venous return from muscle and other structures deep to the deep fascia. The volume of venous blood passing through the deep system far exceeds that through the superficial system, the function of the latter being mainly temperature regulation. The superficial veins communicate with the deep veins at the saphenopopliteal and saphenofemoral junctions and, by way of the perforating veins, through openings in the deep fascia.

The superficial veins

These are the great and small saphenous veins and the tributaries of the perforating veins. The correct anatomical nomenclature is 'great' and 'small' saphenous veins (saphena magna and saphena parva), but 'long' and 'short' are still in common clinical use.

THE GREAT SAPHENOUS VEIN

The great saphenous vein (GSV) arises from the medial end of the dorsal venous arch of the foot (Fig. 3.1), then passes in front of the medial malleolus and along the medial surface of the leg, enclosed in its own 'fascial sheath'.[7,8] Caggiati and Ricci[9] have undertaken detailed studies of this sheath by dissection and ultrasound examination and have demonstrated a connective tissue lamina originating from the lateral part of the inguinal ligament and descending over the anteromedial aspect of the thigh and medial aspect of the calf. The GSV lies in a narrow compartment between this and the underlying muscular fascia, and thick connective tissue strands from the two laminae extend to the saphenous adventitia. The superficial lamina appears to arise from the interlacing of the hypodermal connective sheets in an intermediate plane between the dermis and the muscular fascia and it divides the hypodermis into a superficial and a deep compartment. The dissection demonstrated the subcutaneous lamina lying superficial to the GSV consistently in the upper third of the leg, but in the middle third it appeared in only one-quarter of cases. The importance of the fascial compartment enclosing the GSV to modern

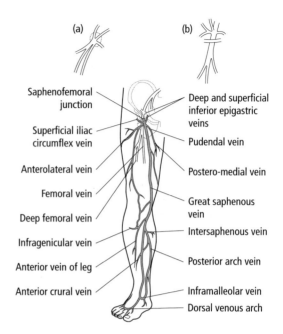

Figure 3.1 *The great saphenous vein and its tributaries. Insets: A, duplication of the great saphenous vein; B, aberrant superficial external pudendal artery.*

phlebology is that this structure is readily seen on ultrasound imaging (inset A, Fig. 3.1) and this allows the main saphenous trunk to be identified and separated from its tributaries. This is helpful in establishing the correct identity of incompetent superficial veins during ultrasonography as well as during ultrasound-guided injection of veins. Fascial sheaths also enclose the anterior accessory saphenous vein in the thigh and the small saphenous vein in the calf.

The GSV lies posteriorly at knee level and then passes up the thigh and through the foramen ovale and the femoral triangle to join the common femoral vein (Plate 3.1). It crosses the superficial external pudendal artery at the lower border of the foramen ovale.

The anatomy of the GSV and its important tributaries can easily be remembered by thinking of two tridents, or three-part pronged forks, one in the thigh and one just below the knee. In the groin, the important tributaries are the anterolateral and posteromedial veins of the thigh. Smaller tributaries are the superficial and deep external pudendal veins, and the superficial epigastric and circumflex iliac veins. Just below the knee, the anterior and posterior prongs of the trident are the anterior vein of the leg and the posterior arch vein. The important medial calf direct perforating veins communicate with the posterior arch vein (first accurately observed and drawn by Leonardo da Vinci) and not directly with the GSV.

The tributaries of the GSV commonly become varicose; the saphenous vein itself is only occasionally dilated and varicose in the lower leg and varicose dilatation of the anterior accessory saphenous vein in the thigh may occur without great saphenous incompetence. The GSV is accompanied by

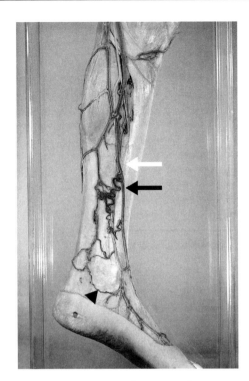

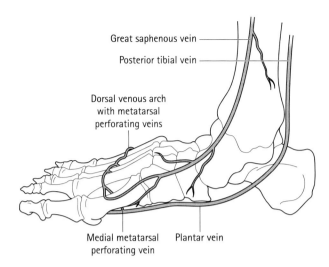

Figure 3.3   *The four metatarsal communicating veins join the superficial system (dorsal venous arch) to the deep system of veins (plantar veins) in the foot.*

Figure 3.2   *The saphenous nerve (white arrow) becomes more closely applied to the great saphenous vein (black arrow) in the lower leg and ankle, where it is more at risk of damage by vein stripping. Also note the inframalleolar vein which joins the great saphenous and posterior arch veins (arrow head).*

the saphenous nerve, which is closely applied to the vein in the lower third of the calf, where it may be damaged by the passage of a vein stripper (Fig. 3.2).

It may seem unnecessary to emphasize that the GSV lies in front of the medial malleolus. The posterior tibial artery passes behind this bony landmark. Failure to remember this very elementary anatomical point has resulted in the femoral artery being stripped on more than one occasion. The GSV is occasionally duplicated, either in part or along the whole of its course. It is also sometimes crossed by the superficial external pudendal artery in the groin, instead of passing superficial (anterior) to it. Surgeons must be aware of these anatomical abnormalities if they are to dissect safely and effectively in this area. The dorsal venous arch of the foot communicates with the plantar veins by way of four perforating veins which pass between the metatarsals (Fig. 3.3) and the GSV, which arises from the medial end of the dorsal venous arch and gives one or two inframalleolar tributaries to the posterior arch vein and its tributaries, the corona phlebectatica network of malleolar veins that drain into the medial calf perforating veins (Figs 3.1, 3.2 and 3.4). These apparently unimportant communications are clinically significant and will be discussed further in Chapter 4.

THE SMALL SAPHENOUS VEIN

The small saphenous vein starts at the lateral end of the dorsal venous arch of the foot and passes behind the lateral

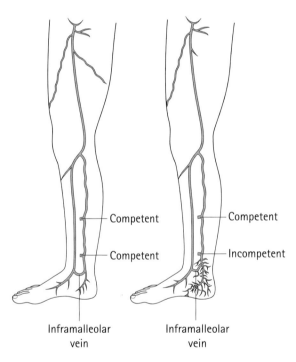

Figure 3.4   *The medial direct perforating veins of the calf and ankle. These are usually found in the following sites: behind the medial vein; 8–10 cm above the malleous; 12–15 cm above the malleous.*

malleolus to join the popliteal vein in the popliteal fossa. This termination is very variable (Fig. 3.5). The high termination occurs in 33 percent of cases;[10] in this variation, the small saphenous vein passes up the posterior surface of the thigh (persistent postaxial vein; Giacomini vein) and either joins the GSV or terminates in muscle veins. The low termination occurs in about 9 percent, the small saphenous vein then joining gastrocnemius veins in the calf.

The paired gastrocnemius veins usually join the small saphenous vein close to its termination. Occasionally they

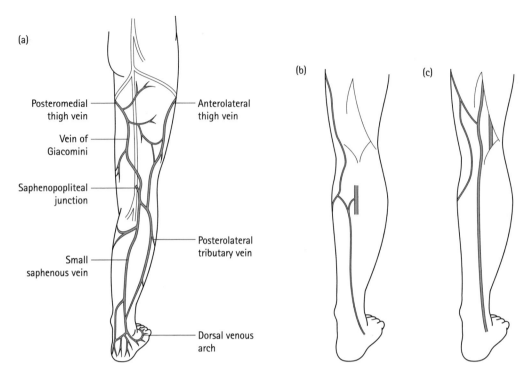

Figure 3.5 *The small saphenous vein. (a) Normal termination; (b) low termination; (c) high termination.*

join the popliteal vein directly, close to the saphenopopliteal junction. Incompetence of the gastrocnemius vein valves and reflux results in calf swelling and discomfort, which can be relieved by ligating these veins.

It is important to realize that the small saphenous vein perforates the deep fascia in the lower or middle third of the calf and lies deep to the deep fascia, between the bellies of gastrocnemius, until it joins the popliteal vein in the popliteal fossa. This feature of the small saphenous vein is described incorrectly in most anatomical textbooks and failure to appreciate this point results in many inadequate operations. Ultrasonography shows that the small saphenous vein is enclosed in a fascial sheath during most of its course in the calf. The description of the external (short) saphenous vein in the 1897 (14th) edition of *Gray's Anatomy*[11] is accompanied by the following footnote: 'Mr. Gay calls attention to the fact that the external saphenous vein often (he says invariably) penetrates the fascia at or about the point where the tendon of the Gastrocnemius commences, and runs below the fascia in the rest of its course, or sometimes among the muscular fibres, to join the popliteal vein. See Gay on Varicose Disease of the Lower Extremities, p. 24, where there is also a careful and elaborate description of the branches of the saphena veins.' The same footnote appears in an American edition 'revised' from the 15th English edition (an original copy of this edition has proved impossible to find), but this footnote has disappeared from the 16th edition and all subsequent editions of *Gray's Anatomy*. As in other aspects of phlebology, Gay appears to have been ahead of his time, and was first grudgingly acknowledged and subsequently ignored by his successors.

In the popliteal fossa, the small saphenous vein continues in the thigh as the 'thigh extension of the small saphenous

vein'. This vein is often referred to as the Giacomini vein, although strictly this vessel is one which ascends the thigh for a variable distance before turning medially to join the GSV. It is sometimes the source of filling of an incompetent GSV where the saphenofemoral junction is competent but the trunk of the GSV is incompetent. The anatomical track of this vein is readily identified on ultrasound imaging.

Ulceration on the lateral surface of the ankle is almost always associated with incompetence of the small saphenous vein. The great and small saphenous veins have relatively thick muscle coats, but the walls of their tributaries are thin and more likely to dilate and become varicose.

The perforating veins

The perforating veins are those veins, other than the long and short saphenous, which penetrate the deep fascia, passing from superficial to deep. Between 50 and 100 unimportant indirect perforating veins enter the muscles before joining the deep veins. These are not normally important to calf muscle pump function, but may dilate and become haemodynamically significant following deep vein thrombosis, recanalization and reflux.

THE CALF AND ANKLE PERFORATING VEINS, THE CORONA PHLEBECTATICA

There are normally three direct perforating veins on the medial surface of the leg and ankle (Fig. 3.4), and one or two laterally. The medial perforating veins communicate with the posterior arch vein, not the GSV itself [although there is an indirect communication by the inframalleolar vein(s) which joins the GSV to the posterior arch vein below the medial malleolus (Figs 3.1, 3.2 and 3.4)]. Each perforating vein contains a valve which directs blood from superficial to deep.[12] An easy way to remember their positions is that the lowest lies behind the medial malleolus, the next a hand's-breadth above this, and the most proximal another hand's-breadth higher (Cockett's hand's-breadth rule).

The direct calf and ankle perforating veins drain the skin over the medial and lateral malleoli by networks of venules and small veins at the distal end of the posterior arch vein; these dilate under increased venous pressure to form the 'ankle venous flare' or 'corona phlebectatica' (Figs 3.4 and 3.6, Plate 3.2).[13] The medial and lateral ankle skin, the 'ulcer-bearing area' of the leg, is not directly drained by either the long or small saphenous vein. The GSV does, however, communicate with the medial perforating veins through the inframalleolar vein(s) and the distal GSV also communicates with the plantar veins through the dorsal venous arch of the foot and the transmetatarsal veins (Figs 3.2 and 3.3). The malleolar venous network which dilates to form the visible 'ankle venous flare' or 'corona phlebectatica' therefore communicates with the deep system by two routes: directly to the posterior tibial vein through the calf perforating veins; and indirectly through the plantar veins by way of the dorsal venous arch. Incompetence of a perforating vein valve results in high pressure in, and dilatation of, the malleolar venules, which results in the ankle venous flare (Fig. 3.6 and Plate 3.2). Calf perforating vein incompetence and an ankle flare are common precursors of venous ulceration; other, more proximal, perforating veins are less often incompetent, and are usually related to primary varicose veins.

THE FOOT PERFORATING VEINS

The foot perforating veins join the plantar veins (distal deep veins) to the dorsal venous arch, which joins the distal long and small saphenous veins (Fig. 3.3). They are therefore able to transmit the high venous pressures in incompetent deep veins to the distal GSV and, by way of the inframalleolar veins, to the malleolar veins (Fig. 3.4).

THIGH PERFORATING VEINS

The Hunterian perforators form communications between the GSV in the lower third of the thigh and the superficial femoral vein in the subsartorial ('Hunter's') canal. Peroperative retrograde saphenography in a series of 60 patients showed at least one Hunterian perforator in 87 percent of 80 saphenograms.[14] Seventy percent of incompetent thigh perforating veins are found in the region of the adductor canal[13] and their incompetence (Fig. 3.7) is a common cause of recurrent varicose veins of the GSV following saphenofemoral ligation without stripping.[15] Other, less common, perforating veins are Boyd's perforator, which joins the great saphenous to the posterior tibial vein on the medial surface of the upper calf at the level of the tibial tubercle, and occasionally a similar perforating vein is found on the lateral surface of the upper calf.

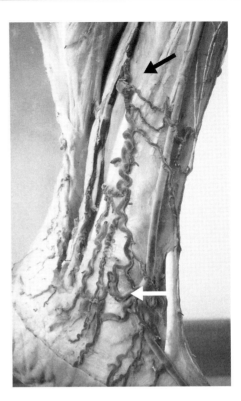

Figure 3.6 *Corrosion cast dissection of the medial surface of the calf showing dilated veins of the 'corona phlebectatica' communicating with the posterior tibial vein through an incompetent perforating vein (black arrow). Note that a number of venules cross the long saphenous vein without communicating with it, but there are two communications below the medial malleolus (white arrow), the inframalleolar veins. (Anatomy Museum, Royal College of Surgeons of England.) See frontispiece for colour photograph.*

The deep veins

The deep veins of the lower leg are the paired venae comitantes of the anterior and posterior tibial and the peroneal arteries, the gastrocnemius veins and the soleus venous arcades. These all join to form the popliteal vein, which receives the small saphenous vein. The main calf veins are profusely valved, but the soleus arcades dilate into large valveless sinusoids. These important vessels, with a total capacity of about 140 mL, act as reservoirs or ventricles for the calf muscle pump. They are a common site of thrombus initiation.

The calf and ankle direct perforating veins penetrate the deep fascia to join the posterior tibial vein medially and the peroneal vein laterally.

Contraction of the calf muscles, enclosed in their tight fascial sheath, forces blood proximally from the soleus sinusoids into the posterior tibial and popliteal veins, reflux being prevented by the numerous valves; during calf muscle relaxation, blood passes from superficial to deep along the direct perforating veins.

The popliteal vein becomes the femoral vein in the lower thigh. This large vein only contains two or three valves and has few tributaries apart from the Hunterian perforator, some muscle veins and the profunda femoris vein, which joins it to form the common femoral vein. The common femoral vein receives the termination of the GSV and often also a deep pudendal branch. The common femoral vein becomes the external iliac vein at the inguinal ligament and this in turn becomes the common iliac vein after receiving the internal iliac vein at the level of the sacroiliac joint. The iliac veins are usually valveless; in 200 cadaver dissections, valves were only found in 54.[6]

THE ILIAC VEINS AND ILIAC COMPRESSION SYNDROME

It has long been recognized that iliac venous thrombosis affects the left leg more commonly than the right. In 1784, White[16]

noticed that the left leg alone was affected by 'white leg of pregnancy' in seven out of nine women and this observation was confirmed by two of his contemporaries. At the time, white leg of pregnancy was thought to be due to the accumulation of milky lymph in the leg and the left leg preponderance was attributed to the fact that most women were delivered lying on their left side. The left-sided predominance of iliac venous thrombosis was later noticed by Welch (1887)[17] and by Aschoff (1924),[18] and compression of the left common iliac vein was described by John Gay in 1867.[19] This phenomenon has been confirmed in several other series, which are shown in Table 3.1.

Post-thrombotic stenosis of the common iliac vein often follows acute thrombosis and is also more common on the left side than the right. A series of 57 patients with post-thrombotic iliac stenosis or occlusion investigated at St Thomas's Hospital in 1967 showed a 67 percent left-sided incidence.[6]

Some degree of anteroposterior narrowing of the termination of the left common iliac vein, with an increase in the lateral diameter, is common. Iliac venograms, performed in 54 patients with no previous history of deep vein thrombosis and essentially normal veins, showed a partially translucent area at the termination of the left common iliac vein (Fig. 3.8). The

Table 3.1 *The incidence of iliofemoral venous thrombosis*

Date	Authors	Total cases	Incidence (%)		
			Left	Right	Bilateral
1784	White[16]	9	65	35	
1941	Barker et al.[25]	210	72	28	
1943	Ehrich and Krumbhaar[23]	16	50	18.7	31.3
1967	Negus[6]	88	53.5	27	19.5
1967	Mavor and Galloway[26]	38	75.3	24.7	

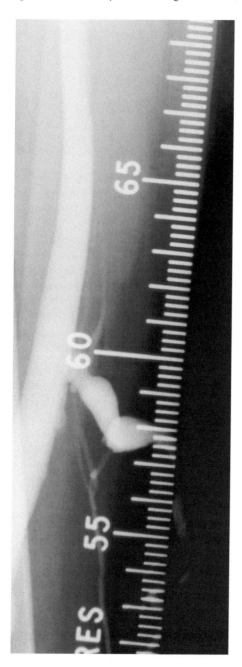

Figure 3.7 *Dilated and incompetent thigh perforating vein.*

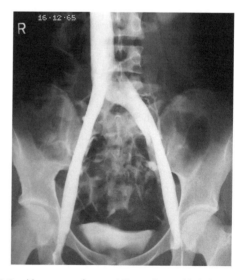

Figure 3.8 *Venogram of normal iliac veins and inferior vena cava showing widening and translucency of the termination of the left common iliac vein as it crosses the body of the fifth lumbar vertebra and is crossed by the right common iliac artery.*

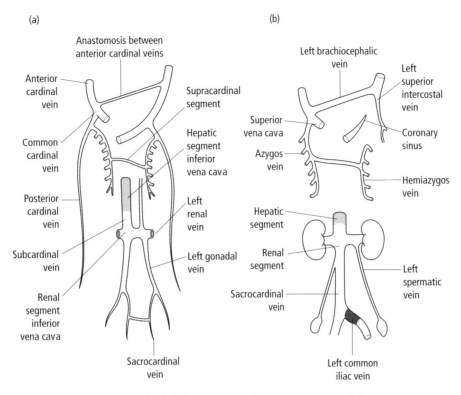

(a)

(b)

Anastomosis between anterior cardinal veins

Anterior cardinal vein

Supracardinal segment

Common cardinal vein

Hepatic segment inferior vena cava

Posterior cardinal vein

Left renal vein

Subcardinal vein

Left gonadal vein

Renal segment inferior vena cava

Sacrocardinal vein

Left brachiocephalic vein

Left superior intercostal vein

Superior vena cava

Coronary sinus

Azygos vein

Hemiazygos vein

Hepatic segment

Renal segment

Left spermatic vein

Sacrocardinal vein

Left common iliac vein

Figure 3.9 *Diagrams showing the development of the inferior vena cava, the azygos systems and the superior vena cava. (a) Seventh week of intrauterine life. Note the anastomoses which have formed between the subcardinal, the supercardinal, the sacrocardinal and the anterior cardinal veins. (b) The venous system at birth. Note that the left common iliac vein is formed from the communication between the two sacrocardinal veins.*

diameter of the common iliac veins was also investigated by preparing corrosion casts of the iliac vessels in nine cadavers. There was marked flattening of the termination of the left common iliac vein in all but one (Plate 3.3).

Compression of the left common iliac vein between the convexity of the lumbosacral spine and the overlying right common iliac artery can best be understood by considering the embryology of the iliac veins and inferior vena cava. The lower part of the embryo body is initially drained by the posterior cardinal vein. During the fifth to seventh weeks of embryonic life, a number of additional veins develop: the subcardinal veins, which mainly drain the kidneys; the sacrocardinal veins, which mainly drain the extremities; and the supracardinal veins, which form the intercostal veins and take over the function of the posterior cardinal veins (Fig. 3.9).[20] The subcardinal veins communicate at the level of the renal veins and the left subcardinal vein then develops into the left

gonadal vein, the inferior vena cava being formed by fusion of the right subcardinal vein and the right sacrocardinal vein. The left common iliac vein therefore joins the inferior vena cava at almost a right angle (Fig. 3.8). The confluence of the

Table 3.2 *Bands at the mouth of the left common iliac vein*

Date	Authors	Dissections	Incidence of bands (%)
1906	McMurrich[22]	31	32.3
1943	Ehrich and Krumbhaar[23]	399	23.8
1957	May and Thurner[24]	430	18.6
1968	Negus et al.[21]	100	14.0

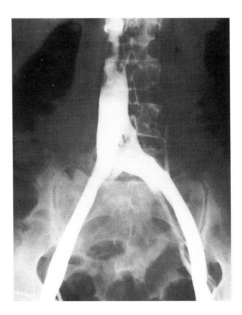

Figure 3.10 *Venogram showing two central bands at the termination of the left common iliac vein.*

(a) 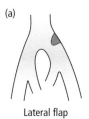 (b) 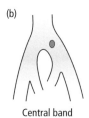 (c)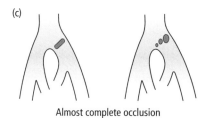

Lateral flap   Central band   Almost complete occlusion

Figure 3.11 *The variety of bands found in 100 dissections of the iliac veins and inferior vena cava.*

common iliac veins with the inferior vena cava is sometimes illustrated as a Y; this is quite inaccurate.

In passing from left to right to join the inferior vena cava, the left common iliac vein has to traverse the forward prominence of the lumbosacral vertebrae. At the same time, it is crossed by the right common iliac artery and these two factors seem responsible for anteroposterior flattening and lateral widening of the termination of the left common iliac vein (Plate 3.3).

Band formation

Bands or spurs joining anterior and posterior walls of the left common iliac vein are not uncommon and appear to be related to extreme degrees of compression of the vein at this point. A typical band is illustrated in Plate 3.4. Bands were found in 14 out of 100 dissections performed at St Thomas's Hospital,[21] and variations in these are illustrated in Figures 3.10 and 3.11. Lateral bands were found in six cases, a central single or double band in six cases, and almost complete occlusion of the lumen of the vein in two cases. No band was found with any other part of the iliac veins or the inferior vena cava. Histologically these bands consist of fibrous tissue and smooth muscle with a surface of normal endothelium. These bands or spurs were first described by McMurrich in 1906[22] and subsequently by Ehrich and Krumbhaar in 1943,[23] and May and Thurner in 1957.[24] Including the author's series,[21] a total of 960 dissections have demonstrated spur formation at the junction of the left common iliac vein and the inferior vena cava in a mean of 22.2 percent. There is no histological support for the view that bands originate from an organized thrombus or embolus and they would appear to be developmental and related to compression of the common iliac vein.

There is little doubt that compression of the left common iliac vein and band formation are responsible for the predominantly left-sided incidence of iliofemoral venous thrombosis.[25–27] The same anatomical anomalies are also responsible for the difficulty in performing left common iliac thrombectomy with a balloon catheter, which often cannot be passed into the inferior vena cava, and also for the failure of this segment of vein to recanalize, resulting in permanent venous occlusion and obstruction to blood flow. This phenomenon has been called the iliac compression syndrome,[28] but is also known as the Cockett and May–Thurner syndromes. Many patients with post-thrombotic iliac vein occlusion develop adequate collaterals which compensate for the main vessel obstruction. The pattern of these collaterals is illustrated in Figure 3.12.

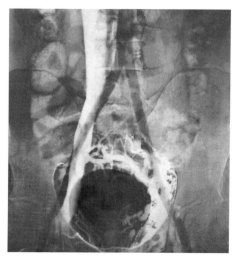

Figure 3.12 *Digital subtraction angiogram showing post-thrombotic occlusion of the termination of the left common iliac vein, with following venous collateral veins: pudendal, presacral and the ascending lumbar vein.*

Congenital abnormalities of the inferior vena cava include paired cavae, a left-sided cava (persistence of the left subcardinal vein), and occasionally complete absence of the inferior vena cava, blood reaching the heart from the lower limbs by way of the azygos and hemiazygos systems.

REFERENCES

1. Williams PL, Warwick R, Dyson M, Bannister LH (eds). *Gray's Anatomy*. Edinburgh: Churchill Livingstone, 1989.
2. Shepherd JT, van Houtte PM. *Veins and their Control*, London: WB Saunders, 1975; 193.
3. Michel CC. Physiology of the skin circulation. *Phlebology* 1991; **6**(Suppl. 1): 1–2.
4. Bauer KA. Management of thrombophilia. *J Thromb Haemost* 2003; **1**: 1429–34.
5. Ackroyd JS, Patterson M, Browse NL. A study of the mechanical properties of fresh and preserved femoral vein wall and valve cusps. *Br J Surg* 1985; **72**: 117–9.
6. Negus D. The sequelae of venous thrombosis in the lower limb. *DM Thesis*. Oxford, University of Oxford, 1967.
7. Dodd H, Cockett FB (eds). *The Pathology and Surgery of the Veins of the Lower Limb*, 2nd edn. Edinburgh: Churchill Livingstone, 1976; 136.
8. Papadopoulos NJ, Sherif MF, Albert EN. A fascial canal for the great saphenous vein: gross and anatomical observations. *J Anat* 1981; **132**: 321–9.

9. Caggiati A, Ricci S. The great saphenous vein compartment. *Phlebology* 1997; **12**: 107–11.

10. Kosinski C. *J Anat London* 1926; **60**: 131. [Quoted in: Dodd H, Cockett FB (eds). *The Pathology and Surgery of the Veins of the Lower Limb*, 2nd edn. Edinburgh: Churchill Livingstone, 1976; 27.]

11. *Gray's Anatomy*, 14th edn. London: Longmans Green, 1897; 689.

12. Van der Molen HR. Taches de stase, corona phlebetica et antres signes de stase veineuse. *Folia Angiol* 1961; **viii**(3).

13. Papadakis K, Christodoulou C, Christopoulous D *et al.* Number and anatomical distribution of incompetent thigh perforating veins. *Br J Surg* 1989; **76**: 581–4.

14. Sutton R, Darke SG. Should the great saphenous vein be stripped? A study of per-operative retrograde saphenography. In: Negus D, Jantet G, eds. *Phlebology '85*. London: Libbey, 1986; 196–9.

15. Munn SR, Morton JB, Macbeth WAAG, McLeish AR. To strip or not to strip the great saphenous vein? A varicose vein trial. *Br J Surg* 1981; **68**: 426–8.

16. White C. An inquiry into the nature and cause of the swelling in one or both of the lower extremities, which sometimes happens to lying-in women. London: C Dilley, 1784.

17. Welch WH (1887) [quoted by Welch WH. In: Allbutt C, ed. *A System of Medicine*. London: Macmillan, 1899; 155.]

18. Aschoff L. *Lecture Notes on Pathology*. New York: Hoeber, 1924.

19. Gay J. On the varicose disease of the lower extremities. *Lettsomian Lectures of 1867*. London: Churchill, 1868.

20. Langman J. *Medical Embryology*. Baltimore: Williams & Wilkins, 1981.

21. Negus, Fletcher EW, Cockett FB, Lea Thomas M. Compression and band formation at the mouth of the left common iliac vein. *Br J Surg* 1968; **55**: 369–74.

22. McMurrich JP. The valves of the iliac vein. *Br Med J* 1906; **2**: 1699–700.

23. Ehrich WE, Krumbhaar EB. A frequent obstructive anomaly of the mouth of the left common iliac vein. *Am Heart J* 1943; **26**: 737–50.

24. May R, Thurner J. The cause of the predominantly sinistral occurrence of thrombosis of the pelvic veins. *Angiology* 1957; **8**: 419–27.

25. Barker NW, Nygaard KK, Walters W, Priestley JT. A statistical study of postoperative venous thrombosis. IV. Location of thrombus. *Mayo Clin Proc* 1941; **16**: 33–7.

26. Mavor GE, Galloway JMD. The ilio-femoral venous segment as a source of pulmonary embolism. *Lancet* 1967; **i**: 871–4.

27. Hurst DR, Forauer AR, Bloom JR *et al.* Diagnosis and endovascular treatment of iliocaval compression syndrome. *J Vasc Surg*, 2001; **34**: 106–13.

28. Cockett FB, Lea Thomas M. The iliac compression syndrome. *Br J Surg* 1965; **52**: 816–21.

4

Venous return from the lower limb: muscle pumps, normal and disordered function

DAVID NEGUS

The veins are the 'capacitance vessels' of the circulation and contain about two-thirds of the total circulating blood volume. Local changes in blood volume are controlled by changes in venous tone mediated by the sympathetic system. The most important function of the superficial veins of the lower limb, as elsewhere in the body, is thermoregulation. Venoconstriction is effected by adrenergic sympathetic nerve endings, and sympathetic stimulation by emotion or pain, or during exercise, also results in superficial vasoconstriction. The deep veins have less powerful muscle coats and mainly act as passive blood conduits.

The veins of the human leg are better adapted to the erect posture than those of other mammals and it is often said that the calf muscle pump is a feature unique to humans and their erect posture. This may not be entirely true as important features of the calf muscle pump, large venous sinusoids in the soleus and gastrocnemius muscles and the direct perforating veins, have been described in dissections of the hindleg of a quadrupedal macaque monkey (*Macaca fascicularis*).[1] It can perhaps be argued that the human calf muscle pump is better developed than that of the macaque and that this development is in keeping with Darwinian theory in being one of many factors which enabled primitive humans to survive and dominate other species.

Blood is returned to the heart against gravity by a number of muscle pumps, most of which are illustrated in Figure 4.1. Three pumps which are not shown in this diagram are the foot pump, the abdominal pump and the respiratory pump. Gardner and Fox[2] have investigated the mechanism of the foot venous pump and have demonstrated that blood is expelled from the plantar veins by their intermittent stretching during foot movement, rather than by pressure of the sole of the foot on the ground. Their book, *The Return of Blood to the Heart*, also contains a chapter by Griffiths, which

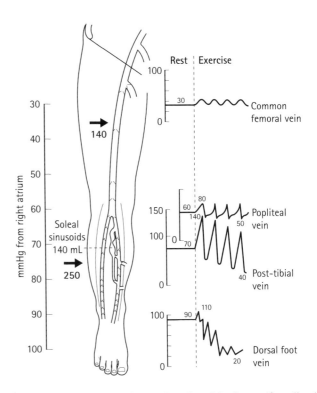

Figure 4.1 *Pressure profiles in the veins of the foot, calf, popliteal fossa and upper thigh at rest and on walking. Foot venous pressure is progressively reduced by contractions of the calf muscle pump whose excursions of pressure are significantly greater than those of the popliteal or 'groin pumps'. The heavy black arrows indicate intramuscular pressures.*

throws considerable doubt on the traditional concept of a respiratory pump. He argues that 'shallow inspiration probably does act to increase the total venous return slightly ... but deep inspiration almost certainly reduces venous return'.

The capacity and pressure profiles of the calf muscle pump are outstandingly greater than all the other pumping mechanisms and its disordered function is the single most important factor in the etiology of venous ulceration.

There are four important components of the calf muscle pump: the dilated valveless sinusoids within the soleus and gastrocnemius muscles; the direct perforating veins; the numerous valves in the communicating and deep veins which direct flow from the superficial to the deep veins and from distal to proximal; and the layer of very tough deep fascia which surrounds the calf muscles. This results in the high intramuscular pressures being transmitted directly to the soleal venous sinusoids as well as all deep veins of the calf.

The calf muscle pump has been described as a 'peripheral heart' and it is interesting to observe that the total blood volume of the lower leg in the erect position is between 100 and 140 mL, very much the same as that of a heart ventricle. The calf muscles constitute a powerful pumping mechanism; intramuscular pressures of 250 mmHg have been measured by Ludbrook[3] and it is likely that venous pressures in the soleal sinusoids are similar, although these have not yet been directly measured.

In the deep veins of the calf, which lie within the deep fascia but between the muscles, the pressures are rather lower: Arnoldi[4] has measured pressures of 140 mmHg in the posterior tibial veins of volunteers. Pressure profiles at rest and during exercise in foot veins, the posterior tibial vein, the popliteal vein and the common femoral vein are shown in Figure 4.1. This is a composite diagram based on the work of Arnoldi and Ludbrook and on personal observation. The greatest pressure swings are seen in the posterior tibial vein. In the normal leg, the foot veins and tributaries of the calf and ankle perforating veins are protected by the integrity of their valves from the high systolic pressures produced by calf muscle contraction. During muscle relaxation (diastole), the valves prevent reflux and the calf muscle sinusoids refill from muscle veins and from the veins draining the medial and lateral surfaces of the ankle and lower leg. These are the malleolar veins (corona phlebectatica) which communicate with the deep calf veins through the direct perforating veins. Note that, in the popliteal and femoral veins, erect resting pressures are significantly lower as the gravitational pressure is lower here. The pressure exerted by the thigh muscles is also significantly lower; unlike the calf, these muscles are not enclosed in a rigid deep fascia.

Calf muscle pump function is traditionally evaluated by foot venous pressure measurement in the erect posture although plethysmographic methods of assessing venous function have been more widely used in recent years. Resting foot venous pressure reflects the height between the right atrium and foot and, in the erect position, is about 80–90 mmHg, depending on the subject's height. Following exercise, by raising the heel repeatedly off the ground, the pressure falls to about 25 mmHg (Fig. 4.2). Standing motionless, the foot venous pressure takes 25–30 s to return to its previous high resting levels. Calf pump failure due to muscle weakness results in a poor exercising fall in the foot venous pressure; venous reflux results in a rapid

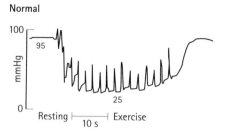

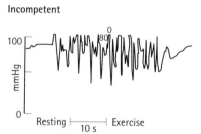

Figure 4.2 *Normal and abnormal foot venous pressure profiles. In the lower trace, deep venous incompetence results in pressure swings with very little fall in mean pressure and a rapid return to high resting pressure.*

return to resting pressure following exercise. In severe venous reflux, exercise produces swings about the mean venous pressure, as shown in Figure 4.2, with very little reduction in mean foot venous pressure and a very rapid return to the resting level.

THE DISORDERED CALF MUSCLE PUMP

The calf muscle pump may become ineffectual due to weakness of the muscles themselves, as may occur in paraplegia, multiple sclerosis or other neurological or muscular disorders. Pump failure usually arises from venous valvular incompetence but may also result from venous obstruction. The effects are markedly different; patients with muscle weakness often develop edema of the lower limb and ankle and this may be due as much to failure to pump tissue fluid along lymphatic trunks as to venous muscle pump insufficiency. Although some degree of edema is usual, ulceration is rare in these patients. Venous ulcers were called 'gravitational' by Dickson Wright,[5] but ambulatory venous hypertension is now considered the most important factor in those with normal muscles but with peripheral venous incompetence.

The venous disorders responsible for reduction in calf muscle pump function include direct calf perforating vein incompetence, superficial (saphenous) incompetence and deep vein incompetence.

The role of direct perforating vein incompetence in venous ulceration

The high venous pressures in the deep veins of the leg, which result from post-thrombotic recanalization and valve incompetence, are unlikely to have any direct effect on the skin or subcutaneous tissues, from which they are separated by muscles and by a rigid deep fascia. There must be pathways for conducting these high venous pressures to the dermal venous plexus of the ankle skin. In 1867 John Gay[6] questioned the relationship between ankle ulceration and varicose veins, and described the ankle and calf perforating veins, and in 1917 John Homans[7] described the relationship of ankle ulceration to previous deep vein thrombosis. He divided leg ulcers into those associated with varicose veins, easily cured by removal of those veins, and post-phlebitic ulcers 'rapid in development, always intractable to palliative treatment, generally incurable by the removal of varicose veins alone, and [which] must be excised to be cured'. Turner Warwick[8] provided the first practical demonstration of flow from deep to superficial in incompetent perforating veins with his 'bleed-back' test, and Cockett[9] coined the descriptive term 'ankle blow-out' for direct perforating vein incompetence. Calf perforating vein incompetence was then considered the most important factor in venous ulceration.

The enthusiasm which followed Linton[10] and Cockett's operations for perforating vein ligation, and the disillusion which subsequently followed, have been described in Chapter 1. The importance of calf perforating vein incompetence in the etiology of venous ulceration continues to be questioned, and Sethia and Darke[11] have shown that, in patients without deep vein incompetence, long-term ulcer healing can be achieved by saphenous ligation without perforating vein ligation. However, incompetent calf perforating veins do play an important role in transmitting high venous flow and pressure in patients with deep venous reflux.

Dodd and Cockett[12] made the important, and often overlooked, point that the direct perforating veins of the lower leg and ankle communicate with the main deep veins of the calf very close to their junction with the soleal arcades, which dilate to form the intramuscular soleal sinusoids (Fig. 4.3). Incompetence of the perforating vein valves will therefore transmit high exercising intramuscular pressures directly to their tributaries, the corona phlebectatica. These regions of the ankle are drained by a network of small tributaries of the posterior arch vein which communicates with the direct perforating veins. These malleolar veins become visible as the ankle venous flare or corona phlebectatica when distended by high venous pressures resulting from perforating vein incompetence (Fig. 3.6, p. 19). This important physical sign is almost invariably seen before the development of lipodermatosclerosis or ulceration. Although these ankle veins communicate primarily with the direct perforating veins, they also communicate with the great saphenous vein by the inframalleolar communicating veins and, by way of the distal great saphenous vein, with the deep veins of the foot and leg through the metatarsal perforating veins[13] (see Ch. 3).

Bjordal, in 1984,[14] performed direct measurements of pressure and flow in the superficial veins of the lower calf and ankle and demonstrated the transmission of high pressures through incompetent perforating veins during muscle contraction,

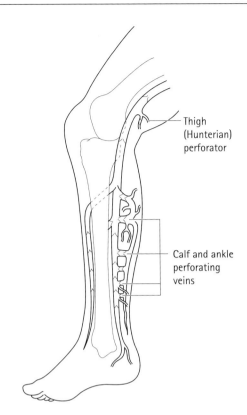

Figure 4.3 *Diagram to demonstrate the close proximity of the direct perforating veins of the calf to the soleal sinusoids.*

blood flow being inward during muscle relaxation and outward during contraction. He recorded a net outward flow of 60 mL/min in a patient with post-thrombotic deep venous incompetence. High pressure and flow in the malleolar veins are responsible for dilatation of the corona phlebectatica, which results in the microcirculatory changes underlying lipodermatosclerosis and ulceration in the overlying skin. The situation can be compared to a leaking bellows (Fig. 4.4). The bellows with a damaged flap valve over its inlet hole continues to eject air through its normal outlet, but air will also escape through the damaged inlet side holes. Substitute venous blood for air and remember that the direct perforating veins communicate with the corona phlebectatica and the effect of perforating vein incompetence can be understood.

Saphenous incompetence without perforating vein incompetence

In 1982, Hoare et al.[15] suggested that saphenous incompetence was more important than perforating vein incompetence in the etiology of venous ulcers in patients without deep vein incompetence, and this was followed by Sethia and Darke's[11] demonstration that great saphenous ligation and stripping improved foot venous pressure profiles in patients with both saphenous and perforator incompetence, but with normal deep veins. Duplex ultrasonography has shown that superficial venous reflux may be the only venous abnormality in up to half of patients with venous ulceration.[16] Surgical treatment

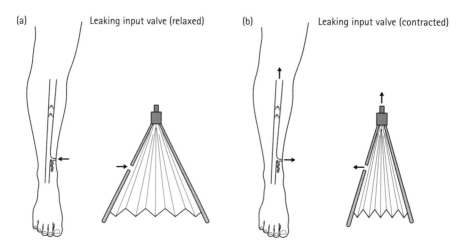

Figure 4.4 *Illustration of the similarity between an incompetent direct calf perforating vein and a broken flap valve in a bellows. (a) In calf muscle relaxation, the reduced pressure in the deep veins 'sucks' blood from the superficial veins through the perforating veins (air is similarly 'sucked' into the bellows when it is expanded). (b) During muscle contraction, the perforating vein valve normally prevents blood refluxing to the superficial system but its incompetence allows reflux and the transmission of high pressures from the deep veins to the superficial (similarly, air will escape through the broken side valve of the bellows as it is closed).*

of incompetent saphenous trunks identified by duplex ultrasonography demonstrated that 82 percent of ulcers had achieved healing and remained healed 18 months afterwards.[17] A randomized controlled trial has recently demonstrated that superficial venous surgery in addition to compression therapy speeds up healing and reduces recurrence of venous ulcers when compared with compression alone.[18]

Saphenous and perforating vein incompetence in venous ulceration

In the Lewisham Hospital Varicose Vein Clinic, the incidence of ulceration was observed in 113 patients with great saphenous incompetence of 153 legs and 24 ulcers were recorded. Calf or ankle perforating vein incompetence was detected in 19 of these 24 legs. Thus, only five ulcers (3.3 percent) were truly 'varicose' in etiology.[19] In a second series of 77 patients with 109 ulcerated legs, saphenous incompetence was found in 36 (47 percent), all of whom had direct perforating vein incompetence.[20]

In 1992, Darke and Penfold,[21] in a series of 213 patients with venous ulcers, found both saphenous and calf perforating vein incompetence in 87 patients with 91 ulcerated legs, deep vein incompetence in 122 patients and perforating vein incompetence alone in only eight. Fifty-three of the first group of 87 patients, with 54 ulcerated limbs, were treated by saphenous ligation, without perforating vein interruption, and 91 percent remained healed at a mean follow-up period of 3–4 years. I have confirmed these observations in a small (unpublished) series and have also confirmed that the perforating veins remain patent and with two-way flow following saphenous ligation. These patients usually do not need to wear compression stockings after the immediate postoperative recovery period. As in the Lewisham Hospital series,[20] the combination of saphenous and perforating vein incompetence has been

shown to be responsible for ulceration in patients without deep vein incompetence, and Darke has also shown that, in most of these patients, it is no longer necessary to ligate the perforating veins as well as ligating and stripping the incompetent saphenous vein in order to obtain long-term ulcer healing.

The series of patients from Lewisham Hospital and that of Darke and Penfold predated the use of duplex ultrasonography, which is now employed almost universally in the assessment of patients with venous disease. The more recently published studies[17,18] which did use duplex ultrasonography to assess the venous system have reached similar conclusions to those from the Lewisham Hospital study and from Darke and Penfold, where phlebography and continuous-wave Doppler ultrasound were employed. In both cases, provided that truncal saphenous incompetence was treated effectively, it proved unnecessary to treat associated incompetent perforating veins.

A THEORETICAL EXPLANATION FOR THE ROLE OF INCOMPETENT PERFORATING VEINS IN ULCERATION RELATED TO SUPERFICIAL VENOUS INCOMPETENCE

The majority of patients with saphenous incompetence and primary varicose veins never develop venous ulcers, even after many years. Ulceration is, however, commonly seen in those with both saphenous incompetence and perforating vein incompetence. How can we explain the apparent contradiction that perforating vein incompetence seems to be necessary for the development of ulceration in patients with saphenous incompetence, but it is usually only necessary to ligate and strip the saphenous vein in order to obtain long-term ulcer healing? A possible explanation involves some elementary hemodynamics, and also depends on the observation that, although the great saphenous vein does not communicate directly with the calf perforating veins, it does communicate with the posterior

(a)   (b)

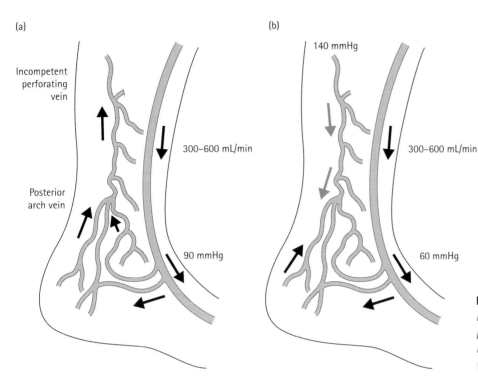

Incompetent
perforating
vein

Posterior
arch vein

140 mmHg

300–600 mL/min

300–600 mL/min

90 mmHg

60 mmHg

Figure 4.5 *(a) Calf muscle relaxation in a patient with saphenous and calf perforating vein incompetence. (b) Calf muscle contraction in the same patient, with distension of the malleolar veins.*

arch vein and the corona phlebectatica, which are tributaries of the perforating veins, through the inframalleolar veins.

Venous distension is related to intraluminal volume and pressure. Initially, as an empty vein is filled, its geometry is restored to cylindrical with little increase in pressure. As the volume is further increased, there is a marked increase in pressure with accompanying distension of the vein segment through increase in its circumference and length.[22] Analysis of the pressure–volume curves of lower limb veins has shown that high-pressure changes in volume are a result of venous wall stretching.[23]

The corona phlebectatica, which underlies the ulcer-bearing area of the leg, communicates with the distal saphenous vein through the inframalleolar veins distally and with an incompetent perforating vein proximally (see Fig. 3.6, p. 19). Distal blood flows of between 300 and 600 mL/min in the saphenous veins of patients with saphenous and calf perforating incompetence have been measured by Bjordal,[14] who also demonstrated normalization of ankle pressures by occlusion of the saphenous vein. The ambulatory mean venous pressure in patients with gross great saphenous and perforating vein incompetence is of the order of 60 mmHg, and systolic pressures of 140 mmHg have been measured in the posterior tibial veins by Arnoldi (see Fig. 4.1, p. 25[4]); this pressure will be transmitted through the deep fascia by an incompetent perforating vein into the posterior arch vein and thus into the corona phlebectatica on calf muscle contraction.

In patients with saphenous and perforating vein incompetence, the following sequence of blood flow and pressure changes in the malleolar veins during walking can be made from the observations of Bjordal and Arnoldi.

During calf muscle relaxation, blood flows distally along the great saphenous vein at a rate of 300–600 mL/min. Some diverges at the knee to flow down the posterior arch vein directly into a dilated calf perforating vein, but most of the distal flow continues down the larger great saphenous vein into the inframalleolar veins and then into the posterior arch vein from below to pass proximally through the dilated calf perforating vein (Fig. 4.5a). When the calf muscles contract, distal flow down the great saphenous vein continues, but proximal flow along the distal posterior arch vein, which is already distended to its elastic limit, is opposed by an outward pressure of 140 mmHg transmitted through the deep fascia from the deep veins by an incompetent perforating vein (Fig. 4.5b). The resulting high pressure and flow are transmitted through the tributaries of the posterior arch vein, which dilate to form the corona phlebectatica. The high venous pressure and flow in this venous network are then transmitted to the venules which drain the skin capillaries and these dilate and elongate, resulting in the microcirculatory changes which underlie lipodermatosclerosis and ulceration.

In patients with deep vein incompetence, the increased blood flow will enter the distal posterior arch vein and the malleolar veins directly through an incompetent perforating vein, and Bjordal has measured a mean outward flow of 60 mL/min in a patient with post-thrombotic deep venous reflux.

Establishing the significance of incompetent perforating veins in practice

In the absence of deep venous incompetence, most incompetent perforating veins are hemodynamically insignificant when the great saphenous vein is occluded. This was demonstrated by Zukowski *et al.*,[24] who used foot venous pressure measurements and serial tourniquets first to occlude the saphenous vein and then the perforating vein and to distinguish incompetent perforating veins into those which were hemodynamically significant (30 percent), moderately significant (35 percent) or of major hemodynamic significance (35 percent). I have repeated these investigations in a small series patients using photoplethysmography as a non-invasive alternative to venous pressure measurement and have found this a simple and useful investigation in clinical practice.

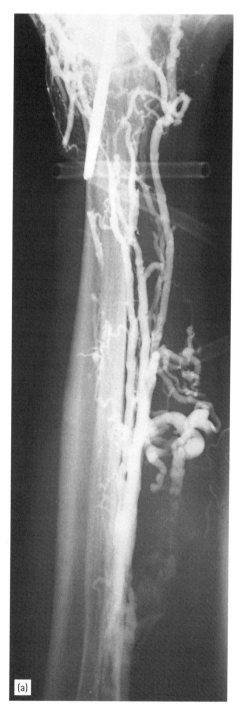

(a)

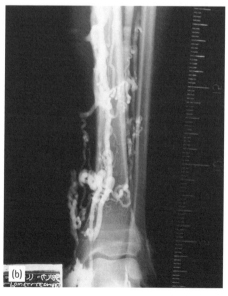

(b)

Deep vein incompetence without perforating vein incompetence

This is an uncommon condition, as most patients with deep vein incompetence rapidly develop perforating vein incompetence, either because the thrombosis responsible for the deep venous incompetence also damages the perforating vein valves, or because the venous hypertension in the deep veins dilates the perforating vein so that their valves become secondarily incompetent. Patients with deep vein incompetence alone suffer from 'heaviness' of the legs on standing or walking, and often from calf swelling and ankle edema. Lipodermatosclerosis or ulceration do not occur until perforating vein incompetence develops, and this can sometimes be delayed for many years by the use of compression stockings.

Deep vein incompetence with perforating vein incompetence

This combination results in the most severe venous ulcers and the most resistant to treatment (Fig. 4.6b). Burnand *et al.*[25] reported 100 percent ulcer recurrence within 5 years in a series of patients with phlebographic evidence of deep vein damage who were treated by direct perforating vein ligation. The same operation achieved very good results in other patients with venous ulcers in whom perforating vein incompetence was accompanied by phlebographically normal deep veins. Neither group of patients wore elastic stockings postoperatively. We have subsequently shown that the addition of class 2 knee-length compression stockings to perforating vein ligation can achieve 80 percent long-term ulcer healing in

Figure 4.6 *(a) Perforating vein incompetence. (b) Perforating and deep vein incompetence.*

Table 4.1 *Results of perforating vein ligation, with saphenous ligation where necessary, and class 2 compression hosiery in patients with deep vein incompetence[a]*

Legs	n	Healed (%)	Not healed (%)
Deep vein incompetence	41	33 (80)	8 (20)
No deep vein incompetence	51	44 (86)	7 (14)
Total	92	77 (84)	15 (16)

[a] 1–11 year review (mean 6 years); 16 patients with rheumatoid arthritis/ischemia excluded.[26]

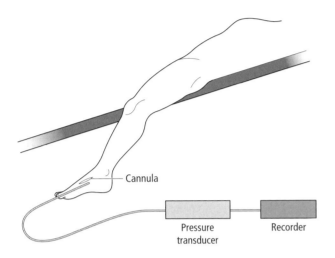

Cannula

Pressure transducer

Recorder

Figure 4.7 *Distal great saphenous pressure measurements at rest and with passive ankle movements.*

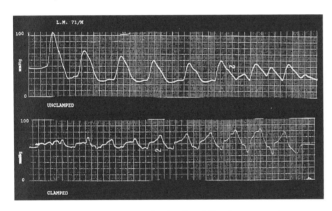

Figure 4.8 *Pressure profiles in the distal (foot) great saphenous vein in a patient with deep vein incompetence and recurrent ulceration following proximal great saphenous ligation and stripping, and calf perforating vein ligation. Top trace: leg-dependent, passive exercise; bottom trace: distal great saphenous patent, distal great saphenous clamped.*

patients with deep vein incompetence (Table 4.1).[26] It is unclear why compression stockings improve the results of perforating vein ligation in patients with deep vein incompetence. They may help by compressing the distal great saphenous vein on the foot and ankle, thus preventing high pressures in the deep veins from being transmitted to the ankle flare veins through the metatarsal perforating veins and the dorsal venous arch (see

Fig. 3.3, p. 17). Compression also has a direct protective effect on the skin in patients with skin changes and leg ulceration. This is the basis of its efficacy in healing leg ulcers. Compression minimizes the transmural pressure in the microcirculation and accelerates flow in these vessels. The reasons why this is effective at reversing the skin changes remain unclear.

DISTAL GREAT SAPHENOUS LIGATION IN THE TREATMENT OF RECURRENT ULCERATION WITH DEEP VEIN INCOMPETENCE

Recurrent ulcers in these patient can be healed by ligating the distal great saphenous vein on the dorsum of the foot,[27] thus cutting off the transmission of high ambulatory venous pressures from the deep veins of the calf to the corona phlebectatica via the plantar and metatarsal perforating veins and the distal great saphenous vein and inframalleolar veins. The significance of these communicating veins has been demonstrated in a small series of four patients with four recurrent medial ulcers and one recurrent lateral ulcer.[27] Venous pressure profiles were measured in the distal great saphenous vein of anesthetized patients, with the operating table in a head-up position and the ulcerated leg hanging down over its side (Fig. 4.7). The calf muscle pump was activated by passive ankle movement.

Resting pressures ranged from 35 to 54 mmHg (Fig. 4.8). During passive exercise, the peak systolic pressures rose to between 85 and 140 mmHg. Following occlusion of the great saphenous vein distal to the canula, the exercising peak systolic pressures fell significantly (38–68 mmHg). The distal great saphenous vein was then ligated and the incision closed. Elastic compression was continued and four of the five ulcers have subsequently healed. Since this study was published,[22] two further patients with recurrent ulceration have been treated by distal great saphenous ligation and these ulcers also remain healed.

This small study has demonstrated that high exercising pressures in incompetent deep veins are transmitted to the corona phlebectatica through its communications with the distal great saphenous vein, the dorsal venous arch of the foot, the metatarsal perforating veins and the plantar veins (see Fig. 3.3, p. 17). It has also demonstrated that recurrent ulcers will often heal following division and ligation of the distal great saphenous vein, and the addition of this simple procedure should be considered before undertaking major surgery for deep venous reconstruction in the surgical treatment of patients whose ulcers are the result of deep and perforating vein incompetence. The study is too small for firm conclusions to be drawn, but it can be asserted that it has demonstrated the importance of considering all communications of the corona phlebectatica in the surgical treatment of venous ulceration and indicates the need for further investigation of this simple procedure.

Deep vein obstruction

Patients with deep vein obstruction, most commonly due to failure of the iliac vein to recanalize following thrombosis

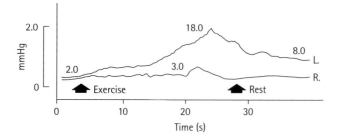

Figure 4.9 *Femoral venous pressure measurement in a patient with post-thrombotic left iliac occlusion. When the pressure reached 18 mmHg, the patient complained of severe 'bursting' calf pain and was no longer able to continue exercising the leg.*

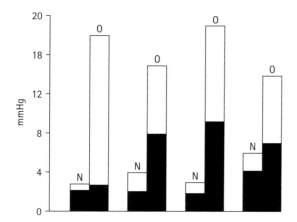

Figure 4.10 *Histogram of resting (■) and exercising (□) femoral venous pressures (supine) in four patients with post-thrombotic obstruction of one iliac vein. N, normal; O, obstructed.*

(see Fig. 3.12, p. 22, and Plate 9.1), suffer from swelling of the affected limb and also from 'bursting pain' on walking. The latter has been called 'venous claudication'.[28] Proximal venous obstruction results in gradual distension of the peripheral deep and perforating veins and eventually in ulceration. This is common in patients with post-thrombotic iliac vein obstruction of 10–15 years' duration (see Fig. 6.13, p. 55), although ulceration is rarely seen in the first few years after iliofemoral thrombosis.

Iliac vein obstruction can usually be diagnosed by Duplex ultrasound scan but, in cases of doubt, this can be confirmed by prefemoral iliac venography with resting and exercising venous pressure measurements (Figs 4.9 and 4.10). An early study of 10 legs in seven patients showed a mean exercising venous pressure rise of 9.9 mmHg (normal controls: 1.4 mmHg).

SUMMARY

The significant factors in the etiology of venous ulceration are high pressure and flow in the corona phlebectatica. This

malleolar venous network communicates with the great saphenous vein through the inframalleolar veins and with the deep veins through the calf perforating veins and the distal saphenous vein via the metatarsal perforating veins.

In patients with deep vein incompetence, each of these communications requires identification and control, and compression stockings or surgery to control deep venous reflux is usually necessary. However, in venous ulceration resulting from superficial venous incompetence alone, it is usually sufficient to control saphenous reflux without perforating vein ligation, and permanent elastic compression is then not necessary.

REFERENCES

1. Chappell CR, Wood BA. Venous drainage of the hind limb in the monkey. *J Anat* 1980; **131**: 157–71.
2. Gardner AMN, Fox RH. *The Return of Blood to the Heart*. London: Libbey, 1989.
3. Ludbrook J. *Aspects of Venous Function in the Lower Limbs*. Springfield: Thomas, 1966.
4. Arnoldi CC. Venous pressure in the leg of healthy human subjects at rest and during muscular exercise in the nearly erect position. *Acta Chir Scand* 1965; **130**: 570–83.
5. Wright AD. Treatment of varicose ulcers. *Br Med J* 1930; **2**: 996–8.
6. Gay J. On varicose disease of the lower extremities. *Lettsomian Lectures of 1867*. London: Churchill, 1868.
7. Homans J. The aetiology and treatment of varicose ulcers of the leg. *Surg Gynecol Obstet* 1917; **24**: 300–11.
8. Turner Warwick W. *The Rational Treatment of Varicose Veins and Varicocele*. London: Faber, 1931.
9. Cockett FB, Elgan-Jones DE. The ankle blow-out syndrome: a new approach to the varicose ulcer problem. *Lancet* 1953; **i**: 1–17.
10. Linton RR. The communicating veins of the lower leg and the operative technique for their ligation. *Ann Surg* 1938; **107**: 582–93.
11. Sethia KK, Darke SG. Great saphenous incompetence as a cause of venous ulceration. *Br J Surg* 1984; **71**: 754–5.
12. Dodd H, Cockett FB. *The Pathology and Surgery of the Veins of the Lower Limbs*, 2nd edn. Edinburgh: Churchill Livingstone, 1976; 38.
13. Kuster G, Lofgren EP, Hollinshead WH. Anatomy of the veins of the foot. *Surg Gynecol Obstet* 1968; **127**: 817–23.
14. Bjordal I. The role of perforating vessels in varicose disease. In: Tesi M, Dormandy JA, eds. *Superficial and Deep Venous Disease of the Lower Limbs*. Turin: Edizione Panminerva Medica, 1984; 91–7.
15. Hoare MC, Nicolaides AN, Miles CR *et al.* The role of primary varicose veins in venous ulceration. *Surgery* 1982; **92**: 450–3.
16. Shami SK, Sarin S, Cheatle TR *et al.* Venous ulcers and the superficial venous system. *J Vasc Surg* 1993; **17**: 487–90.
17. Bello M, Scriven M, Hartshorne T *et al.* Role of superficial venous surgery in the treatment of venous ulceration. *Br J Surg* 1999; **86**: 755–9.
18. Vascular Surgical Society of Great Britain and Ireland. The ESCHAR ulcer study: a randomised controlled trial assessing venous surgery in 500 leg ulcers. Belfast: Vascular Surgical Society of Great Britain and Ireland, 2002.
19. Negus D. Perforating vein interruption in the post-phlebitic syndrome. In: Bergen JJ, Yao JST, eds. *Surgery of the Veins*. New York: Grune and Stratton, 1985; 195.

20. Negus D, Friedgood A. The effective management of venous ulceration. *Br J Surg* 1983; **70**: 63–5.

21. Darke SG, Penfold C. Venous ulceration and saphenous ligation. *Eur J Vasc Surg* 1992; **6**: 4–9.

22. Shepherd JT, van Houtte PM. *Veins and their Control*, London: WB Saunders, 1975; 102.

23. Clarke GH. Venous elasticity. MD *Thesis*. London: University of London, 1989; 158.

24. Zukowski AJ, Nicolaides AN, Szendro G *et al*. Haemodynamic significance of incompetent calf perforating veins. *Br J Surg* 1991; **78**: 625–9.

25. Burnand KG, Thomas MC, O'Donnell T, Browse NL. Relationship between post-phlebitic changes in the deep veins and results of surgical treatment of venous ulcers. *Lancet* 1976; **ii**: 936–8.

26. Holme TE, Negus D. The treatment of venous ulceration by surgery and elastic compression hosiery; a long-term review. *Phlebology* 1990; **5**: 125–8.

27. Negus D. The distal great saphenous vein in venous ulceration: a preliminary report. In: Raymond-Martimbeau P, Prescott R, Zummo M, eds. *Phlebologie '92*. Paris: Libbey Eurotext, 1992; 1291–3.

28. Negus D. Calf pain in the post-thrombotic syndrome. *Br Med J* 1968; **2**: 156–8.

5

Venous thrombosis: etiology, pathology, diagnosis, prevention and treatment

M. MATTHIAS, S. J. MACHIN

INTRODUCTION

Venous thromboembolism (VTE) involves health professionals in all medical specialties, and in an era of increasing medical sophistication it continues to have significant morbidity and mortality. The incidence of VTE increases with age, being about 1 per 10 000 patients per year below the age of 40 years, increasing to 1 per 100 patient-years over 70 years of age. Untreated, about 5–10 percent of deep vein thrombosis (DVT) cases progress to form a pulmonary embolism (PE), of which 1–2 percent are fatal. Numerous clinical conditions predispose to thrombosis but, although understanding of these has improved considerably in recent years, it remains very difficult to predict which patients will succumb, even within known 'at risk' groups. Diagnostic imaging techniques and well-defined treatment protocols are becoming universal, but identification of specific risk factors, and hence preventative measures, should continue to be a goal for those involved in the management of venous thrombosis.

Venous thrombosis is a pathological excess of the normal physiological process that is hemostasis. To understand the factors that bring about thrombosis, it is first necessary to outline the mechanism of normal hemostasis and fibrinolysis.

Primary hemostasis results initially in the formation of a platelet plug which is brought about by the activation of platelets by factors such as exposure to collagen in damaged endothelial cells. Once activated, the platelets change their physical conformation and adhere to the vessel wall and to each other via platelet membrane glycoproteins interacting with von Willebrand factor and fibrinogen. The change in conformation results in an increased platelet surface area composed of exposed negatively charged phospholipids, which provide an optimal environment for the activation of the coagulation cascade. It has become increasingly clear in recent years that the extrinsic pathway, in which activated factor VIIa and tissue factor bring about the activation of factor X, is crucial in the initiation of thrombin generation (Fig. 5.1), while the intrinsic pathway initiated by contact factor activation provides an essential amplification loop.

Thrombin, once generated, converts fibrinogen into a fibrin clot which is stabilised by cross-linking by factor XIIIa. Fibrin seals its own fate by binding plasminogen and tissue plasminogen activator, which allows the process of fibrinolysis to proceed locally (Fig. 5.1). This process results in the gradual

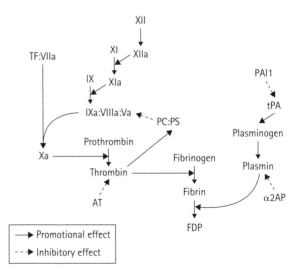

Figure 5.1 *Thrombin generation.*

lysis of the stable clot, re-establishment of vascular patency and the release of fibrin degradation products of varying size, including D-dimers.

In order to prevent uncontrolled clot propagation, there are inherent checks on the hemostatic process. These are inhibitory proteins of the coagulation cascade such as protein C, protein S and antithrombin, which are activated by thrombin generation. The fibrinolytic pathway is similarly checked by proteins such as α_2-antiplasmin (α2AP) and plasminogen activator inhibitor (PAI-1), whereas platelet activation is limited by vessel wall prostacyclin and nitric oxide release. Venous thrombosis generally results from a disruption of the delicate balance of these opposing forces.

ETIOLOGY

Virchow observed in 1856 that three basic pathological abnormalities are commonly associated with the formation of venous thrombosis: an abnormal pattern of blood flow; an abnormality in the vessel wall; and an abnormality in the constituents of the blood, leading to an increased overall coagulability. This classical triad still applies. In most cases of VTE, it is a combination of these factors that results in the formation of clinical thrombosis.

Abnormal blood flow

It has long been recognized that prolonged immobility is associated with an increased risk of venous thrombosis. This results from the absence of the normal pumping action of the calf muscles leading to a relative stasis of the blood, which in turn encourages thrombin generation, platelet activation and clot formation. The relative hypoxia secondary to reduced blood flow also inhibits the natural antithrombotic properties of the vascular endothelial cells. Any other cause of sluggish venous blood flow, such as congestive cardiac failure, varicose veins, obstructing tumors or increased blood viscosity, will also be associated with an increased risk of venous thrombosis. Raised plasma viscosity may be secondary to an increased hematocrit (above 50 percent), e.g. in polycythemia rubra vera, or to excess production of circulating proteins such as immunoglobulins or fibrinogen.

Abnormal vessel wall

When either trauma or surgery occur, they result in increased exposure of tissue factor on the endothelial cell surface to the flow of venous blood. Tissue factor is a potent stimulus for the generation of factor Xa, which then leads to the production of thrombin, and hence fibrin, by positive feedback and amplification. Acute-on-chronic damage to endothelial cells also reduces their capacity to exert an antithrombotic effect which would normally be brought about by the production

of factors such as prostacyclin, nitric oxide and heparan sulfate, which is an endogenous antagonist to thrombin.

Abnormal blood composition

There are numerous specific inherited and acquired deficiencies in the hemostatic process that are associated with an increased incidence of VTE. These so-called inherited thrombophilia conditions are present in about 10–15 percent of the Caucasian population (the incidence varies in different racial groups) and in up to 50 percent of patients under the age of 40 years with proven, recurrent episodes of VTE (Box 5.1). More generalized multiple hemostatic activation changes occur during pregnancy, associated with hormonal preparations such as the combined oral contraceptive and hormone replacement therapy and with other specific medical conditions (Box 5.2). These conditions result in excess thrombin generation (manifest by raised levels of D-dimer, thrombin–antithrombin complexes and prothrombin fragment 1.2) and platelet activation (which can be demonstrated by flow cytometry and exposure of platelet membrane neoantigens such as CD62 and 63). Some of these thrombophilia conditions, either because they

---

Box 5.1 Specific inherited risk factors for venous thromboembolism

- Factor V Leiden
- G20210A prothrombin gene mutation
- Antithrombin deficiency
- Protein C deficiency
- Protein S deficiency
- High FVIII:C (<150 IU/mL)
- Hyperhomocysteinemia

Box 5.2 Acquired risk factors for venous thromboembolism

- Trauma
- Inflammation
- Malignancy
- Pregnancy and puerperium
- Oral contraceptive/hormone replacement therapy
- Surgery
- Sepsis
- Antiphospholipid syndrome
- Immobility
- Hyperviscosity
- Dehydration
- Congestive cardiac failure
- Nephrotic syndrome
- Previous DVT

are strongly associated with venous thrombosis or because they occur frequently, require further discussion.

ANTITHROMBIN DEFICIENCY

Antithrombin deficiency was the first inherited thrombophilic defect to be described. Antithrombin belongs to the family of serine protease inhibitors and acts by forming inhibitory complexes with the activated clotting factors thrombin, IXa, Xa and XIa. The heterozygous deficiency occurs in about 1 percent of young patients with a first spontaneous DVT and the odds ratio for venous (and rarely arterial) thrombosis is increased 10- to 20-fold in heterozygous individuals. Homozygous antithrombin deficiency is not thought to be compatible with life. Once the diagnosis is established, most heterozygous patients who have had a thrombosis will remain on lifelong warfarin. Antithrombin concentrate is now available for use at times of particular thrombotic risk and when anticoagulation is contraindicated, such as during major surgery or in the puerperium.

PROTEIN C AND PROTEIN S DEFICIENCY

In addition to the procoagulant generation of fibrin, thrombin also exerts a negative feedback effect by activating protein C, which, in the presence of its activated cofactor, protein S, inhibits the complex of aFVIII.V.IX. An inherited deficiency of either protein results in an increase in the background risk of venous thrombosis. As these proteins are vitamin K-dependent and have a short half-life, the initial effect of warfarin is to cause a procoagulant effect unless it is covered by concurrent heparin therapy. The most hazardous, but fortunately rare, manifestation of this is warfarin-induced skin necrosis which can occur in protein C- or S-deficient patients started on relatively high loading doses of warfarin alone. Homozygous deficiency of either of these proteins is fortunately rare and presents in the neonatal period with purpura fulminans, requiring lifelong replacement therapy with protein C concentrate or fresh frozen plasma (FFP) in the case of protein S deficiency.

FACTOR V LEIDEN AND THE PROTHROMBIN GENE MUTATION

Studies in the 1990s revealed that some families with venous thrombosis showed a resistance to activated protein C, which was later shown by the Leiden group to equate to a polymorphism in the FV gene. This is a common variation in northern Europe, affecting 1 in 20 people, many of whom will never have a thrombotic event. However, those heterozygotes who have the gene have a two- to eightfold increased risk, increasing to approximately 80-fold in homozygotes. It has become apparent that additional risk factors, such as smoking or taking the combined oral contraceptive, have a synergistic effect rather than an additional effect on the development of VTE, so that a heterozygote woman who is taking the combined oral contraceptive has an increased risk of around 25-fold.

Paradoxically there is some evidence that this risk only applies to DVT, with little increased risk of PE.

The G20210A prothrombin gene mutation (PGM), which was described in 1996, is also relatively common (around 1 in 100 of the population of northern Europe are affected), is associated with raised prothrombin levels and increases the background risk of thrombosis by two- to sixfold. The PGM and FV Leiden quite often cosegregate in families, which appears to increase their risk further than would be expected by addition alone.

ANTIPHOSPHOLIPID ANTIBODIES

Antiphospholipid antibodies (APLAs) are an acquired autoimmune thrombotic risk factor which can occur in many clinical situations but which are only significant if they are detectable on at least two separate occasions and 6 weeks apart. These APLAs may cause an *in vitro* prolongation of the activated partial thromboplastin time (APTT) and the majority of them will be detectable by either a positive confirmatory lupus anticoagulant test (such as dilute Russell viper venom time – DRVVT) or an enzyme-linked immunosorbent assay (ELISA) for anticardiolipin or anti-β_2 glycoprotein 1 antibodies – screens which must form part of routine thrombophilia testing.

Patients with persistently positive APLA and recurrent venous or arterial thrombosis or recurrent early pregnancy loss have the primary antiphospholipid syndrome, whereas secondary antiphospholipid syndrome occurs in people with persistently positive APLA and other autoimmune diseases, such as systemic lupus erythematosus (SLE). Those who suffer from venous thrombosis often develop DVTs in atypical sites or at a particularly young age.

OTHER ACQUIRED ABNORMALITIES

It is well recognized that other medical conditions are associated with an increased risk of venous thrombosis, particularly malignancy, which is linked to VTE in up to 20 percent of cases. In some conditions this can be traced to expression of tissue factor on the surface of the malignant cells, but in most cases it is likely to be multifactorial, e.g. in the case of a woman with a gynecological tumour who may have partial occlusion of her leg veins and a secondary raised fibrinogen. Nephrotic syndrome is also associated with an increased risk, which is thought to be due to loss of inhibitory proteins such as antithrombin in the urine. Pregnancy and the puerperium times of particular vulnerability to venous thrombosis because of the physiological procoagulant changes which include a decrease in protein S and slight increase of factors II, VII, VIII, IX, X and fibrinogen, but with some compensatory hyperfibrinolysis. Patients with a variety of medical conditions are at greater than the background risk of venous thrombosis although defining risk stratification is more difficult than for surgical patients. Congestive heart failure with resulting venous stasis, diabetes, hyperlipidaemia and myocardial infarction with its inflammatory aftermath are all triggers for hypercoagulability. It is now generally accepted that air travel is associated with an increased risk of DVT, though the precipitating factors are not fully understood.

PATHOLOGY

As discussed, venous thrombosis results from an inappropriate excess of a physiological process. The process is perhaps most easy to understand in situations where trauma or surgery have occurred: exposure of the platelets to collagen in the damaged vessel wall brings about platelet activation and subsequent aggregation, while the interaction between factor VII and tissue factor initiates the clotting cascade. The normal self-limiting mechanisms are overcome either due to the degree of trauma or because there are additional risk factors such as prolonged immobility and obesity, and the thrombosis is allowed to propagate.

Thrombus formation often begins in the cusp of a valve in a calf deep vein (Fig. 5.2 and Plate 5.1), where slower flow increases contact between blood cells and the vessel wall leading to thrombin generation, which in turn brings about platelet activation and aggregation.

Although about 50 percent of DVTs are completely asymptomatic, thrombus propagation leads to the cardinal signs of venous thrombosis: swelling, pain, erythema, and warmth in the affected limb. These may be accompanied by dilatation of the superficial veins, superficial thrombophlebitis or cyanosis.

Notoriously, however, venous thrombosis cannot be diagnosed with any accuracy from the presence or absence of clinical signs or symptoms and must be confirmed or excluded by invasive or non-invasive imaging techniques. If there is delay in confirming the diagnosis, for the purpose of clinical management decisions the patient must be assumed to have a thrombosis until proven otherwise.

DIAGNOSIS

With the advent of venography in the 1960s, Haeger showed that 46 percent of patients receiving anticoagulation for venous thrombosis had normal venous systems. There are a wide range of common clinical pathologies which mimic lower limb thrombosis (arterial occlusion, ruptured Baker's cyst, superficial thrombophlebitis, lymphedema and torn muscles), necessitating accurate diagnostic procedures.

Venography

The gold standard for the diagnosis of venous thrombosis is still venography, and it remains the most reliable method of detecting isolated calf vein, iliac or inferior vena cava thromboses.[1] In addition, it has been shown to be the most useful method for diagnosing asymptomatic DVT in high-risk groups, such as postoperative patients. A positive scan shows an intraluminal filling defect and a negative scan shows no

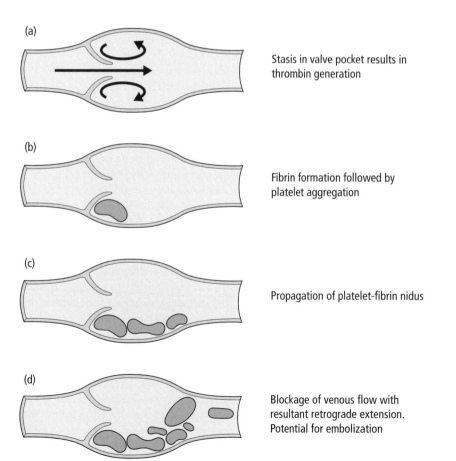

(a)   Stasis in valve pocket results in thrombin generation

(b)   Fibrin formation followed by platelet aggregation

(c)   Propagation of platelet-fibrin nidus

(d)   Blockage of venous flow with resultant retrograde extension. Potential for embolization

Figure 5.2   *Thrombus formation.*

filling defect; non-filling of a venous segment is inconclusive. The disadvantage of the procedure is that the patient must stand in a semi-erect position and must have adequate venous access in the foot of the affected leg. There are potential complications from the use of contrast media, such as allergic reactions, renal impairment, localized skin necrosis secondary to extravasation, nausea, vomiting, dizziness and a small incidence of recurrent thrombosis.

Compression ultrasonography

The advent of compression ultrasonography has provided a non-invasive alternative to venography which has been shown by numerous studies to be sensitive and specific in diagnosing proximal *de novo* venous thrombosis. By applying gentle pressure to the veins of the deep venous system from the groin to the calf bifurcation, the presence or absence of compressibility is assessed. In the absence of thrombosis, the lumen should collapse and the anterior and posterior walls of the vein become superimposed; if a thrombus is present the vein will remain uncompressed even if enough pressure is applied to occlude the artery. Compression ultrasonography for upper limb thrombosis seems to be equally useful, although it has not been as widely assessed.

Ultrasound cannot be relied upon to diagnose an asymptomatic or below-knee DVT; this is important as about 20 percent of asymptomatic isolated calf DVTs extend above the knee if left untreated. Patients with a high clinical probability of DVT and a negative ultrasound at presentation should have a follow-up scan at 5–7 days to exclude extension of a calf thrombosis if anticoagulation therapy is initially withheld. Ultrasound scanning is also not reliable in the diagnosis of recurrent thrombosis: scans remain abnormal post-DVT in 80 percent of cases at 3 months and 50 percent of cases at 12 months,[2] so it can only be used reliably to diagnose a new thrombosis if a patient with a previous thrombosis has had a normal follow-up scan documented prior to the recurrent symptoms (an unusual situation in the UK).

Color duplex ultrasonography

Ultrasound imaging machines currently available often have color Doppler blood flow measurement included in their capabilities. This is commonly used in the assessment of the peripheral vascular system, including the diagnosis of deep vein thrombosis. The use of colour flow assessment may be helpful in the diagnosis of DVT, facilitating the detection of regions of veins without blood flow and possibly increasing the sensitivity of ultrasound in detecting DVT.[3]

Impedance plethysmography

Impedance plethysmography (IP) is less commonly used in the UK and most studies have shown it to be less reliable than ultrasound. It is based on the measurement of changes in calf blood volume in response to inflation and deflation of a pneumatic thigh cuff.[4]

Clinical pre-test probability assessments

Both IP and ultrasound have recently been shown to have better positive and negative predictive values when used in combination with simple clinical predictive indices such as the one described by Wells *et al.*[5] (Box 5.3). This was used to divide patients into those with high, intermediate and low risk of thrombosis based on easily ascertainable factors such as

---

Box 5.3 Clinical model for predicting pre-test probability for deep vein thrombosis. (Adapted from Wells *et al.*[5])

Major points

- Active cancer (treatment ongoing/within previous 6 months/palliative)
- Paralysis, paresis or recent plaster immobilization of lower extremities
- Recently bedridden >3 days and/or major surgery within 4 weeks
- Localized tenderness along the distribution of the deep venous system
- Thigh and calf swollen (should be measured)
- Calf swelling 3 cm > symptomless side (measured 10 cm below the tibial tuberosity)
- Strong family history of DVT (≥two first-degree relatives with history of DVT)

Minor points

- History of recent trauma (≤60 days) to the symptomatic leg
- Pitting edema (symptomatic leg only)
- Dilated superficial veins (non-varicose) in symptomatic leg only
- Hospitalization within previous 6 months
- Erythema

Clinical probability

- High
- ≥three major points and no alternative diagnosis
- ≥two major points and two minor points with no alternative diagnosis
- Low
- One major point + ≥two minor points + has an alternative diagnosis
- One major point + ≥one minor point + no alternative diagnosis
- No major points + ≥three minor points + has an alternative diagnosis
- 0 major points + ≥two minor points + has no alternative diagnosis
- Moderate
- All other combinations

diagnosis of cancer, history of recent immobility or family history of thrombosis. The positive predictive value of abnormal ultrasound scan in the high-, intermediate- and low-risk groups was 100, 96 and 63 percent, respectively.[5]

D-dimer

The place of D-dimer measurement in the diagnosis of venous thrombosis remains controversial. A negative D-dimer assay, with a clearly defined cut-off level, when measured by a sensitive ELISA technique and in combination with a negative ultrasound scan or IP study has a high negative predictive value. Many hematology laboratories in the UK are now introducing automated rapid latex-based ELISA D-dimer tests: these tests are of sufficient sensitivity that, in the accident and emergency setting, a negative result, in conjunction with a low probability score with a clinical screening index, may avoid the need for expensive, time-consuming imaging techniques. A positive D-dimer assay by any method does not have a good positive predictive value because of the numerous causes of raised D-dimer, including infection, malignancy and pregnancy, and it should not be used in isolation for the diagnosis of venous thrombosis.[6]

Computed tomography (CT) and magnetic resonance venography (MRV)

Computed tomography scanning has a role in the diagnosis of an isolated iliac DVT presenting with a swollen leg but negative ultrasonography. Magnetic resonance venography has the advantages over conventional venography of not requiring intravenous contrast injection or exposure to ionizing radiation. However, at present, it has not been evaluated in a management study and is not a first-line investigation.

Diagnosis of pulmonary embolism

The mainstay of diagnostic imaging for pulmonary embolism is ventilation/perfusion scanning, with high-resolution CT scanning, magnetic resonance angiography and pulmonary angiography reserved for equivocal cases or those where V/Q scanning is unreliable, e.g. in those patients with chronic pulmonary disease. As with DVT diagnosis, various strategies have evolved for diagnosing pulmonary embolism which vary from center to center but tend to involve a combination of imaging with either pre-test probability scoring or a sensitive D-dimer test.

PREVENTION OF DEEP VEIN THROMBOSIS

In many cases, venous thrombosis occurs spontaneously without clear precipitating factors. In hospital practice, the risk of DVT may be increased during admission of patients for both medical and surgical treatment. Some operations, such as hip or knee arthroplasty as well as operations in the pelvis, result in the risk of postoperative DVT rising to as much as 70 percent. General surgical operations of greater than 30 min duration increase the risk to 25 percent. Patients being treated in hospital for myocardial infarction and stroke are also at risk. A series of 'risk factors' are recognized, which, when present, increase the likelihood of DVT. These include increasing age, history of previous venous thrombosis, long operations (over 1 h in duration) and complex surgery, treatment for malignant tumours, obesity and presence of a thrombophilia.

A series of measures can be taken to prevent postoperative DVT and protect patients receiving medical treatment in hospital from developing DVT. These can be categorized into mechanical and pharmacological methods.

Mechanical prophylactic devices

The most widely used method of prevention of DVT is graduated elastic compression stockings. These minimize the diameter of deep veins in recumbent patients and increase venous flow velocity. In 1972, Scurr et al.[7] showed that, in patients undergoing abdominal operations, an elastic stocking applying 18 mmHg compression at the ankle and 8 mmHg at the thigh resulted in a considerably reduced rate of DVT compared with control patients who wore no stocking.[7] Subsequent work has shown that compression stockings reduce the risk of DVT by 60–70 percent and also that knee-length stockings are as effective as those of thigh length.[8] Compression stockings are widely used as a preventive measure either alone or in combination with other techniques.

Pneumatic compression sleeves applied to the legs during and after surgery have been shown to be an effective preventive measure. These inflate periodically (usually once per minute) and promote blood flow in the deep veins, reducing venous stasis. A pneumatic foot pump has also been devised to simulate the effect on the foot of walking. This too has been found to reduce the risk of postoperative venous thrombosis in orthopedic patients.

In the past, a series of other mechanical devices intended to move the lower limb in bed-bound or anesthetized patients has been devised. Few are currently in use.

The advantage of mechanical devices in the prevention of venous thrombosis is that they do not increase the risk of hemorrhage, which can be a problem with the pharmacological techniques. In patients considered to be at very high risk of venous thrombosis, mechanical and pharmacological methods may be combined to maximize the protection against DVT.

Pharmacological prophylaxis

A more detailed description of the mechanism of action of anticoagulant drugs is given in the section on 'Treatment' below. The most widely used drug for the prevention of DVT is heparin. This was originally used in its unfractionated form at a low dose, given subcutaneously by injection two or three times per day. The introduction of low-molecular-weight heparins (LMWHs) has allowed a one-dose-per-day regime to be used in the majority of patients. More recently, the pentasaccharide fondaparinux has been introduced and this too allows a once per day injection to prevent DVT.

Warfarin has also been shown to be effective in the prevention of postoperative DVT, but its long duration of onset and action make it less convenient for the management of patients undergoing surgical treatment and this drug is not widely used for this purpose.

Aspirin is a widely used antiplatelet drug which reduces the risk of stroke and myocardial infarction in patients who have previously suffered an ischemic event. It probably has little effect on the development of DVT, but it has been advocated in the prevention of DVT following air travel, despite the lack of evidence of efficacy. It carries the risk of gastrointestinal bleeding if taken by patients with a history of peptic ulceration and should not be taken by asthmatics.

All antithrombotic drugs increase the risk of bleeding to some extent and should be used with this in mind during surgical procedures.

Which preventive measures should be used in which cases?

A range of measures is available but which treatment should be used in which patient? It has been suggested in a consensus document that the risk of developing a DVT should be assessed in each patient and appropriate prophylactic measures taken according to the likelihood of postoperative DVT.[9] Patients at low risk are considered to be those under the age of 40 years, undergoing minor procedures lasting less than 30 min with no other risk factor. The risk of a DVT developing is small (about 1 percent) in such patients and graduated elastic compression stockings would be sufficient protection. Medium-risk patients are considered to be those between 40 and 60 years undergoing surgery lasting more than 30 min without additional risk factors. Here the risk of DVT is about 10 percent and it is suggested that the combination of graduated elastic compression stockings and low-dose heparin or fondaparinux would be appropriate. The patients at highest risk are those over the age of 60 years undergoing operations such as hip or knee arthroplasty or pelvic operations or complex surgical procedures. Patients with a known thrombophilia or previous history of venous thrombosis also fall into this group. Here, combinations of graduated elastic compression, intermittent pneumatic compression and low-dose heparin or fondaparinux should be considered. Clearly, this description is not exhaustive and it may not be feasible to use all modalities of prophylaxis in every case. However, in every patient undergoing surgical treatment in hospital, the postoperative risk should be considered and appropriate prophylactic measures implemented. Ideally this should be part of a hospital policy.

TREATMENT

The treatment of venous thrombosis should encompass prevention of propagation and embolization, pain relief, and measures to minimize long-term complications. The use of class II medical compression stockings should reduce the incidence and severity of the post-phlebitic limb syndrome.

Surgical intervention and thrombolysis

In the vast majority of venous thromboses, rapid treatment with effective anticoagulation is all that is required to prevent extension or embolization occurring. However, there are cases which require more aggressive intervention in the form of surgical embolectomy or thrombectomy or in the form of thrombolysis if the thrombus is less than 3 days old and venous infarction is potentially developing. Surgical intervention is usually reserved for patients with pulmonary embolism who have significant cardiovascular compromise or who have suffered a cardiorespiratory arrest or, in the case of thrombosis, whose arterial supply is compromised by the extent of the venous thrombosis. The place for thrombolysis in the management of venous thrombosis is not as clear-cut as in the management of arterial thrombosis.[9] Randomized controlled data show more rapid clot lysis with thrombolytics but no reduction in the incidence of post-phlebitic syndrome. While the increased risk of serious bleeding with thrombolysis can be justified in the treatment of life-threatening pulmonary embolism or limb-threatening DVT, it would be difficult to justify in the setting of an uncomplicated thrombosis.

In patients with serious hemorrhage, the potential for serious bleeding (e.g. thrombocytopenia associated with chemotherapy or the requirement for urgent surgery) or failed therapeutic anticoagulation, insertion of a temporary or permanent venacaval filter is possible. The nature of the indications has not allowed collection of randomized data on outcome but filters are likely to remain one of the available clinical options. Only one study has looked at the prophylactic use of filters in proximal DVT in patients who were also receiving anticoagulation and this did not show a survival benefit at 2 years, and indeed the patients with filters had an increased risk of recurrent DVT.

Heparins

Heparins are the anticoagulant of choice for the initial treatment of suspected venous thrombosis while the diagnosis is confirmed. Treatment can be started immediately, ensuring effective anticoagulation within 2 h.

Over the last 10 years the initial anticoagulation of patients with venous thrombosis has been revolutionized by the widespread introduction of LMWHs. There are at least seven such products licensed in the UK, with Xa to IIa ratios between two- and four-fold, all of which have similar efficacy for treatment and prophylaxis of VTE. Administered by subcutaneous injection once or twice daily, these products have a far more predictable bioavailability than unfractionated heparins (with a longer half-life of 4 h), which means that the dose can be calculated according to the patient's weight and levels do not ordinarily need to be monitored. The alternative method of anticoagulation is an intravenous infusion of unfractionated heparin following a bolus dose, which requires regular measurement of the APTT and dose adjustments to keep the APTT within the required range (usually 2–3). The latter method is more labour-intensive and subject to human error and laboratory variability. However, it is sometimes necessary in order to achieve safe anticoagulation. Patients with impaired renal function, a significantly elevated body mass index or who are in the second or third trimester of pregnancy may respond atypically to weight-adjusted doses of LMWH. The dosing of the drug is unpredictable in the last two situations, and in the case of renal impairment, dangerous accumulation of the drug can occur because of its renal excretion. Such accumulation of LMWH is not easily monitored because the standard heparin monitoring test, the APTT, is not affected by therapeutic doses of LMWH; in the exceptional circumstances when monitoring is necessary, it is done by chromogenic assays of anti-Xa activity, with the blood test being performed 4 h after a dose of heparin and aiming for anti-Xa levels of between 0.6 and 1.0 units/mL.

Both unfractionated and LMW heparins have the same potential side-effects: hemorrhage, heparin-induced thrombocytopenia (HIT) and osteoporosis. Hemorrhage is more likely in overdose but is well recognized at therapeutic doses. Osteoporosis is only a significant issue when treatment continues for many weeks, as is the case with pregnant women who receive LMWH following a venous thrombosis in early pregnancy. The bone-thinning effects are generally reversible when heparin is stopped but, nonetheless, patients on longer-term heparin should be warned of the possibility of pathological fracture.

Heparin-induced thrombocytopenia is a potentially life-threatening complication resulting in a dramatic fall in the platelet count which may be associated with widespread rebound thrombosis. It occurs 4–14 days after heparin is started, although it may occur more rapidly if the patient has previously been exposed to heparin. Antibodies are formed to heparin bound to the platelet-specific protein platelet factor 4 and the resulting immune complexes trigger platelet activation by binding to platelet Fc receptors, bringing about activation and then consumption of the circulating platelets. Some patients only become thrombocytopenic, but others have progression of existing thromboses or additional thrombotic events. Both unfractionated and LMW heparins have been associated with HIT, with an incidence of about 5 and 1 percent, respectively. All patients remaining on either unfractionated heparin or LMWH for more than 4 days should have a platelet count performed to check for HIT and this must be considered if there is progression of thrombosis despite adequate anticoagulation.

The treatment of HIT is immediate cessation of heparin and its replacement with an alternative anticoagulant such as hirudin.

Pentasaccharides

Pentasaccharides have been recently developed and are now licenced agents which are administered subcutaneously and specifically inhibit factor X and which, unlike LMWHs, do not exert any anti-IIa activity. Their introduction for the prevention of postoperative thrombosis in orthopedic surgery has been shown to be more effective than LMWH in reducing VTE, with no significant difference in bleeding. There is some *in vitro* evidence that the risk of HIT may be negligible with pentasaccharides. Newer forms of pentasaccharide are being developed which have a longer half-life and only require once-weekly administration.[10]

Danaparoid and hirudin

Danaparoid is a heparinoid which is administered intravenously and monitored by anti-Xa activity. There is a low but documented cross-reactivity with the antibodies present in patients with HIT, and renal metabolism limits its use in renal impairment, but it is useful in certain resistant cases with extensive ongoing thrombosis. Hirudin is a recombinant thrombin inhibitor derived from leeches which can also be used in patients with HIT. It is monitored by the APTT or an ecarin clotting time, but the dose–response relationship is unpredictable at high and low doses and the dose must also be adjusted for renal impairment.

Warfarin

Once a definitive diagnosis of venous thrombosis has been made, some form of oral anticoagulation is usually indicated. Warfarin is the most widely used oral anticoagulant in the UK. It antagonizes vitamin K, resulting in reduced effective biological levels of the vitamin K-dependent coagulation factors II, VII, IX and X, by preventing gamma carboxylation of their terminal glutamic acid residues. Warfarin is usually commenced as soon as venous thrombosis is confirmed and takes 3–4 days to become fully effective. Current British Society of Haematology Guidelines recommend a minimum of 4 days of heparin therapy concurrent with the warfarin[11] and an international normalized ratio (INR) >2 should be achieved on two consecutive days before the heparin is stopped. A stable INR is usually achieved within 14 days, with initial testing occurring every 2–3 days and then with decreasing frequency. Doses are adjusted according to the INR and in many hospitals the adjustment is made according to a computer algorithm, reducing dosing inconsistencies. The INR can be measured using either venous blood or capillary blood from a finger-prick test, and the latter means that there are now a number of devices available which allow appropriately selected patients to monitor their INR at home.

A target INR of 2.5 (2.0–3.0) is recommended for the treatment of DVT and pulmonary embolism, the former requiring anticoagulation for a minimum of 3 months and the latter requiring a minimum of 6 months' anticoagulation. Recommendations for the duration of anticoagulation vary according to the presence or absence of precipitating factors or contraindications such as a bleeding history. The recurrence rate of VTE after warfarin is stopped is up to 10 percent, but prolonging the length of anticoagulation in a first spontaneous thrombosis only delays recurrence rather than reducing the rate of recurrence.[12] Recurrent DVT in patients who are effectively anticoagulated requires the target INR range to be increased to 3.0–4.5.

The most frequent and significant side-effect of warfarin is hemorrhage which, as with heparin, occurs more commonly at supratherapeutic levels, but can occur when the INR is well controlled at a lower range. Warfarin is contraindicated in pregnancy because of its teratogenicity. Alopecia and rashes sometimes occur but rarely justify switching to an alternative anticoagulant. Alternatives are other coumarin derivatives or phenindione, an indane 1:3 dione derivative.

The future

Although a very effective anticoagulant, use of warfarin is labour-intensive and expensive to health care providers and inconvenient for patients because of the need for regular INR monitoring. In addition, it has a very narrow therapeutic index and patients on long-term warfarin therapy have an estimated 3 percent chance of a bleeding episode per annum.[13] The ideal oral anticoagulant would have a low risk of hemorrhage, be effective at a regular dose and not require monitoring. The development of direct oral thrombin inhibitors may place us closer to this ideal, and one such drug, ximelagatran, is undergoing phase III trials for the treatment of DVT. Such an approach may allow safe, extended oral anticoagulation with minimal impact on patient lifestyle and quality of life whilst reducing long-term recurrence of VTE.

REFERENCES

1. Fraser JD, Anderson DR. Deep venous thrombosis: recent advances and optimal investigation with US. *Radiology* 1999; **211**: 9–24.
2. Kearon C, Julian JA, Newman TE, Ginsberg JS. Noninvasive diagnosis of deep venous thrombosis. McMaster Diagnostic Imaging Practice Guidelines Initiative. *Ann Intern Med* 1998; **128**: 663–77.
3. Noren A, Ottosson E, Rosfors S. Is it safe to withhold anticoagulation based on a single negative color duplex examination in patients with suspected deep venous thrombosis? A prospective 3-month follow-up study. *Angiology* 2002; **53**: 521–7.
4. Chunilal SD, Ginsberg JS. Advances in the diagnosis of venous thromboembolism a multimodal approach. *J Thromb Thrombolysis* 2001; **12**: 53–7.
5. Wells PS, Hirsh J, Anderson DR *et al.* Accuracy of clinical assessment of deep-vein thrombosis. *Lancet* 1995; **345**: 1326–30.
6. Kelly J, Rudd A, Lewis RR, Hunt BJ. Plasma D-dimers in the diagnosis of venous thromboembolism. *Arch Intern Med* 2002; **162**: 747–56.
7. Scurr JH, Ibrahim SZ, Faber RG, Le Quesne LP. The efficacy of graduated compression stockings in the prevention of deep vein thrombosis. *Br J Surg* 1977; **64**: 371–3.
8. Porteus LJ, Le F, Nicholson EA *et al.* Thigh length versus knee length stockings in the prevention of deep vein thrombosis. *Br J Surg* 1989; **76**: 296–97.
9. Thromboembolic Risk Factors (THRIFT) Consensus Group. Risk of and prophylaxis for venous thromboembolism in hospital patients. *Br Med J* 1992; **305**: 567–74.
10. Ludlum CA, Bennett B, Fox KA *et al.* Guidelines for the use of thrombolytic therapy. Haemostasis and Thrombosis Task Force of the British Committee for Standards in Haematology. *Blood Coagul Fibrinolysis* 1995; **6**: 273–85.
11. Hirsh J, Lee AY. How we diagnose and treat deep vein thrombosis. *Blood* 2002; **99**: 3102–10.
12. BCSH Guidelines on oral anticoagulation: third edition. *Br J Haematol.* 1998; **101**: 374–87.
13. Agnelli G, Prandoni P, Santamaria MG *et al.* and Warfarin Optimal Duration Italian Trial Investigators. Three months versus one year of oral anticoagulant therapy for idiopathic deep venous thrombosis. Warfarin Optimal Duration Italian Trial Investigators. *N Engl J Med* 2001; **345**: 165–9.

6

The pathology of leg ulcers and venous disorders

DAVID NEGUS, PHILIP D. COLERIDGE SMITH, S. S. ROSE

METHODS OF CLASSIFICATION AND GRADING OF LOWER LIMB CHRONIC VENOUS DISEASE

Previous methods of classification of lower limb venous disease include that of Widmer,[1] which categorized limbs, based on their clinical appearance. In 1994, an international consensus report under the auspices of the American Venous Forum presented the latest method of classification and grading of lower limb chronic venous disease, which was as a result of significant progress made in the field of non-invasive investigation of venous pathology with the use of electronic and computer-aided technology. This system requirement was similar to those for diagnosing peripheral arterial disease, which had long been in use.

The CEAP method classifies lower limb chronic venous disease according to the clinical signs and symptoms (C), the etiology (E), the anatomic distribution of the pathology (A) and the pathophysiologic dysfunction (P) resulting in a multiaxial system.[2] The clinical classification differentiates telangiectases from truncal varicose veins, and healed ulcers from open ulcers, in a seven-stage description. In addition to the classification of disease, the CEAP method also allows one to score the disease.

The CEAP method of classification is discussed below (and summarized in Box 6.1):

Clinical classification (C_0–C_6). C is for clinical signs (grade 0–6) graded in increasing order of severity according to the objective clinical signs of disease listed in Box 6.1. Limbs with more severe signs of chronic venous disease will be placed in the higher categories and may have some or all of the findings defining a less severe clinical category. Each limb will be further characterized as symptomatic (S) or asymptomatic (A).

Therapy may alter the clinical category of a limb therefore it was recommended that limbs should be reclassified after any form of medical or surgical intervention at least 6 months after.

Etiologic classification (E_C, E_P, E_S). E is for etiologic classification, i.e. whether the venous dysfunction is congenital, primary or secondary.

Anatomic classification (A_S, A_D, A_P). A is for anatomic distribution, i.e. whether the vein(s) affected by venous disease is in the superficial, deep or perforator systems. One, two or three systems may be involved in any combination. Box 6.1 lists the anatomic segments in the superficial, deep and perforator systems that may be involved.

Pathophysiologic classification (P_R, P_O). P is for pathophysiologic dysfunction, which may result from reflux (P_R), obstruction (P_O) or both ($P_{R,O}$).

It is now recommended that in the investigation of patients with chronic venous disease, sufficient objective measurements of venous hemodynamics and anatomy by either invasive or non-invasive means must be carried out to document adequately the individual pathophysiologic changes, reflux, and/or obstruction accompanying chronic venous disease. Phlebographic or vascular laboratory investigations can objectively assess the presence of venous outflow obstruction (P_O) as well as the presence of venous reflux (P_R) in the superficial, deep and perforating systems.

The anatomic segments that are involved with either reflux or obstruction are reported using the venous segments outlined in Box 6.1, as the severity of venous dysfunction is influenced by the anatomic location and extent of the reflux and/or obstruction present.[3,4]

Scoring of venous dysfunction

Another feature of the CEAP method of classification of lower limb chronic venous disease is the scoring system of chronic venous dysfunction that is incorporated into the system. This provides a numerical base for the scientific comparison of limb condition and evaluation of results of treatment. The scoring system is based on three elements:

- the number of anatomic segments affected (anatomic score)
- grading of symptoms and signs (clinical score)
- disability (disability score).

This method of scoring and grading is thought to be more accurate as the grading of signs is objective whereas the grading of symptoms is subjective.

CLINICAL SCORE

The clinical score is the sum of the values assigned to the signs and symptoms listed in Box 6.2.

ANATOMIC SCORE

The anatomic score is the sum of the anatomic segments affected by either reflux, obstruction or both, each scored as one point, as listed in Box 6.1.

DISABILITY SCORE

The disability score is the sum of the values assigned to the signs and symptoms listed in Box 6.3.

Box 6.1   CEAP classification of lower limb chronic venous disease

C for **Clinical** signs (grade 0–6), supplemented by (A) for asymptomatic and (S) for symptomatic presentation
E for **Etiologic** classification – congenital (E_C), primary (E_P), secondary (E_S)
A for **Anatomic** distribution – superficial (A_S), deep (A_D), or perforator (A_P), alone or in combination
P for **Pathophysiologic** dysfunction – reflux (P_R) or obstruction (P_O), alone or in combination

Clinical classification

Class 0   No visible or palpable signs of venous disease
Class 1   Telangiectases or reticular veins
Class 2   Varicose veins
Class 3   Edema
Class 4   Skin changes ascribed to venous disease (e.g. pigmentation, lipodermatosclerosis, venous eczema)
Class 5   Skin changes as in class 4 with healed ulceration
Class 6   Skin changes as in class 4 with active ulceration

Etiologic classification

- Congenital (E_C)
- Primary (E_P) – with undetermined cause
- Secondary (E_S) – with known cause
  - post-thrombotic
  - post-traumatic
  - other

Anatomic classification

Superficial veins (A_{S1-5}):
Segment 1   Telangiectases/reticular veins
                  Great saphenous vein

Segment 2   Above knee
Segment 3   Below knee
Segment 4   Small saphenous vein
Segment 5   Non-saphenous vein

Deep veins (A_{D6-16}):
Segment 6   Inferior vena cava
                  Iliac
Segment 7   Common
Segment 8   Internal
Segment 9   External
Segment 10   Pelvic – gonadal, broad ligament, other
                  Femoral
Segment 11   Common
Segment 12   Deep
Segment 13   Superficial
Segment 14   Popliteal
Segment 15   Crural – anterior tibial, posterior tibial, peroneal (all paired)
Segment 16   Muscular – gastrocnemial, soleal, other

Perforating veins ($A_{P17,18}$):
Segment 17   Thigh
Segment 18   Calf

Pathophysiologic classification

- Reflux (P_R)
- Obstruction (P_O)
- Reflux and obstruction ($P_{R,O}$)

LEG ULCERS

An ulcer has been defined as a 'discontinuity of an epithelial surface'.[5] A simpler definition is that of Sir Roy Cameron in *Pathology*:[6] 'An ulcer is a local defect, or excavation, of the surface of an organ or tissue, which is produced by the sloughing [shedding] of inflammatory necrotic tissue'.

Box 6.2 Clinical scoring of the signs and symptoms of lower limb venous disease

Pain	0, none; 1, moderate, not requiring analgesics; 2, severe, requiring analgesics
Oedema	0, none; 1, mild/moderate; 2, severe
Venous claudication	0, none; 1, mild/moderate; 2, severe
Pigmentation	0, none; 1, localized; 2, extensive
Lipodermatosclerosis	0, none; 1, localized; 2, extensive
Ulcer	
– size (largest ulcer)	0, none; 1, <2 cm diameter; 2, >2 cm diameter
– duration	0, none; 1, <3 months; 2, >3 months
– recurrence	0, none; 1, once; 2, more than once
– number	0, none; 1, single; 2, multiple

Box 6.3 Disability score

0   Asymptomatic
1   Symptomatic, can function without support device
2   Can work 8-hour day *only* with support device
3   Unable to work even with support device

The base of an ulcer consists of necrotic tissue and inflammatory exudate with variable degrees of fibroblastic proliferation and scarring. The surface always contains some bacteria and, in an acutely infected ulcer, these may proliferate to produce a purulent exudate. The base of a healing ulcer consists of bright red granulation tissue, the surface of the capillary loops arising from the dermal blood vessels (Fig. 6.1).

The edges are composed of epidermal cells attempting to migrate inwards to cover the granulation tissue and effect healing. Chronic ulceration occurs where epithelialization of the edge and fibroblast proliferation in the base are opposed by factors preventing healing; in the leg, these factors are usually vascular. Healing will be slow or non-existent when the arterial blood flow is insufficient to provide adequate metabolites for growth of the epithelial edge and the granulation tissue of the base; it will equally be deficient where venous hypertension opposes the process of tissue repair. Healing may also be inhibited by other factors, such as infection, diabetes or the anti-inflammatory effect of steroid therapy, as well as vitamin C deficiency, anemia and malnutrition.

Common leg ulcers: clinical features

ISCHEMIC ULCERATION

The base of an ischemic ulcer has poorly formed, pale granulation tissue usually covered by necrotic slough (Fig. 6.2). In the most severe cases, removal of this slough and debris will reveal the deep fascia or ankle tendons, with little or no granulation tissue. The edges are poorly epithelialized and there may be no visible epithelialization at all, the base of the ulcer sharply demarcating into the surrounding ischemic skin. Ischemic ulceration is characterized by its site, in areas of poor blood supply, and, where ulceration is secondary to major arterial disease, it is usually accompanied by ischemic rest pain. Ischemic ulceration most commonly results from atherosclerotic main vessel occlusion, but it can also arise from insufficiency of the small vessels, as in thromboangiitis obliterans (Buerger's disease), which is related to heavy cigarette smoking.

Small-vessel insufficiency also occurs in diabetic arteriopathy and vasculitis. Ulceration in patients suffering from these disorders, particularly diabetes, may result from a

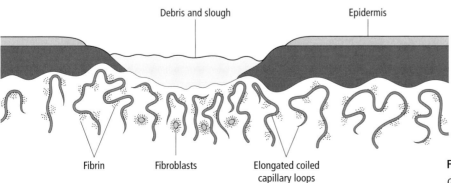

Debris and slough   Epidermis

Fibrin   Fibroblasts   Elongated coiled capillary loops

Figure 6.1 *Diagrammatic cross-section of a healing venous ulcer.*

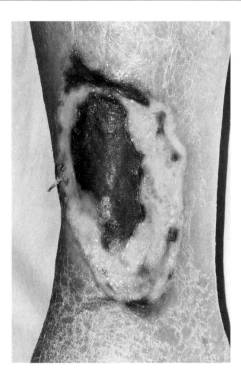

Figure 6.2 *Ischemic leg ulceration showing central gangrenous slough.*

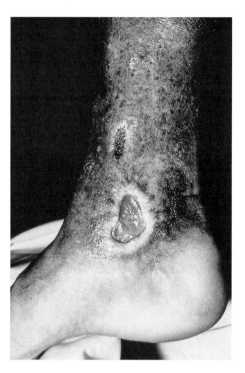

Figure 6.3 *Venous ulcer.*

combination of large- and small-vessel disease. Care must be taken to detect peripheral pulses by palpation or by Doppler ultrasound in such patients, rather than dismissing them from consideration for arterial reconstructive surgery on the grounds that their arterial insufficiency is confined to small vessels and is therefore not suitable for surgical intervention. Care must also be taken to exclude arterial insufficiency in patients presenting with ulceration of predominantly venous origin. Concomitant arterial insufficiency is common in the elderly and attention must therefore be paid to treating both venous and arterial causes. Apparent foot ulceration may result from a sinus arising from underlying osteomyelitis and this possibility should be checked by X-ray.

VENOUS ULCERS

Venous ulcers most commonly occur over the medial malleolus and less frequently over the lateral surface of the ankle. A true varicose ulcer may lie anterior or posterior to these sites, usually directly over a large varix. However, anterior leg ulcers are much more likely to be ischemic in origin and those on the dorsum of the foot are almost invariably ischemic.

Venous ulcers vary in size from only a few centimetres (Fig. 6.3) to giant ulcers which may be circumferential and involve the whole of the gaiter area of the lower leg. They are often infected when first seen but the infection responds rapidly to daily cleaning, non-irritant dressings, firm compression bandaging and appropriate antibiotics. Although antibiotic treatment can address clinically apparent infection, these drugs do not directly promote leg ulcer healing. In contrast, infected ischemic ulcers usually fail to respond to antibiotics

until the ischemia is successfully corrected. A clean venous ulcer has a base composed of healthy pink granulations covered perhaps by a little debris, and the edges consist of sloping pink epithelium. The granulation tissue represents the surface of capillary loops. A venous ulcer is usually surrounded by pigmented, indurated skin (lipodermatosclerosis), the result of pericapillary fibrin and hemosiderin deposition.

Bacteriology of leg ulcers

Most leg ulcers are infected when first seen. Infection is usually secondary to the underlying venous or arterial disorder. Minor skin abrasions are invariably accompanied by the entry of a few skin bacteria whose colonization can proceed unimpeded in the presence of ischemia or venous hypertension.

The organisms cultured are mostly Gram-positive skin organisms. A random survey of the bacteriological findings in 30 leg ulcers in patients attending clinics at Lewisham Hospital between May and September 1989 is shown in Table 6.1. *Streptococcus aureus* was the most commonly cultured organism. Coliforms were never cultured alone, but were always found in combination with a Gram-positive organism, usually *S. aureus*. Coliforms were occasionally found with other organisms, *Streptococcus* in three cultures and *Staphylococcus albus* in one. Anaerobic organisms were not looked for in these bacteriological examinations, but Browse et al.[7] did investigate their presence and found them in 44 percent of the ulcers cultured. For this reason, it is always wise to prescribe metronidazole in addition to antibiotics specific for aerobic organisms where there is clinical evidence of infection.

Table 6.1 *Bacteriological findings in 30 leg ulcers*

Organism cultured	Number of cases
Single	
Staphylococcus aureus	9
Pseudomonas aeruginosa	4
Streptococcus faecalis	1
Diphtheroids (+ *Staphylococcus albus*)	1
Coliforms (+ *Staphylococcus albus*)	1
Multiple	
Staphylococcus aureus + coliform	5
Staphylococcus aureus + diphtheroids	1
Staphylococcus aureus + *Streptococcus faecalis*	1
Staphylococcus aureus + β-hemolytic *Streptococcus*	1
Staphylococcus aureus + β-hemolytic *Streptococcus* + *Pseudomonas*	1
Staphylococcus aureus + E. coli + group B *Streptococcus*	1
β-haemolytic *Streptococcus* + *P. aeruginosa* + coliform	1
Streptococcus faecalis + coliform	1
Streptococcus viridans + coliform + diphtheroids	1

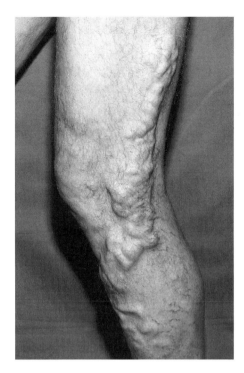

Figure 6.4 *Gross varicose veins of the great saphenous system.*

Most microorganisms are relatively innocuous but beta-hemolytic streptococci have been shown to be severely pathogenic[8] and must be treated rigorously.

A detailed review of the use of antibiotics in chronic wounds finds no support for the routine use of antibiotics in the management of venous leg ulcers.[9] Naturally, clinical infection of an ulcer must be treated, but this is best done by local ulcer toilet, unless cellulitis or septicemia supervene. Intravenous antibiotics are indicated when severe infection is present.

Venous disorders responsible for ulceration

Venous ulcers may occasionally occur over a large distended varix on the lower leg, without perforating vein incompetence; these are true 'varicose' ulcers. More commonly, one or more perforating veins are incompetent in ulcerated limbs with saphenous incompetence, although it is usually unnecessary to ligate these perforating veins (see Ch. 4). The most difficult ulcers to treat are those which result from post-thrombotic deep vein incompetence, which were described by Homans[10] as 'rapid in development, always intractable to palliative treatment, generally incurable by the removal of varicose veins alone and [which] must be excised to be cured'.

VARICOSE VEINS

Varicose veins are defined as distended, elongated, tortuous superficial veins with incompetent valves (Fig. 6.4). Rare among rural Africans and Indians, primary familial varicose veins are very common indeed in industrialized Western society.

A number of studies from Europe and North and South America have described an incidence of about 50 percent in the middle-aged and elderly, with about a 10 percent greater incidence in women.[11] The Edinburgh Vein Study found a slightly higher incidence of varicose veins in men.[12]

It has been supposed that valvular incompetence starts at the saphenofemoral junction and may be the result of pressure from a gravid uterus or even from pressure produced by the constipated sigmoid colon. The statement that 'varicose veins are the penalty that man pays for assuming the upright posture' ignores the fact that there are many mammals with longer legs and therefore potentially greater foot venous pressures than humans.

It is unlikely that primary varicose veins occur as the result of valve defects, as varicose blowouts are often found distal to intact valves.[13,14] Tensiometer studies have demonstrated that the valve is the single strongest part of the vein.[15] High venous pressure resulting from primary valve failure also seems less likely as a cause of varicosity when it is remembered that the saphenous vein used as an arterial conduit becomes thick-walled and arterialized, rather than thin-walled and varicose. The most recent convincing argument contradicting primary valve failure in the etiology of varicose veins is the observation that saphenous vein reflux has been detected by duplex scan in the absence of saphenofemoral or saphenopopliteal incompetence.[16,17] This suggests that a problem with the vein itself leads to the development of varicose veins rather than the effects of gravity.

Patients with primary varicose veins usually have a strong family history (usually in the mother), and these observations provide a more acceptable hypothesis for the etiology of varicose veins than dubious explanations based on 'the penalty for assuming the upright posture', 'constipation', or 'pressure of the gravid uterus'. However, they fail to explain why the long and short saphenous systems may become varicose independently of each other or why one leg is often affected but not the other.

Secondary varicose veins may follow valve destruction by thrombosis and may also result from arteriovenous fistula formation.

Histological observations: vein, valve or venous wall

Following the discovery of the circulation by William Harvey, it was assumed that the varicose condition was the result of valvular incompetence (Plate 6.1) and gravitational pressure would be the cause of varicosity. Although this is a logical argument, there are certain aspects of the development of varicosities which suggest that the part played by the condition of the vein wall cannot be ignored.[14]

Exactly how do valves become incompetent? Do valves atrophy? Normally atrophy is a phenomenon which occurs with advancing age, yet varicose veins can develop in the young, and in the majority of cases they develop in middle life.

Pregnancy provides a clinical model of how veins become varicose. The evidence against atrophy of the valves is that many varicose veins disappear within 3 months after delivery, i.e. incompetent valves, if these are the cause of the varicosities, become competent again. Are varicose veins of pregnancy the result of back pressure from the gravid uterus? No, for the varicosities of pregnancy often develop during the first 6 weeks, before the uterus is large enough to cause back pressure. Varicose veins of pregnancy are related to the effect of estrogens and progesterone on the vein wall.[18] It is known that estrogens cause relaxation of smooth muscle and our attention must be directed to the muscle fibres of the vein wall. The physiological effect on the muscle cell results in loss of elasticity or tone and this results in the valve ring becoming so enlarged that the cusps are prevented from closing, although the cusps themselves are not affected. When the hormonal cocktail returns to normality the tone will usually recover following a first pregnancy and the valves become competent again (Fig. 6.5). Following subsequent pregnancies, varicose veins will usually persist and enlarge, due to permanent loss of tone following repeated stretching.

Taking pregnancy as an example, it is obvious that the evidence is in favour of examining the pathology of the vein wall in varicose veins.

To return to the question of venous tone. In the past, veins were regarded as conduits through which blood is returned to the heart and little attention was paid to the muscle coat. It is now generally accepted that venous tone plays an important part in assisting venous return and is complementary to the vis a tergo. Most of the strength of the vein wall is thought to lie in the elastic and collagen tissue. Vascular surgeons who use the saphenous vein as a bypass graft have often noted that a large

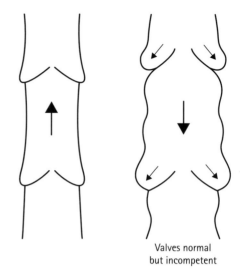

Valves normal
but incompetent

Figure 6.5   *Competent and incompetent venous valves.*

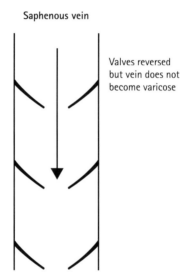

Saphenous vein

Valves reversed
but vein does not
become varicose

Figure 6.6   *Reverse saphenous vein for arterial bypass. Valves reverse, but vein does not become varicose.*

vein can contract to an uncomfortably small size on handling and it is evident that the muscle wall is capable of exerting considerable tone (Fig. 6.6).

In the development of varicose veins, if the basic lesion is in the muscle cell, the cycle of loss of tone, followed by venous dilatation accompanied by dilatation of the valve ring with prevention of closure of the valve cusps will be sufficient to produce varicosity. This is then aggravated by gravitational back pressure.

This theory explains how lateral blowouts occur with or without incompetent proximal valves, how fusiform dilatations occur, how varicosity occurs below competent valves and why simple proximal ligation of the long saphenous vein (without stripping) or ligation of the deep perforators will only produce a temporary effect. It also explains why stripping that does not eradicate the individual varicosities will be a failure.

All these arguments have stimulated us to examine the structure of the vein wall with special reference to the muscle cell. This has been carried out by light and electron microscopy and the following findings have been consistent in all the varicose vein sections examined.

LIGHT MICROSCOPY

The sections were first examined by light microscopy using an H&E stain, a Van Gieson elastic stain and a Masson trichrome muscle stain, using a normal vein as a control.[14]

The control (Plate 6.2) showed that the circular muscle layer consisted of cells arranged in regular whorls in a fine connective tissue matrix. The connective tissue tended to be condensed subintimally immediately deep to an internal elastic lamina and it again became condensed in the outer coat where it formed the adventitia.

In the varicose vein, the most marked change was the considerable increase of fibrous tissue which especially invaded the muscle layer and caused the break-up of the regular pattern with separation of the muscular bundles. The intima was mainly intact and there was no evidence of an inflammatory response (Plate 6.3). Plate 6.3(a) shows an early localized change and Plates 6.3(b) and (c) show advanced change.

ELECTRON MICROSCOPY

Transmission electron microscopy was carried out as follows.[19] The tissue was fixed in glutaraldehyde buffered at pH 7.4 for 4–24 h. Post-fixation it was immersed in osmium tetroxide buffered at pH 7.4 for 1–2 h. It was embedded in epoxy resin (Agar 100). Uranyl acetate and Reynold's lead citrate formed the post-staining medium. The examination was carried out by a Philips 301 transmission electron microscope with photographic enlargement.

The findings were as follows: in the normal vein the muscle cells showed well marked nuclei with a clearly defined chromatin network. The cells were in close proximity to each other surrounded by a fine layer of amorphous fibrous tissue and in places separated by regularly arranged collagen fibre bundles both vertically and horizontally disposed. The cytoplasm of the cell appeared to be quite normal with the occasional appearance of what looked to be vacuole formation. Some of these 'vacuoles' contained granular material (Fig. 6.7a).

In the varicose vein there was a completely different picture (Fig. 6.7b). The muscle cells appeared to be separated from each other by a marked increase in fibrous tissue which in part consisted of grossly irregular collagen fibres,[13,20] which had in the main lost their bundle formation although some bundles were vestigially present. There were also isolated groups of elastic tissue in between the muscle cells completely unconnected with the recognized elastic layers.

On examination of the individual cells under extremely high power, the normal cell (Fig. 6.8a) shows a well marked nucleus regular in shape surrounded by a granular cytoplasm containing numerous vacuoles. The cytoplasm is surrounded by a fine layer of amorphous fibrous tissue.

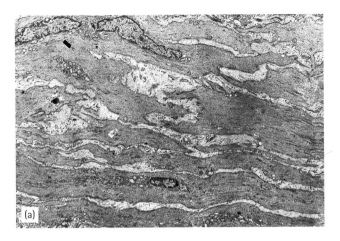

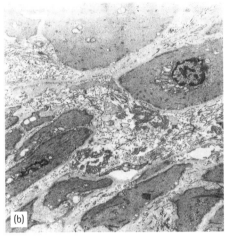

Figure 6.7 *(a) Normal vein wall electron microscopy (× 12 500). (b) Varicose vein electron microscopy (× 12 500).*

In the varicose cell (Fig. 6.8b) this pericellular layer is much more marked and looks as though it has been secreted by the muscle cell itself. The nuclear membrane is irregular and shows a well marked chromatin skein. There is an increase in 'granule' formation in the cytoplasm. Some of the vacuoles appear to contain vacuoles and others appear to be empty. It is tempting to think that the vacuoles are secreting the amorphous fibrous tissue but they may be artifacts.

Figure 6.9 shows the relationship of two adjacent cells in the wall of a normal vein. The basement membrane of the left-hand cell shows hemidesmasomes distributed along its length at well spaced intervals. There are small protoplasmic protrusions into the intercellular space. It has been suggested that it is through these structures that the contractile condition of the muscle cell is communicated to its neighbours. However the communication is mediated it is reasonable to suppose that the wider the cells become separated the more difficult it becomes for this contact to be established, resulting in loss of tone.

We are all aware of the danger of misreading an electron microscopy section and the problems of interpretation, but many studies have been carried out and other authors have achieved similar results. It is reasonable to suggest that the basic

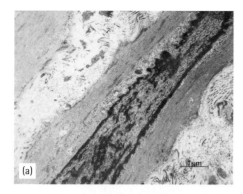

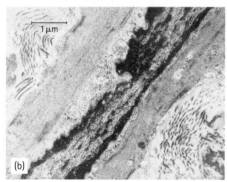

Figure 6.8   *Electron microscopy (×25 000) (a) showing normal muscle cell; (b) varicose vein muscle cell.*

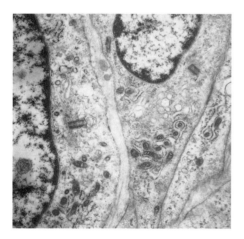

Figure 6.9   *Cells of normal vein wall, electron microscopy (×30 000).*

lesion is in the muscle cell where an abnormal metabolic process is taking place. The result of this is twofold: in the first place the muscle cells separate, lose contact and the normally tightly knit muscular grid sags, stretches and eventually is so disorganized that it loses its tone. At the same time the stretched intermuscular space is filled with an increase of interstitial collagen tissue with some elastic tissue. It seems likely that the increase in the pericellular amorphous layer is an essential part of the basic lesion. It may be argued, however, that the lesion is in the fibrous tissue itself which, by its overgrowth, strangulates the muscle cells and impedes their activity. In this case the fibrosis and abnormality of the collagen network, and the

infiltration of elastic tissue may be primary rather than secondary. This view is supported by the observations of Svejcar *et al.*[21] in Russia, who described deficient collagen in the walls of varicose veins and showed that the same defect was present in undilated leg veins and in the arm veins of the same subject.

Smooth muscle disorganization has been confirmed by Haardt,[22] and Lees *et al.*[23] have shown that, in spite of the disorganization, there is no significant difference in the level of smooth muscle-derived myosin between normal and varicose veins. The disorganization of the vein wall architecture appears to be responsible for the decrease in elasticity observed in the walls of varicose veins.[24]

Biochemical observations

Catabolism of connective tissue in patients with primary varicose veins is greater than in normal controls.[25] This is associated with increased lysosomal activity,[25,26] and an increase in serum levels of these enzymes.[27] Haardt,[22] in addition to demonstrating the histological features of varicose veins, has also undertaken elegant histochemical studies in which he has demonstrated not only an increase in the collagen-splitting enzymes in the connective tissue of the vein wall, but also a decrease in phosphatases in the muscle coats, and this has subsequently been confirmed by Ascády *et al.*[28] These observations suggest that the weakness of the walls of varicose veins is the result not only of structural disorganization, but also of muscle weakness from lack of energy-producing enzymes in the Krebs cycle, and this hypothesis is supported by the finding of a primary defect in α-adrenergic responsiveness in varicose veins.[29] Varicose veins result from a combination of vein wall weakness and gravitational pressure.

Varicose veins in pregnancy: increase in plasma volume

The effect of hormone-related weakness of the vein wall in pregnancy is exacerbated by an increase in plasma volume, which reaches a maximum of 49 percent of the non-pregnant plasma volume between the 68th and the 5th day before parturition.[30] Two-thirds of the circulating blood volume is contained in the veins, the capacitance vessels. The combination of vein wall weakness and an increase in the contained volume would seem to be responsible for the varicose dilatation, which often persists after pregnancy, particularly after the second pregnancy. Pregnancy is occasionally complicated by vulval varices which can prevent vaginal delivery. They usually resolve after parturition.

Varieties of varicose veins

Varicose veins may present as small local varices without evidence of either great or short venous incompetence. Much more common are those associated with truncal saphenous incompetence and reflux. The great saphenous vein itself is only rarely dilated and incompetent in the lower leg. Most calf varices are dilated tributaries which join the great saphenous vein at knee level. Ankle varices may be related to calf perforating vein incompetence, but incompetent perforating veins are often without varicose tributaries; they are more frequently demonstrated only by a malleolar venous flare (corona phlebectatica).

THE POST-THROMBOTIC SYNDROME AND PERFORATING VEIN INCOMPETENCE

Primary deep vein incompetence, the 'valveless syndrome', is rare. Tibbs[31] quotes an incidence of 8 percent, but most authorities would dispute this figure and this author has only encountered three patients with proven deep venous reflux and without evidence of post-thrombotic damage in over 20 years' experience of dealing with venous disorders. This diagnosis must never be made without confirmation by duplex ultrasonography or descending venography.

Following thrombosis, fibroblasts, mast cells, polymorphs and histiocytes invade the vein wall and the occluded lumen is usually restored by a combination of thrombus retraction and recanalization (Fig. 6.10). Post-thrombotic deep venous incompetence, often accompanied by perforating vein incompetence and secondary varices, results from pathological changes of the vein wall entirely different from those of varicose veins. Instead of the vein wall becoming thin and weak, as in primary varicose veins, the walls of previously thrombosed veins are thicker and less distensible than those of normal veins, due to collagen deposition by fibroblasts in the process of recanalization. The lumen is usually patent but irregular. In the process of recanalization, the delicate valves are either destroyed or become permanently adherent to the adjacent vein wall (Fig. 6.11). Venous incompetence is therefore the direct result of valve incompetence, rather than vein

wall dilatation resulting in incompetence of normal valves, as in varicose veins.

Homans'[10] description of the post-phlebitic syndrome was an important step in directing attention away from the concept of varicose ulceration but it has subsequently become clear that by no means all patients with venous ulceration have a past history of deep vein thrombosis. In 1942 Bauer[32] found that 87 percent of 38 patients with venous ulcers gave a definite history of previous thrombosis, but Dodd, in 1954 (cited in Dodd and Cockett[33]) found such a history in only 30 percent of 121 cases of venous ulceration. In the Lewisham Hospital series of 77 patients with venous ulcers, a past history of venous thrombosis was found in 45 (58 percent).[34] In the last 10 years a considerable improvement in our understanding of conditions predisposing to venous thrombosis has been achieved. It is now recognized that many patients presenting with venous ulceration attributable to deep vein incompetence have a recognizable thrombophilia and these may be an important factor leading to valve damage in the deep veins.[35] Although previous deep vein thrombosis has

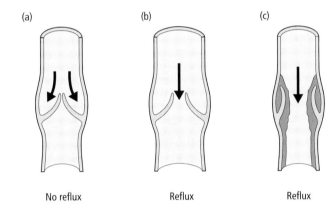

No reflux   Reflux   Reflux

Figure 6.11 *(a) Normal venous valve, no reflux. (b) Dilated varicose vein, normal valve cusps but fail to meet, reflux. (c) Post-thrombotic recanalization with adherent valve cusps, reflux.*

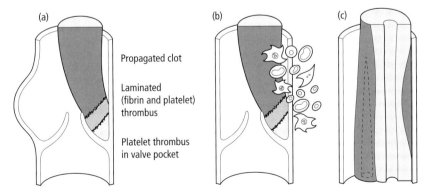

Propagated clot

Laminated (fibrin and platelet) thrombus

Platelet thrombus in valve pocket

Figure 6.10 *The natural history of venous thrombosis. (a) Thrombus formation in a valve pocket; the lines of Zahn (fibrin) are separated by platelet accumulations and these together form the 'white head', which is followed by the tail of propagated clot. (b) Organization: infiltration by histiocytes, mast cells and fibroblasts. (c) Post-thrombotic thrombus retraction and recanalization, resulting in valve incompetence.*

been discounted as an inevitable cause of venous ulceration, perforating vein incompetence is usually found in such cases. In 1953, Cockett[36] explored the perforating veins of 135 limbs with lipodermatosclerosis and ulceration and, using the Turner Warwick bleed back test, found 96 of these to be incompetent. The incidence of saphenous and perforating vein incompetence was investigated in the Lewisham Hospital series of 77 patients;[34] incompetent direct calf and ankle perforating veins were demonstrated by Doppler ultrasound and confirmed at operation in 108 of 109 ulcerated legs. In this series, deep venous incompetence was diagnosed in only 32 (42 percent). It is now recognized that about half of all venous ulcers result from a combination of saphenous incompetence and perforating vein incompetence, although it is usually only necessary to ligate and strip the saphenous vein in these cases (see Ch. 4).

Direct perforating vein incompetence may arise from one (or a combination) of the following causes:

- Long-standing primary varicose veins with long or short saphenous incompetence – the varicose perforating vein dilates and its valve becomes incompetent in the same way as in other primary varicose veins.
- Following deep vein thrombosis and recanalization – the perforating veins are very often involved in such thrombosis and recanalization and their valves are damaged in this process. Alternatively, even if the individual perforating vein is not thrombosed, incompetence of and reflux down the deep veins with which it communicates may lead to dilatation of its valve ring and therefore to secondary incompetence. Ulcers resulting from the combined effects of perforating vein and deep vein incompetence are the most difficult to treat and the most likely to recur.[37]
- Following local thrombophlebitis, with recanalization and valve damage, which in turn usually follows local trauma. Isolated calf perforating vein incompetence is very rarely seen.

Post-thrombotic venous occlusion

Post-thrombotic recanalization occasionally fails, leaving permanent venous stenosis or occlusion. This most commonly affects the left common iliac vein (Fig. 6.12) and is related to the anatomic anomalies which are described in Chapter 3. Venous occlusion occasionally occurs elsewhere, particularly in the superficial femoral vein. Main vessel occlusion is often adequately compensated by the development of numerous collateral veins, but failure of adequate collateral vein development results in functional obstruction to the venous return. Venography will show the site of venous occlusion, but cannot indicate its functional significance, and physiological investigations by femoral venous pressure measurements,[38] plethysmography or duplex scanning are required for full evaluation.

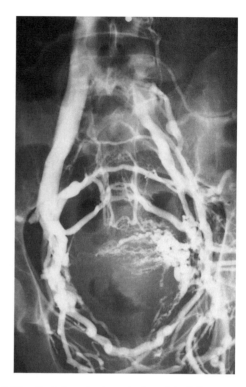

Figure 6.12 *Post-thrombotic occlusion of the left common and external iliac veins; collateral flow through pudendal and presacral tributaries of the internal iliac veins.*

The high exercising venous pressure which follows proximal venous obstruction causes distension of the deep veins. Intramuscular pressure in the calf muscles is elevated during exercise in legs with outflow obstruction,[39] and muscle water content is also increased, probably due to increased transudation of fluid.[40] An increased interstitial pressure may lead to compression of the distal end of the capillaries, resulting in the increased fluid transudation and increase in muscle water content. Capillary compression would also seem to be the reason for the reduced exercising muscle blood flow and increase in lactate content in the gastrocnemius muscles of legs with iliac occlusion and outflow obstruction.[39] These changes are responsible for pain on exercise (venous claudication) which can be disabling in its severity.[33,41]

Patients with post-thrombotic iliac vein obstruction rarely develop ulceration in the first 5 years following thrombosis. Ulceration becomes much more common after 10 or 15 years (Fig. 6.13) and results from the development of secondary incompetence of the peripheral deep and perforating veins and, often, also of the saphenous veins.

Important collaterals in common iliac occlusion have been described in Chapter 3. In the thigh, the collateral pathways which usually compensate for occlusion of the superficial femoral vein are the profunda femoris vein and the great saphenous vein. Care must be taken not to ligate the latter in patients with post-thrombotic stenosis or occlusion of the superficial femoral vein.

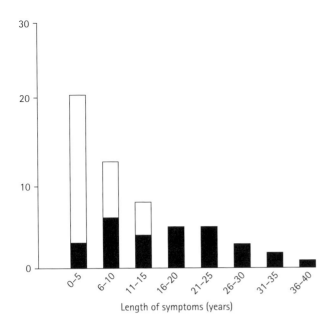

Figure 6.13 *The relationship of ulceration to post-thrombotic iliac occlusion. □, total patients in each group; ■, number of patients with ulcers.*

REFERENCES

1. Widmer LK. Classification of venous disorders. *Peripheral Venous Disorders*. Basle III. Bern: Hans Huber, 1978.
2. Beebe HG, Bergan JJ, Bergqvist D *et al*. Classification and grading of chronic venous disease in the lower limbs: a consensus statement. *Phlebology* 1995; **10**: 42–5.
3. Gooley NA, Sumner DS. Relationship of venous reflux to the site of venous valvular incompetence: implications for venous reconstructive surgery. *J Vasc Surg* 1988; **7**: 50–9.
4. Hanrahan LM, Araki CT, Rodriguez AA *et al*. Distribution of valvular incompetence in patients with venous stasis ulceration. *J Vasc Surg* 1991; **13**: 805–11.
5. Harding Rains AJ, Mann CV (eds). *Bailey and Love's Short Practice of Surgery*. London: Lewis, 1988; 113.
6. Robbins SL. *Pathology*. Philadelphia: Saunders, 1967; 56.
7. Browse NL, Burnand KG, Lea Thomas M. *Diseases of the Veins; Pathology, Diagnosis and Treatment*, London: Arnold, 1988; 406.
8. Schraibman IG. The bacteriology of leg ulcers. *Phlebology* 1987; **2**: 265–70.
9. O'Meara SM, Cullum NA, Majid M, Sheldon TA. Systematic review of antimicrobial agents used for chronic wounds. *Br J Surg* 2001; **88**: 4–21.
10. Homans J. The operative treatment of varicose veins and ulcers, based on a classification of these lesions. *Surg Gynecol Obstet* 1916; **22**: 143–58.
11. Franks PJ, Wright DDI, McCollum CN. Epidemiology of venous disease: a review. *Phlebology* 1989; **4**: 143–151.
12. Fowkes FG, Lee AJ, Evans CJ *et al*. Lifestyle risk factors for lower limb venous reflux in the general population: Edinburgh Vein Study. *Int J Epidemiol* 2001; **30**: 846–52.
13. Cotton L. Varicose veins; gross anatomy and development. *Br J Surg* 1961; **48**: 589.
14. Rose SS. The aetiology of varicose veins. In: Negus D, Jantet G, eds. *Phlebology '85*. London: Libby, 1986; 6–9.
15. Ackroyd JS, Patterson M, Browse NL. A study of the mechanical properties of fresh and preserved human femoral vein wall and valve cusps. *Br J Surg* 1985; **72**: 117–9.
16. Abu-Own A, Scurr JN, Coleridge Smith PD. Saphenous reflux without saphenofemoral junction incompetence. *Br J Surg* 1994; **81**: 1452–4.
17. Cooper DG, Hillman-Cooper CS, Barker SG, Hollingsworth SJ. Primary varicose veins: the sapheno-femoral junction, distribution of varicosities and patterns of incompetence. *Eur J Vasc Endovasc Surg* 2003; **25**: 53–9.
18. Wooley DE. On the sequential changes in levels of oestradiol and progesterone during pregnancy and parturition. In: Piez KA, ed. *Extracellular Matrix Biochemistry*. New York: Elselvier, 1984; 138.
19. Mashiah A, Rose SS, Hod I. The scanning electron microscope in the pathology of varicose veins. *Med Sci* 1991; **27**: 202–8.
20. Jurakova Z, Milenkov C. Ultrastructural evidence of collagen degradation in the walls of varicose veins. *Exp Mol Pathol* 1982; **37**: 37–47.
21. Svejcar J, Prerovsky I, Linhart J *et al*. Content of collagen, elastin and hexosamine in primary varicose. *Clin Sci* 1953; **24**: 325–30.
22. Haardt B. A comparison of the histochemical enzyme pattern in normal and varicose veins. *Phlebology* 1987; **2**: 135–58.
23. Lees TA, Mantle D, Lambert D. Analysis of the smooth muscle content of the normal and varicose vein wall via analytical electrophoresis. In: Raymond-Martimbeau P, Prescott R, Zummo M, eds. *Phlebologie '92*. Paris: Libbey Eurotext, 1992; 56–8.
24. Thulesius O, Gjores JE, Berlin E. Valvular function and venous distensibility. In: Negus D, Jantet G, eds. *Phlebology '85*. London: Libby, 1986; 26–8.
25. Buddecke E. Alters Veranderungen der Proteoglykane verh deutsch. *Ges Pathol* 1975; **59**: 43.
26. Niebes P, Lazst L. Influence *in-vitro* d'une serie de flavinoids sur des enzymes de metabolism des mucopolysaccharides de veines saphenes humaines et bovines. *Angiologia* 1971; **8**: 297–302.
27. Niebes P, Berson I. *Determination of Enzymes and Degradation*. London: Churchill Livingstone, 1976; 35.
28. Ascády G, Lengyel I, Solti F. A possible theory explaining the pathochemical background of varicosity. In: Raymond-Martimbeau P, Prescott R, Zummo M, eds. *Phlebologie, '92*. Paris: Libbey Eurotext, 1992; 64–7.
29. Schuller-Petrovic S, Blöcul-Daum B, Woltz M *et al*. Primary defect in α-adrenergic responsiveness in patients with varicose veins. In: Prescott R, Zummo M, Raymond-Mertimbeau P, eds. Phelobologie '92 Paris, Libbey Eurotext, 1992; 64–7.
30. Diem K (ed.). *Documenta Geigy. Scientific Tables*. Macclesfield: Geigy, 1962.
31. Tibbs DJ. *Varicose Veins and Related Disorders*. Oxford: Butterworth-Heinemann, 1992; 146–51.
32. Bauer G. A roentgenological and clinical study of the sequels of thrombosis. *Acta Chir Scand* 1942; **86**(Suppl. 74).
33. Dodd H, Cockett FB. *The Pathology and Surgery of the Veins of the Lower Limb*, 2nd edn. Edinburgh: Churchill Livingstone, 1976; 247.
34. Negus D, Friedgood A. The effective management of venous ulceration. *Br J Surg* 1983; **70**: 623–7.
35. Bradbury AW, MacKenzie RK, Burns P, Fegan C. Thrombophilia and chronic venous ulceration. *Eur J Vasc Endovasc Surg* 2002; **24**: 97–104.

36. Cockett FB. Pathology and treatment of venous ulcers. MS *Thesis.* London: University of London, 1953.

37. Burnand KG, Lea Thomas M, O'Donnell P, Browse NL. Relationship between post-phlebitic changes in the deep veins and results of surgical treatment of venous ulcers. *Lancet* 1976; ii: 936–8.

38. Negus D, Cockett FB. Femoral vein pressures in post-phlebitic iliac vein obstruction. *Br J Surg* 1967; **54**: 522–5.

39. Qvarfordt P, Eklof B, Ohlin P *et al.* Intramuscular pressure, blood flow and skeletal muscle metabolism in patients with venous claudication. *Surgery* 1984; **95**: 191–5.

40. Zelis R, Lee G, Mason DT. Influence of experimental oedema on metabolically determined blood flow. *Circ Res* 1974; **34**: 482–9.

41. Negus D. Calf pain in the post-thrombotic syndrome. *Br Med* 1968; **2**: 156–8.

7

Microcirculation and venous ulcers

LUIGI PASCARELLA, GEERT W. SCHMID SCHÖNBEIN

Although the term chronic venous insufficiency (CVI) is in common usage and is becoming increasingly used, the older term, venous stasis, is predominant. This is a tribute to John Homans of Harvard who introduced the concept that venous stasis was the ultimate cause of venous ulceration.

Homans believed that there was a causal relation between venous ulceration of the legs and blood stasis in patients with severe chronic venous insufficiency.[1] Blood stasis, as proposed by Homans, was determined by a shortage of oxygen content in the skin, and it was this that led to a condition of tissue hypoxia, necrosis and ulceration.[1] Many more recent observations have demonstrated that shortage of oxygen is not the main cause of venous ulcers.

It has been hypothesized that the presence of cutaneous arteriovenous fistulas might cause a further deprivation of oxygen in an already hypoxic skin. Such arteriovenous connections have been demonstrated in limbs with severe CVI.[2]

However, Coleridge Smith and others have shown that the content of oxygen in the skin and in varicose veins of limbs with venous ulcers is not decreased but is instead increased.[3] In addition, the oxygen diffusion defects suspected by histological findings of pericapillary fibrin cuffs have been refuted by studies such as clearance of Xenon-133 through liposclerotic skin which has shown no significant oxygen barrier.[4]

Histology and immunocytochemistry have suggested recently that lesions observed in the different stages of CVI may be related to an inflammatory process. It is this inflammatory process that leads first to fibrosclerotic remodeling of the skin and then to ulceration. The vascular network of the most superficial layers of the skin appears to be the target of this inflammatory reaction.[5]

Capillary density may vary in liposclerotic skin. Some areas with white atrophy (atrophie blanche) may show a complete loss of capillaries in some areas, while in others, the capillaries appear dilated, elongated, coiled and tortuous.[5] Endothelial lesions in the capillaries include irregularity of the luminal surface, intracellular edema and increased intracytoplasmic vesicles. Basement membranes appear to be completely fused with the surrounding tissue. Pericapillary spaces are filled with a fluid that is rich in cellular fragments and proteins. Pericytes and fibrin cuffs have been observed in the pericapillary spaces and around the capillaries. T-lymphocytes, plasma cells, elements of the monocyte–macrophage system and neutrophils have been seen to adhere to endothelial surfaces. Transmigration into the surrounding cutaneous tissue has been observed.[5] Red cell packing and platelet aggregates may fill the capillary lumen and may be found in the pericapillary tissue.

Granulation tissue, composed of lymphocytes, plasma cells, macrophages, histiocytes and fibroblasts have been identified in the subepithelial layer of the epidermis.[5] Deposition of collagen fibers, which appear to have completely lost their normal orientation, has also been described.

These lesions account for an inflammatory and post-inflammatory process of tissue fibrosclerosis: liposclerosis.

The studies of Moyses et al.[6] and Thomas et al.[7] have shown leukocyte trapping to occur in limbs with venous dysfunction and this observation constitutes further proof of the importance of this inflammatory process (Fig. 7.1).

Leukocyte activation and its relationship to venous hypertension has been studied extensively by Coleridge-Smith et al.[8] They have shown an increase in neutrophil elastase and lactoferrin, markers of neutrophil activation, in patients under transient conditions of venous hypertension and with chronic venous insufficiency.[9,10]

In addition to venous hypertension, many other factors which lead to leukocyte activation have been investigated in recent years. For example, leukocytes are able to respond to shear stress.[11] Retraction of leukocyte pseudopods has been observed under conditions of higher wall shear stress.

Wall shear stress is defined as the tangential force produced by moving blood, acting on the endothelial surface. It is a function of the velocity gradient of blood near the endothelial surface. Its magnitude is directly proportional to blood flow and blood viscosity and inversely proportional to the cube of the radius of the vessel. Blood flow cessation, blood stasis that implies lower shear stress, may activate leukocytes, as shown by emission of pseudopodia and lamellipodia[11,12] (Fig. 7.1). These protoplasmatic cell expansions allow leukocytes to adhere to endothelial cells and eventually transmigrate into surrounding tissue. Intercellular adhesion molecules (ICAM-1), vascular cell adhesion molecules (VCAM-1), E and L-selectins on the endothelial surface potentially act as intermediaries in the adhesion process, binding specific leukocyte receptors [very late antigen-4 (VLA-4), lymphocyte function-associated antigen-1 (LFA-1)] (Plate 7.1). These leukocyte receptors belong to a family of proteins called β-integrins whose activation state and ligand affinity seem to be enhanced by a lower shear stress. The expression of these markers has been found in almost every stage of the 'venous dermatitis' (Plate 7.1 and Fig. 7.2).

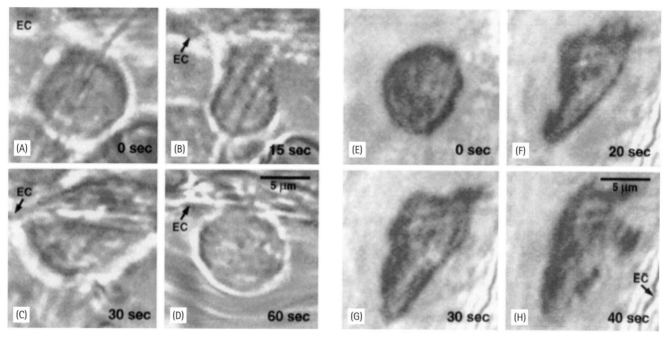

Figure 7.1 *Selected frames during the time course of pseudopod formation of a neutrophil in a rat mesentery venule. (A–D) Adhering neutrophil. (A) The leucocyte shape is spherical without pseudopods immediately after occlusion of the vessel with a micropipette; (B and C) leucocyte spreading on the endothelium (EC) by active pseudopod formation during stasis; (D) retraction of pseudopods upon restoration of flow. (E–H) Freely suspended neutrophil. (E) The cell is initially spherical; (F) pseudopod projection shortly after flow stoppage, and continuation throughout stasis (G and H). The cell is carried away from the observation field upon return of flow. [Reproduced with permission from Moazzam et al. Copyright (1997) National Academy of Sciences, USA.][12]*

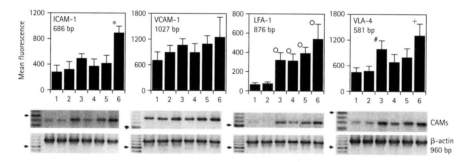

Figure 7.2 *High levels of intercellular adhesion molecule-1 (ICAM-1), vascular cell adhesion molecule-1 (VCAM-1), lymphocyte function-associated antigen-1 (LFA-1) and very late antigen-4 (VLA-4) messenger RNA (mRNA) are detected in stasis dermatitis, lipodermatosclerosis and venous leg ulcers. Expression of ICAM-1, VCAM-1, LFA-1 and VLA-4 mRNAs was examined in biopsies by reverse transcriptase polymerase chain reaction (RT-PCR). Healthy skin (lane 1, n = 5), telangiectases (lane 2, n = 4), stasis dermatitis (lane 3, n = 4), hyperpigmentation (lane 4; n = 4) lipodermatosclerosis (lane 5, n = 4), and venous leg ulcer (lane 6, n = 4). Mean fluorescence intensity was determined semi-quantitatively. Beta-actin was used as control. Arrow indicates 800-bp fragment in the 100-bp DNA ladder. Statistically significant increase in ICAM-1 expression compared with lanes 1, 2, 3, 4 and 5. No statistically significant increase was found in VCAM-1 expression. Statistically significant increase in LFA-1 expression compared with lanes 1 and 2. Statistically significant increase in VLA-4 expression compared with lanes 1 and 2. Statistically significant increase in VLA-4 expression compared with lanes 1, 2, 4 and 5. (mean ± SD; statistically significant at P < 0.05, Student–Newman–Keuls Method, SigmaStat; Jandel Scientific Software, Corte Madern CA, USA). Reproduced with permission from Peshen et al.[13]*

Clearly, hemodynamic forces appear to play an important role in leukocyte activation and in the inflammatory reaction of the pathogenesis of chronic venous insufficiency, venous dermatitis and venous ulceration.[13]

Leukocyte activation is characterized by synthesis and release of many inflammatory molecules such as leukotrienes, prostaglandin, bradykinin, free oxygen radicals and cytokines. Cytokines act to regulate and perpetuate the inflammatory reaction by paracrine and autocrine mechanisms.

Tumor necrosis factor-alpha (TNF-α) is a well known chemokine, whose expression is enhanced in many inflammatory reactions. It stimulates the expression of inflammatory adhesion molecules, the synthesis and release of other cytokines and the chemotaxis of neutrophils and macrophages. The expression of TNF-α appears to be upregulated in patients with venous ulcers, and healing of the ulcer may reduce the level of TNF-α.[14]

Vascular endothelial growth factor (VEGF), by definition, is a potent angiogenetic factor.[15] It enhances endothelial proliferation and the vascular permeability. VEGF is also known to induce the expression of adhesion molecules, such as ICAM-1, VCAM-1 and E-selectin.[16] Both VEGF expression and its receptor expression (Flk-1/KDR) are upregulated under variations of blood shear stress and during the inflammatory reaction.[15,17] Patients with chronic venous insufficiency and skin changes (CEAP 4, see Box 6.1, p. 46) exhibit higher levels of VEGF than those in CEAP classes 2 and 3 and normal individuals.[15] The expression of VEGF and other growth factors does not seem to be related to the capillary density of liposclerotic skin or to the slow or poor healing of venous ulcers. Venous ulcer exudates have been found to inhibit the growth of human endothelial cells.[18] Possible degradation of VEGF and other growth factors may be related to these observations.[18] Probably an enzymatic factor, such as urokinase plasminogen activator (uPA), and its direct product, plasmin, or other lythic enzymes released by leukocytes may act to inhibit angiogenesis and ulcer healing (Figs 7.3 and 7.4).

Transforming growth factor beta (TGFβ) is another cytokine whose expression has been found to be upregulated in patients with venous ulcers.[14,15,19] TGFβ is related to tissue remodeling by stimulating the formation of the granulation tissue, proliferation of fibroblasts and synthesis of collagen fibers.[14,19]

The role of anti-endothelial antibodies in patients with venous leg ulcers has been investigated by comparing the expression of these antibodies in patients with venous leg ulcers to patients with autoimmune disease [lupus, Sjögren's syndrome], calcinosis, Raynaud's disease, esophageal motility disorders, scleroderma, telangiectasia (CREST).[20] This work suggests that patients with venous leg ulcers show an increased level of anti-endothelial cell antibodies compared with autoimmune disease patients and controls. These findings may be seen as the consequence of a chronic inflammatory reaction and may be an important factor in its perpetuation.

As in autoimmune diseases, antibody binding with endothelial cells mediates the activation of leukocytes, the expression of inflammatory adhesion molecules and the release of many proinflammatory cytokines.[15,20] Their role may also have been implicated in an overactivity of the coagulation system leading to the thromboses of capillaries and to deposition of fibrin in the pericapillary spaces.[20]

The importance of matrix metalloproteinases (MMPs) has also been considered because of their involvement in both the inflammatory reaction and the remodeling of cutaneous tissue.[21]

This interest has been focused on MMP2, MMP9, tissue inhibitor of metalloproteinase 1 (TIMP1) and TIMP2. Recent studies showed an increased expression of MMP2 and TIMP1 in liposclerotic skin.[21,22] Expression of MMP9 has been observed to be upregulated on the edges of intractable venous ulcers.[22]

The presence of uPA and tissue plasminogen activator (tPA) has also been investigated,[23] and uPA activity but no tPA activity has been found at the margin of venous ulcers. The role of these enzymes in the venous ulcer formation remains obscure. Probably, as explained above, uPA participates in the breakdown of growth factors slowing and/or inhibiting the ulcer healing process.[18]

In light of the newly proposed mechanisms of venous ulcer formation, future therapy might be directed against leukocyte activation in order to diminish the involvement of the inflammatory response.

With this in mind, the attention of many investigators has been drawn to two different drugs: pentoxifylline and flavonoids. The pharmacodynamics of pentoxifylline in the treatment of venous ulcer seems to be related to:[24]

- inhibition of synthesis of proinflammatory cytokines
- inhibition of leukocyte activation by reducing their adhesion
- inhibition of platelet aggregation.

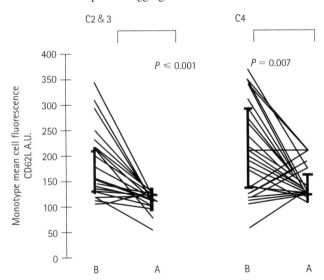

Figure 7.3 *Comparison of changes in monocyte mean cell fluorescence (arbitrary units, AU) for CD62L before (B) and following oral flavonoid therapy (A) in 20 patients with simple chronic venous disease (C2/C3) and those with dermatological changes (C4). This decrease was the highest in magnitude (c. 40 percent). (Reproduced with permission from Jantet, 2005[25].)*

Recent randomized controlled trials of pentoxifylline therapy alone and combined with elastic compression in patients with venous leg ulcers suggests that this drug is effective in ulcer healing. Monotherapy with pentoxifylline may also have some benefits in patients with venous ulcers of lesser severity.[24]

Flavonoids are natural compounds that act at many levels of endothelial physiology and inflammatory response. They may act by protecting cells from the effects of hypoxia, decreasing the permeability and fragility of the vein valves and venous wall, and increasing venous tone. They also affect leukocyte adhesion and free radical formation.

The results of the RELIEF study[25] show that the therapy with twice-daily micronized purified flavonoid fraction (MPFF) (450 mg of micronized diosmin and 50 mg hesperidin), given over 6 months is related to a decrease of CVI symptoms, including pain, leg heaviness, sensation of swelling, and cramps. This has been demonstrated in limbs classified by CEAP as from C0 to C4. The greatest benefits have been seen in the 57 percent of CVI patients who did not show valve reflux. Another randomized trial confirms that 60 days' therapy with Daflon (Servier, Paris, France) at the dose of 500 mg/day orally is effective in addition to the elastic compression by accelerating the healing process in patients with ≥10 cm diameter severe ulcers.[26]

Other studies point out the unique peculiarity of flavonoids to act on microcirculation. Daflon at a dose of 1 g/day over 60 days downregulates the expression of CD62L, ICAM-1 and VCAM-1 on neutrophils and monocytes in patients with CVI in CEAP stage C2–C5 (Fig. 7.4).[27]

The expression of soluble endothelial adhesion molecules has been found to be reduced in animal models of ischemia/reperfusion with a Daflon pretreatment.[28]

CONCLUSION

The development of venous dermatitis and venous ulceration has as its pivotal point an inflammatory reaction that originates in hemodynamic forces such as venous hypertension, circulatory stasis and modified conditions of shear stress. This inflammatory reaction perpetuates itself, leading to a liposclerotic skin tissue remodeling.

REFERENCES

1. Homans J. The etiology and treatment of varicose ulcer of the leg. *Sur Gynecol Obstet* 1917; **24**: 300–11.
2. Brewer AC. Arteriovenous shunts. *Br Med J* 1950; **ii**: 270.
3. Coleridge Smith PD. Treatment of microcirculation disorders in venous leg ulcer. In: Messmer K. *Microcirculation in Chronic Venous Insufficiency. Progress In Applied Microcirculation*, Vol. 23. Basel: Karger, 1999; 121–41.
4. Cheatle TR, McMullin GM, Farrah J *et al.* Three tests of microcirculatory function in the evaluation of treatment for chronic venous insufficiency. *Phlebology* 1990; **5**: 165–72.
5. Leu AJ, Leu H-J, Franzeck UK, Bollinger A. Microvascular changes in chronic venous insufficiency – a review. *Cardiovasc Surg* 1995; **3**: 237–45.
6. Moyses C, Cederholm-Williams SA, Michel C. Hemoconcentration and the accumulation of white cells in the feet during venous stasis. *Int J Micro Circ Clin Exp* 1987; **5**: 311–20.
7. Thomas PRS, Nash GB, Dormandy JA. White cell accumulation in the dependent legs of patients with venous hypertension: a possible mechanism for trophic changes in the skin. *Br Med J* 1988; **296**: 1693–5.
8. Coleridge Smith PD, Thomas P, Scurr JH, Dormandy J. Causes of venous ulceration: a new hypothesis. *Br Med J* 1988; **296**: 1726–7.
9. Shields DA, Andaz SK, Abeysinghe RD *et al.* Neutrophil activation in experimental ambulatory venous hypertension. *Phlebology* 1994; **9**: 119–24.
10. Shields DA, Andaz SK, Sarin S *et al.* Plasma elastase in venous disease. *Br J Surg* 1994; **81**: 1496–9.
11. Marschel P, Schmid-Schönbein GW. Control of fluid shear response in circulating leucocytes by integrins. *Ann Biomed Eng* 2002; **30**: 333–43.
12. Moazzam F, Delano FA, Zweifach BW, Schmid-Schönbein GW. The leucocyte response to fluid stress. *Proc Natl Acad Sci USA* 1997; **94**: 5338–43.
13. Peshen M, Lahaye T, Hennig B *et al.* Expression of the adhesion molecules ICAM-1, VCAM-1, LFA-1 and VLA-4 in the skin is

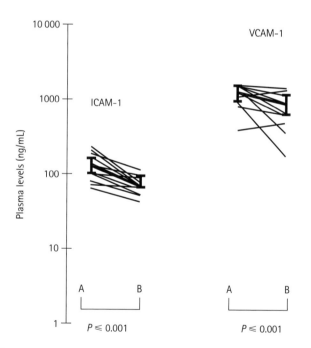

Figure 7.4 *Changes in plasma levels of intercellular adhesion molecule-1 (ICAM-1) and vascular cell adhesion molecule-1 (VCAM-1) in patients with chronic venous disease before (A) and after (B) 60 days of treatment with micronized purified flavonoid fraction. A logarithmic scale has been used because of the differences in the absolute levels of the two molecules. The P levels are from Wilcoxon's ranked sum test. The thick lines join the respective median levels. Vertical lines represent the interquartile range. (Reproduced with permission from Jantet 2002[25].)*

modulated in progressing stages of chronic venous insufficiency. *Acta Derm Venereol (Stockh)* 1999; **79**: 27–32.

14. Murphy MA, Joyce WP, Condron C, Bouchier-Hayes D. A reduction in serum cytokine levels parallels healing of venous ulcers in patients undergoing compression therapy. *Eur J Vasc Endovasc Surg* 2002; **23**: 349–52.

15. Coleridge Smith PD. Leg ulcers: biochemical factors. *Phlebology* 2000; **15**: 156–61.

16. Kim I, Moon SO, Kim SH *et al*. Vascular endothelial growth factor expression of intercellular adhesion molecule 1 (ICAM-1), vascular cell adhesion molecule 1 (VCAM-1), and E-selectin through nuclear factor-κB activation in endothelial cells. *J Biol Chem* 2001; **276**: 7614–20.

17. Abumiya T, Sasaguri T, Taba Y *et al*. Shear stress induces expression of vascular endothelial growth factor receptor Flk-1/KDR through the CT-rich Sp1 binding site. *Arterioscler Thromb Vasc Biol* 2002; **22**: 907–13.

18. Drinkwater SL, Smith A, Sawyer BM, Burnand KG. Effect of venous ulcer exudates on angiogenesis in vitro. *Br J Surg* 2002; **89**: 709–13.

19. Pappas PJ, You R, Rameshawar P *et al*. Dermal tissue fibrosis in patients with chronic venous insufficiency is associated with increased transforming growth factor-beta 1 gene expression and protein production. *J Vasc Surg* 1999; **3**: 1129–45.

20. Guillet G, Garcia C, Sassolas B *et al*. Anti-endothelial cell antibodies in chronic leg ulcers: prevalence and significance. *Ann Dermatol Venereol* 2001; **128**: 1301–4.

21. Herouy Y, May AE, Pronschlegel G *et al*. Lipodermatosclerosis is characterized by elevated expression and activation of matrix metalloproteinase: implications for venous ulcer formation. *J Invest Dermatol* 1998; **111**: 822–7.

22. Tarlton JF, Bailey AJ, Crawford E *et al*. Prognostic value of markers of collagen remodeling in venous ulcers. *Wound Repair Regen* 1999; **7**: 347–55.

23. Rogers AA, Burnett S, Lindholm C *et al*. Expression of tissue-type and urokinase-type plasminogen activator activities in chronic venous leg ulcers. *Vasa* 1999; **28**: 101–5.

24. Jull A, Waters J, Arroll B. Pentoxifylline for treatment of venous leg ulcers: a systematic review. *Lancet* 2002; **359**: 1550–4.

25. Jantet G. Chronic venous insufficiency. worldwide results of the RELIEF study. Reflux assEssment and quaLity of lIfe improvEment with micronized Flavonoids. *Angiology* 2002; **53**: 245–56.

26. Guilhou JJ, Dereure O, Marzin L *et al*. Efficacy of Daflon 500 mg in venous leg ulcer healing: a double-blind, randomized, controlled versus placebo trial in 107 patients. *Angiology* 1997; **48**: 77–85.

27. Shoab SS, Porter J, Scurr JH, Coleridge Smith PD. Effect of oral micronized purified flavonoid fraction treatment on leucocytes adhesion molecule expression in patients with chronic venous disease: a pilot study. *J Vasc Surg* 2000; **31**: 456–61.

28. Korthius RJ, Gute DC. Post-ischemic leucocyte–endothelial cell interactions and microvascular barrier dysfunction in skeletal muscle. Cellular mechanisms and effect of Daflon 500 mg. *Int J Microcirc: Clin Exp* 1997; **17**: 11–7.

8

The differential diagnosis of leg ulcers

DAVID NEGUS, PHILIP D. COLERIDGE SMITH

INTRODUCTION

The successful treatment of leg ulcers depends on accurate diagnosis, which itself depends on the examination and investigations described in Chapters 9–11. As in all branches of clinical medicine, experience is helpful, but a spot diagnosis can often be inaccurate and sensible clinicians will arrange confirmatory investigations, even when they are 90 percent sure of the underlying cause of the ulcer. Most leg ulcers seen in the UK are venous or ischemic in origin. Infectious ulcers are more commonly seen in tropical countries; neoplastic ulcers are less frequent, but it is most important always to be aware of this possibility and there are a number of less common causes which are difficult to classify (Box 8.1). Ulceration associated with rheumatoid disease and diabetes is also frequently encountered. Examination must be directed to the site of the ulcer and the appearance of its base and edge, before examining the leg veins and pedal pulses.

Box 8.1 The differential diagnosis of leg ulcers

- Vascular – venous, ischemic, mixed arterial and venous, arteriovenous fistulae, venous malformations, rheumatoid disease, vasculitis, steroids, hypertensive ulcers, diabetic ulcers
- Traumatic – accidental, injection sclerotherapy, surgery
- Edema – lymphedema (rare), cardiac or renal
- Infection – tropical sores, tuberculosis, syphilis, yaws, leprosy, parasites, fungal infections
- Malignant – Marjolin's ulcer, primary squamous carcinoma, sarcoma, lymphoma, basal cell carcinoma, malignant melanoma
- Others – nutritional, immunodeficiency, contact dermatitis

ULCERATION RELATED TO VENOUS DISORDERS

The varicose ulcer

The true varicose ulcer, i.e. an ulcer overlying a superficial varicosity, is extremely rare.

SITE AND APPEARANCE

Varicose ulcers often occur on the anterior or lateral surface of the lower leg or ankle rather than in the malleolar regions.

They may occur anywhere on the lower leg or ankle; their one constant feature is that they are related to a large dilated varicose vein. Varicose ulcers are usually small, shallow and painless, with a well epithelialized edge and a base of healthy granulation tissue. They often arise in an area of varicose eczema.

Venous ulceration

Venous ulceration is defined as ulceration related to perforating, saphenous or deep venous incompetence, or a combination of these. The original description of post-phlebitic ulceration has now been largely abandoned as many patients with chronic lipodermatosclerosis and ankle ulceration have no history of deep vein thrombosis or evidence of post-thrombotic damage to the deep veins. The term 'venous ulcer' is less specific and allows a variety of causes. In these patients, deep vein reflux is usually associated with calf perforating vein incompetence. Saphenous (superficial) vein reflux commonly accompanies this combination.

Ulcers entirely arising from saphenous incompetence may occur in up to half of patients presenting venous leg ulcers.[1] In the recently published ESCHAR study, patients with combined superficial and deep vein reflux were considered for surgical intervention.[2] In this study, 1418 patients were assessed and about half (765) were considered as possible candidates for superficial venous surgery. Perforating vein incompetence was disregarded in this study as far as eligibility for surgery was concerned. However, perforating vein ligation was frequently performed in combination with saphenous stripping in the surgical group. Careful examination of patients with varicose veins and ankle ulceration will often demonstrate perforating vein incompetence which may play a significant role in the development of ulceration.

HISTORY

A history of local trauma is common; the supermarket trolley is often responsible. A past history of deep vein thrombosis is common but not universal. In the Lewisham Hospital series, only 45 of 77 patients with 109 ulcerated legs (58 percent) gave a history of previous deep vein thrombosis. More recently, in a group of 88 patients with venous ulceration, 35 percent were found to have a history or duplex ultrasound evidence of previous venous thrombosis and 41 percent were found to have a thrombophilia.[3]

If patients give a history of previous iliofemoral thrombosis, particularly in the left leg, there may be chronic iliac vein occlusion with obstruction to venous outflow from the limb. Patients should be asked whether they have experienced any calf swelling (as opposed to ankle edema, which is common in varicose veins and perforating vein incompetence) and, most importantly, whether there are any symptoms suggestive of venous claudication. This is severe calf pain (sometimes described as 'bursting' in nature), which occurs on walking 100 or 200 metres.[4] This is much more severe than the dull ache on prolonged standing experienced by many patients with venous incompetence.

EXAMINATION

The ulcer

Venous ulcers are most commonly found over the medial malleolus (see Fig. 6.3, p. 48), less commonly over the lateral malleolus; these are usually in association with small saphenous incompetence. Occasionally, these ulcers may meet posteriorly or even become completely circumferential. They vary in depth from 1 or 2 mm to extending down to the deep fascia. They are much deeper than varicose or vasculitic ulcers.

Venous ulcers are almost invariably accompanied by an ankle venous flare at the medial malleolus of fine superficial venules and usually by pigmentation and lipodermatosclerosis. These physical signs are likely to be seen accompanying smaller ulcers; very large ulcers may include all the skin normally occupied by the venous flare or lipodermatosclerosis. Unlike 'varicose' ulcers, patients with venous ulceration may have no visible varicose veins, or only very few.

Most venous ulcers are infected when the patient first presents to the clinic and the ulcer base may be obscured by purulent debris and slough. Once this has been removed, the base is seen to consist of healthy pink granulation tissue. If this is not obviously pink, suspect ischemia. The ulcer edge is also pink and slopes gently to the ulcer base. The edge may be punched out in an infected ulcer, but this appearance should rapidly change following appropriate treatment. Undermined edges suggest tuberculosis or other chronic infection.

The limb

Examination of the limb with venous ulceration has two main purposes: first, to identify all points of venous reflux and possible venous obstruction; and, second, to exclude arterial insufficiency as a contributory factor.

The patient is examined lying flat and the site and appearance of the ulcer are noted. Particular note is taken of the presence or absence of surrounding lipodermatosclerosis and also whether an ankle venous flare is visible. The latter is usually present and indicates direct calf perforating vein incompetence, but may be completely obscured by a very large ulcer. In the absence of lipodermatosclerosis, there is doubt that the ulcer is of venous origin. Signs of iliac vein obstruction are looked for, small dilated groin collateral veins (Fig. 8.1), and an increase in calf circumference on the affected side. Abdominal and rectal examination must be performed in all patients with a swollen limb.

With the patient standing on an 18 cm mounting block, the leg is re-examined after a delay of about 30 s to allow for venous filling. The presence of varicose veins is noted and their communication with long or small saphenous systems identified by examination and the percussion and tourniquet tests, as necessary. An ankle venous flare may become more obvious in the erect position.

The patient's toes and forefoot must be examined for evidence of ischemia, e.g. cyanosis and slow capillary refilling

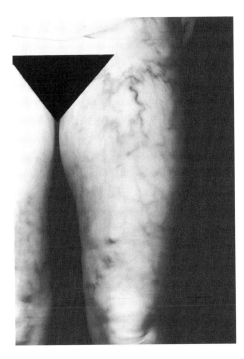

Figure 8.1 *Infrared photograph showing dilated collateral veins in the groin of a patient with post-thrombotic obstruction of the left common iliac vein.*

time. Ankle and foot pulses must be palpated, and ankle pulse pressures are measured by Doppler ultrasound assessment of the ankle:brachial systolic pressure index.

INVESTIGATIONS

Doppler ultrasound examination may be helpful in identifying great and small saphenous incompetence as well as in identifying sites of perforating vein incompetence. However, the most effective method of evaluating the venous system of the lower limb is by duplex ultrasonography and this should be undertaken in all cases of venous ulceration in order to establish the extent of the venous problem. This technique will demonstrate which veins are incompetent and whether there are any occluded venous segments, including chronic iliac vein obstruction. Plethysmographic methods of assessing the venous system may also be useful and these are described in Chapter 11.

Venography

In the absence of Duplex ultrasound, venography is an acceptable alternative, provided that this is performed by an experienced vascular radiologist.

Ascending venography (Fig. 8.2) will localize incompetent perforating veins and also demonstrate deep venous occlusion. Venographic evidence of iliac vein occlusion must be further investigated by femoral venous pressure measurements at rest and on exercise (see Ch. 11), as venography alone cannot evaluate the effectiveness of the collateral venous circulation in bypassing the obstructed iliac vein.

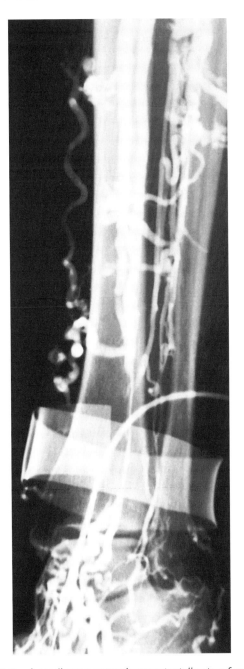

Figure 8.2 *Ascending venogram: incompetent direct perforating vein communicating with superficial veins.*

ISCHEMIC ULCERATION

SITE AND APPEARANCE

Ischemic ulcers may be situated on the toes or forefoot in an area of cyanosed and obviously pre-gangrenous skin. Another common site is the heel, particularly in bedridden patients. These ulcers are usually accompanied by severe rest pain and there is no difficulty in making a diagnosis.

Ischemic ulcers may also present on the dorsum of the foot or on the anterior surface of the leg or may mimic venous ulcers by being situated over the medial or lateral malleolus.

Box 8.2 Case history: ischemic ulcer

A 56-year-old man was referred with a doctor's letter asking for treatment of the 'venous ulcer' over his left medial malleolus. This had been treated unsuccessfully by tight medicated compression bandaging for 2 years. Examination showed a shallow ulcer over the medial malleolus. There was no obvious evidence of venous abnormality but further examination also showed that his second and third toes had been amputated and the amputation site was ulcerated and obviously ischemic.

Further questioning revealed that this patient had been involved in an accident some 5 or 6 years previously and this had been followed by the amputation of two toes. The amputation sites had failed to heal and he was subsequently referred to a vascular clinic elsewhere for lumbar sympathectomy. Temporary healing was followed by further breakdown and then development of the ankle ulcer.

Neither femoral pulse could be palpated and arteriography demonstrated atherosclerotic occlusion of both iliac arteries. The patient was treated by the insertion of an aortobifemoral graft and the ankle ulcer and amputation sites rapidly healed.

The latter may be no more painful than venous ulcers and the diagnosis is then by no means easy.

The base of a typical ischemic ulcer is usually obscured by pale yellow purulent exudate and necrotic debris, often with islands of gangrenous skin. Removal of the necrotic debris is likely to reveal deep fascia or tendon, with little or no granulation tissue. The edges are very poorly epithelialized and may be punched-out (see Fig. 6.2, p. 48).

HISTORY

A history of ischemic rest pain is common in the more severe cases, and lesser degrees of ischemia are usually associated with intermittent claudication. Patients are often heavy cigarette smokers. Many patients are old and bedridden. This is particularly true of heel ulcers, which are usually described as pressure sores; sheepskin pads under the heels or water-filled rubber gloves under the ankles are useful methods of prevention.

EXAMINATION

Ischemic ulceration usually occurs in an area of obviously ischemic skin, which may be cyanosed or pale and shiny.

All pulses must be palpated: femoral, popliteal and ankle. Edema may make the last of these difficult to feel, in which case Doppler ultrasound should be used. It is not sufficient simply to palpate one ankle pulse, e.g. the dorsalis pedis,

and then assume that there must be adequate arterial perfusion of the lower leg and foot; both must be palpated.

The ankle pulse pressures of diabetic patients with ischemic ulceration may appear normal. This is due to increased stiffness of the walls of arteries in patients with diabetes attributable to heterotopic calcification, which make pulse pressure measurements unreliable. Ischemic ulcers can also result from small-vessel insufficiency, particularly in thromboangiitis obliterans (Buerger's disease) and the vasculitides. Ankle pulse pressures may then be normal. The diagnosis depends on clinical examination of the toe capillary refilling time, which is greatly increased in ischemia. The measurement of toe pulse pressures using photoplethysmography (PPG) and a miniature sphygmomanometer cuff may also be useful. The pressure gradient between ankle and toes should not normally exceed 30 mmHg.

INVESTIGATIONS

A duplex examination of the lower limb arteries is the most effective method of establishing the presence and distribution of arterial stenosis and occlusion. This technique can be used to evaluate the aorta and iliac vessels as well as the femoral, popliteal and calf vessels. The severity of any stenosis can be evaluated by measuring the peak flow velocity at the stenosis in comparison with the peak flow velocity in the non-stenotic adjacent vessel. The ratio of these measurements (the peak systolic velocity ratio) accurately assesses the severity of a stenosis. The length of the stenosis can also be assessed. This information is essential when establishing whether an arterial lesion is suitable for management by an endovascular technique.

Angiography is usually reserved for confirmation of the ultrasound findings prior to angioplasty or surgery.

ULCERATION OF MIXED ARTERIAL AND VENOUS ORIGIN

Ankle ulceration resulting from a combination of arterial and venous insufficiency is not uncommon, particularly in the elderly. Callam et al.[5] found evidence of peripheral arterial insufficiency in 176 (21.3 percent) out of 827 ulcerated legs. In a recent study, Moffatt et al.[6] reported that in 21/138 ulcerated limbs (15 percent) ulceration was principally attributable to arterial disease. In the past it was often not recognized that there is an ischemic element until months or even years of conventional dressings and compression bandaging had failed to achieve satisfactory healing. There is now much more emphasis on the assessment of the arterial system in the management of leg ulcers. Much of the workload of managing leg ulcers falls on community nurses, and modern training courses teach the skills required to measure the ankle:brachial systolic pressure ratio in order to detect this problem. This avoids incorrect patient management by avoiding the adverse effects of applying a high compression bandage to a severely ischemic limb.

HISTORY AND EXAMINATION

These patients are more likely to give a history of varicose veins or previous deep vein thrombosis than a history suggestive of arterial insufficiency. Examination is also likely to suggest that the ulcer is purely venous in origin. There is often no obvious cyanosis or other physical sign indicative of a diminished arterial supply. Careful examination of foot pulses is therefore most important in all patients with venous ulceration.

INVESTIGATIONS

Doppler ultrasound measurement of ankle pulse pressures is essential. Doppler ultrasound may be used to identify the sites of venous incompetence, as in the investigation of uncomplicated venous ulcers. Complete evaluation of the patient includes duplex ultrasound evaluation of the arterial and venous system of the lower limb in order to plan effective treatment in these patients.

Arteriovenous fistulae

Arteriovenous fistulae may cause skin ulceration anywhere in the body. Dodd and Cockett[7] describe a patient with ulceration of the shoulder due to a traumatic arteriovenous fistula. Congenital arteriovenous fistulae usually affect the leg and the dilated surface veins may be mistaken for simple varices until their pulsation is noted. Extensive congenital arteriovenous fistulae of one or both limbs, associated with increased blood flow and limb hypertrophy, is known as the Parkes–Weber syndrome.

HISTORY

The patient or parents may have been aware of increased limb growth. This is not invariable and superficial venous dilatation is usually thought to be due to simple varicose veins.

EXAMINATION

The ulcer is usually indistinguishable in its features from a typical venous ulcer. Careful examination of the surrounding skin will show pulsation of the dilated veins and their bruits can be heard with a stethoscope. Arteriography is necessary to demonstrate the site of the fistula and to evaluate the possibility of therapeutic embolization.

Traumatic arteriovenous fistulae may be surgically induced. Ulceration of the hand occasionally develops after the formation of a Brescia–Cimino arteriovenous fistula for dialysis in the arm or leg. Arteriovenous fistula formation may also follow inadequate ligation of tributaries of the great saphenous vein when the latter is used for an *in situ* femoropopliteal vein graft. This omission will lead to tender inflammatory induration of the overlying skin, followed by ulceration if the offending tributary is not immediately ligated.

> **Box 8.3   Case history: Klippel–Trenaunay syndrome**
>
> A 54-year-old woman presented with a long history of atypical varicose veins, with a capillary hemangioma (port-wine stain) on the lateral surface of the thigh, but without the limb enlargement typical of the true Klippel–Trenaunay syndrome. She had developed extensive ulceration along the posterior surface of the calf. This eventually healed after venographic demonstration of the feeding points of the venous malformation, followed by ligation of these and treatment of the varices by avulsions and injection sclerotherapy.

VENOUS MALFORMATIONS

Klippel–Trenaunay syndrome

The Klippel–Trenaunay syndrome[8] is a congenital disorder, usually affecting one limb only and consisting of a cutaneous nevus ('port-wine stain') on the lateral surface of the thigh, extensive varicose veins, also predominantly on the lateral surface of the thigh, and limb hypertrophy. It is distinct from, although often confused with, the Parkes–Weber syndrome. Some patients present with all the features of the Klippel–Trenaunay syndrome apart from limb hypertrophy (see Box 8.3). This has been described as the 'Klippel-type syndrome'. Venous ulceration may develop in unusual sites in patients with the Klippel–Trenaunay syndrome or venous hemangiomas (Plate 8.1).

The management of patients with Klippel–Trenaunay syndrome and other mainly venous angiomas is often difficult, especially if they widely infiltrate the muscles. Surgical excision of these vessels is technically complex and risks considerable hemorrhage as well as damage to adjacent structures. Recently Cabrera has reported a series of 50 patients managed by ultrasound-guided foam sclerotherapy. He reported considerable reduction in size of the angioma in 46 patients with complete disappearance in 18 patients. This technique is worthy of consideration in these difficult cases.

RHEUMATOID AND OTHER VASCULITIC ULCERS

If there is a clear history of rheumatoid arthritis, scleroderma, polyarteritis nodosa or other condition with a known tendency to vasculitis, there should be no difficulty in diagnosis. Difficulty does arise when the patient presents with an apparent venous ulcer and without any other obvious manifestations of vasculitis.

Rheumatoid ulceration

Rheumatoid ulcers are usually serpiginous and shallow (Plate 8.2). Frequently multiple, they may affect the lateral or posterior surfaces of the lower leg, but not infrequently appear in the malleolar regions and mimic venous ulceration, although usually without surrounding lipodermatosclerosis. The base of a rheumatoid ulcer is usually covered by rather pale granulation tissue, often covered by yellow slough, and the edges are poorly epithelialized. A rheumatoid ulcer may look ischemic but the appearance of ischemia is usually less marked than ulcers which are secondary to main vessel obstruction. Careful examination of the hands and other joints will usually show evidence of rheumatoid arthritis. The difficult diagnosis is when the ulcer is in malleolar skin and is accompanied by evidence of great or small saphenous incompetence or perforating vein incompetence. If the patient has few or no physical signs of arthritis, a diagnosis of venous ulceration is almost inevitable and, in the authors' practice, the rheumatoid component to these ulcers is often overlooked until they fail to respond to conventional venous ulcer treatment.

The diagnosis may be confirmed by serological testing for rheumatoid factor. Other systemic inflammatory markers (e.g. erythrocyte sedimentation rate, ESR) may also be elevated.

Vasculitic ulceration

Vasculitic ulcers are usually small, multiple and painful (Plate 8.3). These may be on the lower leg or foot. Unlike rheumatoid ulcers, they do not normally mimic venous ulceration, and, once it is recognized that the ulceration is vasculitic in origin, specific investigations will provide a precise diagnosis.

Patients with scleroderma may have the typical tightness of facial skin, resulting in a fixed expression and shiny, tapered fingers. Polyarteritis nodosa may present with a patchy reticular livido on the legs or elsewhere and is often accompanied by muscle tenderness. Systemic lupus erythematosus (SLE) may present with reticulate telangiectatic erythema on the toes and lateral borders of the feet and heels. There may be a butterfly rash across the nose and cheeks. Dilatation of the nail-fold capillaries may occur in either condition. Examination of the veins and of the peripheral pulses is unlikely to show any abnormality.

INVESTIGATION OF THE VASCULITIDES

Doppler ultrasound examination is likely to be normal; PPG may demonstrate a damped toe pulse waveform. Specific investigations include the ESR which is likely to be very high. However, it must be remembered that a raised ESR may accompany any infected ulcer, whether of venous, arterial or vasculitic origin. Specific investigations for the vasculitides include the Rose–Waaler and latex tests for rheumatoid antibodies and tests for autoantibodies. Anti-double-stranded DNA binding capacity is elevated in SLE (normal: 6–8 mg/L).

Antineutrophil cytoplasmic antibody (ANCA) is elevated in polyarteritis nodosa and in Wegener's granuloma. If scleroderma is suspected, a barium swallow may provide confirmatory evidence; patients with scleroderma typically have uncoordinated esophageal peristalsis. Smooth muscle incoordination is not necessarily confined to the esophagus and investigation of a patient in our clinic by barium studies showed normal esophageal peristalsis, the diagnosis of scleroderma being made by observation of abnormal jejunal peristalsis. In many cases of vasculitis, no specific cause can be identified.

Biopsy of the ulcer edge may be useful in these cases. Specialist histology departments may be able to search for immune complexes in the vessel walls using immunohistochemistry. The presence of these is indicative of a vasculitic syndrome resulting in leg ulceration.

If vasculitis is suspected, help in diagnosis and treatment should be sought immediately from a dermatologist or rheumatologist.

Erythrocyanosis

Although not strictly a vasculitis, it is convenient to consider this condition here. Erythrocyanosis frigida occurs in young women with fat legs. Areas of skin are mottled and cyanotic and small painful ulcers occasionally occur in these areas. Examination will normally show no arterial or venous disorder and investigations for vasculitis will be negative. These patients may be helped by warm stockings and calcium antagonists, and chemical sympathectomy may occasionally be indicated.

STEROID ULCERS

Patients undergoing long-term steroid treatment for rheumatoid arthritis, asthma, ulcerative colitis or other conditions are liable to develop ulceration of the leg (see Box 8.4). These are

---

Box 8.4   Case history: steroid ulcer

This typically difficult case involved a 56-year-old diabetic woman with rheumatoid arthritis requiring steroid treatment, with saphenous and perforating vein incompetence and absent foot pulses. Investigation and treatment of each causative lesion was undertaken in turn. The diabetes was controlled as precisely as possible by insulin and diet. Arteriography showed superficial femoral arterial occlusion, which was treated by femoropopliteal bypass. The points of venous incompetence were ligated and the steroid therapy was reduced as far as possible. Ulcer healing eventually took place and although there were minor recurrent ulcers in subsequent years, these were smaller than before treatment.

usually large, shallow, serpiginous ulcers with very poorly epithelialized edges, and the surrounding skin is thin and fragile. They are often similar to rheumatoid ulcers and are notoriously slow to heal. There is usually no difficulty in diagnosis as patients are known to be undergoing steroid therapy. Occasionally a steroid ulcer may mimic a venous ulcer in site and appearance or may coexist with venous insufficiency. There is then likely to be some confusion in diagnosis.

HYPERTENSIVE ULCERS

Martorell[9] described painful leg ulcers in severely hypertensive patients. Most were situated on the posterior surface of the lower leg, in contrast to typical ischemic ulcers which are usually on the dorsum of the foot or anterior surface of the leg. It has been suggested that most, if not all, of these ulcers are caused by the embolization of atherosclerotic debris into small skin vessels. However, Martorell described 'hyalinosis' of the tunica intima with stenosis of the arteriolar lumen, and arteriography in Cockett's[10] series of eight patients showed small localized occlusions of the peroneal artery with no obstruction of the posterior tibial or foot arteries.

DIABETIC ULCERS

Diabetic ulcers may be the result of peripheral neuropathy, ischemia or infection, or often a combination of all three factors.

SITE AND APPEARANCE

Ischemia diabetic ulcers may affect the toes or forefoot (Plate 8.4) or the heel, particularly as pressure sores in bedridden patients. Neuropathic diabetic ulcers are the result of pressure on the sole of a Charcot foot (Plate 8.5).

Diabetic ulcers often result from both ischemia and neuropathy, with ischemic slough and surrounding anesthesia. Less common is necrobiosis lipoidica, ulceration resulting from infection and fat necrosis of the lower leg skin of diabetic patients (Plate 8.6). These ulcers are most likely the result of failure of the skin and subcutaneous tissues of diabetics to respond to minor infection. The infecting organisms are often synergistic, aerobic and microaerophilic organisms combining to cause skin necrosis, as in the synergic ulceration described by Meleney.[11]

HISTORY

A history of diabetes is usual, but some patients present to an ulcer clinic with previously undiagnosed diabetes. It is therefore essential that urine examination is carried out in all patients. Any patient with glycosuria must be referred immediately to the diabetic clinic for investigation and treatment.

EXAMINATION

After examining the site and appearance of the ulcers, a neurological examination may show no evidence of peripheral neuropathy. Venous disorders must be excluded by examination and investigations, as has been described, and all leg pulses must be palpated, using Doppler ultrasound examination where necessary.

INVESTIGATIONS

Glycosuria must be further investigated in the diabetic clinic. Absent ankle pulses or reduced pulse pressures must be investigated by arteriography. Peripheral ischemia in diabetes is often attributed solely to small-vessel disease and it is important to remember that diabetic patients have a higher than normal incidence of atherosclerosis, which may result in stenosis or occlusion of the main leg vessels. Arteriography is necessary, even if ankle pressures are apparently within normal limits, as the increased stiffness of diabetic arteries may lead to abnormally high pulse pressures.

NEUROPATHIC ULCERATION

Patients with paraplegia or peripheral neuropathies may be referred to the ulcer clinic. A diagnosis has usually already been made. However, neuropathy may occasionally be diagnosed for the first time in the ulcer clinic. Pressure from poorly fitted calipers may sometimes cause local ulceration. Treatment is usually simple, consisting of healing the ulcer by standard cleaning and dressings followed by appropriate padding to prevent further pressure. Other devices may produce local ischemia: in one case, a young paraplegic patient was referred with toe ulceration; examination showed that his indwelling urethral catheter was attached to his leg by an excessively tight strap. The ulcer healed when this was removed.

Patients with long-standing peripheral neuropathy may also develop peripheral vascular disorders and these must always be excluded by careful examination and investigations (see Box 8.5).

Box 8.5   Case history: occlusion of calf arteries

An elderly woman with a long history of muscle wasting due to Charcot–Marie–Tooth disease and with ankle ulceration was found to have absent ankle pulses. Arteriography showed multiple occlusions of the calf arteries.

The message is clear: do not assume that leg or foot ulceration in a patient with peripheral neuropathy is necessarily neuropathic in origin. Always exclude arterial or venous causes by careful examination and investigations.

TRAUMATIC ULCERATION

Traumatic ulcers may be the result of accidental trauma, self-induced trauma, injection sclerotherapy or operative surgery. Many patients with venous or ischemic ulceration give a history of precipitating trauma. Supermarket trolleys have now largely taken over from the steps of buses as causative agents. All patients presenting to an accident and emergency department with abrasions or lacerations of the lower leg should be carefully examined for signs of venous reflux or arterial insufficiency. Urine should be tested for the presence of glucose if healing is slow. These simple investigations are frequently omitted by busy casualty officers and the initial laceration may then develop into chronic ulceration. It should be remembered that abrasions and lacerations of the lower leg and ankle are always slow to heal, particularly in the elderly, even in the presence of normal arteries and veins. A tight bandage or plaster-of-Paris cast may cause skin necrosis and ulceration, particularly in the elderly and those with minor ischemia.

Injection sclerotherapy may cause subcutaneous fat necrosis and ulceration of the overlying skin following extravasation of the sclerosing solution. Sodium tetradecyl sulfate (STD), which is used for the injection sclerotherapy of varicose veins, may produce indolent and painful ulceration if the sclerosing solution extravasates outside the vein lumen. Avoidance of this complication is by very careful attention to certain details:

- Avoid injecting very small varicose veins with strong solutions of STD; extravasation of sclerosant is likely. It is better to inject small varices with low concentrations of polidocanol (e.g. Sclerovein). This sclerosant does not cause ulceration when accidentally injected outside a vein at low concentrations.
- Use a meticulous technique for injection: (i) after inserting the needle into the vein, pull back the syringe plunger and make certain that dark venous blood is aspirated; (ii) before injecting the solution, place one finger in front of and another behind the needle so as to localize the injection. Watch the skin over the point of the needle carefully and stop injecting should any swelling appear.

With these simple precautions, ulceration should not occur. In the event that an ulcer does occur, it should be sufficiently small to allow simple excision and suture under local anesthetic.

Foam sclerotherapy has been widely used by French phlebologists to treat reticular varices and dermal flares. Foam is probably less likely to cause skin ulceration since it contains less sclerosant per unit volume than liquid sclerosants. Henriet[12] has a series of 10 000 patients with reticular varices and telangiectases of the lower limb treated with polidocanol foam. The concentration of polidocanol for use in small veins should be in the range 0.25–0.5 percent. Few complications of this technique have been reported. Foam sclerotherapy is described in more detail in Chapter 18.

An alternative to the use of polidocanol for the treatment of telangiectases and reticular varices is the use of low concentrations of STD (0.2 percent STD is licenced in the UK for this purpose). It may be used as liquid or foam but care should be taken to avoid extravasation during injection.

Scleremo, a solution of chromated glycerol, is both effective in sclerosing telangiectasia and also remarkably free of complications. This is widely used in France but elsewhere glycerol alone is used at high concentration (72 percent). This is an osmotic sclerosant and is safe even when extravasation occurs. It is only effective in the smallest veins. A possible disadvantage to the chromated version of this solution is that a number of patients are allergic to heavy metals such as nickel and chromium and anaphylactic reactions have been described.

Factitious ulceration

Traumatic ulcers may be self-induced. It has become a platitude among those who are responsible for ulcer clinics that failure to heal is often the fault of the patient who continually tampers with the ulcer, and it has been said that 'the ulcer is the elderly patient's best friend', intimating that elderly and lonely people may have their only social contact at ulcer clinics or through the district nurse visiting to perform dressings. This attitude is probably an exaggeration of the truth. In one of the authors' series of 77 patients with 109 ulcerated legs, there was one elderly lady whose ulcers mysteriously broke down after a week or two at home, having been perfectly healed after treatment in hospital. She admitted to enjoying the company of others in the ulcer clinic and her chats with doctors and nurses, between which she wrote frequent and very long letters to the surgeon responsible for her treatment. Apart from this lonely woman, the authors cannot recall any patient in whom personal interference seemed to be responsible for retarding healing.

Factitious ulcers may be quite bizarre in site and appearance, due to being inflicted by such agents as rubber bands tied tightly around the calf. The possibility of self-interference must always be borne in mind in patients whose ulcers are excessively slow in healing, or which recur repeatedly, but conscientious surgeons will first ask themselves whether there is any possible aspect of diagnosis or treatment which could have been overlooked before accusing the patient of self-injury.

LYMPHEDEMA ULCERS

SITE AND APPEARANCE

Ulceration is extremely rare in lymphedema, whether this is primary or secondary to filariasis or malignant involvement of lymph nodes. When they do occur, these ulcers are usually small, indolent and painless and appear on the anterior surface of the ankle or lower leg.

HISTORY

Patients will normally give a long history of swelling of the dorsum of the foot and ankle. The condition is often inherited, and primary familial lymphedema is known as Milroy's disease.

EXAMINATION

The limb shows the typical appearances of lymphedema with marked edema of the dorsum of the foot. This dorsal foot swelling may sometimes be seen in cardiac edema but rarely, if ever, in edema of purely venous origin. Examination will show no evidence of venous disorder and ankle pulses will normally be present. The edema may make these difficult to palpate and Doppler ultrasound examination must then be used.

INVESTIGATIONS

Lymphedema results in swelling of the limb in the presence of a normal venous system. This can be readily established by undertaking duplex ultrasonography. Failure to demonstrate a venous cause in a patient with lower extremity edema does not prove that the patient has lymphedema, but greatly limits the possible range of diagnoses. Doppler ultrasound examination of ankle pulses is important in any case of doubt as ischemic ulceration and lymphedema can coexist.

The most appropriate method for studying the lymphatic function in order to confirm the diagnosis is quantitative isotope scintigraphy. A recent review details current methods of investigation and management of this disease.[13]

Edema of other causes

Ulceration may occur in the grossly distended skin of severely edematous legs in patients with congestive cardiac or renal failure. Examination will usually show no evidence of venous insufficiency, although some impairment of arterial supply is likely to be present in these elderly patients. The ulcers are usually scattered over all surfaces of the leg; they are shallow and may be serpiginous in outline. Treatment must be directed principally at correcting the congestive failure and reducing leg edema.

TROPICAL SORES AND OTHER INFECTIONS

Tropical sores or ulcers, which are colonized by a variety of pathogenic bacteria, occur more commonly in underdeveloped tropical countries than in the industrialized north.

Tropical ulcers

A. D. Landra,[14] a consultant plastic surgeon in Nairobi, defines tropical ulcers as chronic ulcers of the lower leg or dorsum of the foot which occur among the poor populations of tropical countries and are of mixed bacteriology. He excludes those ulcers where *Mycobacterium buruli*, *Mycobacterium leprae*, *Mycobacterium tuberculosis* and Guinea worms have been identified. Anaerobes (fusobacteria) are present in 35 percent and coliform bacilli in 60 percent of tropical ulcers. According to Landra, the most common pathogens are *Pseudomonas aeruginosa* and *Proteus mirabilis vulgaris*, but MacGraith[15] states that *Treponema vincenti* and *Bacillus fusiformis* are most frequently cultured and can be identified in 80 percent of smears. The diagnosis of tropical ulcers should exclude ulceration with a specific underlying cause such as ischemia, diabetes or the hemoglobinopathies.

Tropical ulcers are more common in males, with an approximate male:female sex ratio of 2:1. The ulcers are usually single, occasionally multiple, with well-defined raised edges and surrounding edema. The surface is covered by a greenish-grey foul slough, which pulls away easily to reveal a bleeding granulating base. Predisposing factors are: tropical environment, poverty, malnutrition, chronic anemia, poor educational standards, lack of hygiene and poor medical facilities. Lack of washing facilities and incentive to keep clean seems to be important; tropical ulceration is less common among Muslim communities in Indonesia, where daily or twice-daily washing is practiced, than among similar socioeconomic groups who do not practice this discipline.

Long-standing ulcers may be complicated by periostitis, osteomyelitis or lymphedema. Malignant change (squamous cell carcinoma) is common in ulcers of between 12 and 15 years' duration, particularly in West Africa and New Guinea.

Other infectious ulcers

Leg ulcers resulting from specific infections are also more common in tropical countries. Tubercular skin ulcers (scrofula) may occur on the legs, but are more common elsewhere. Tuberculous ulcers are characterized by an undermined edge which is irregular, bluish and friable. The ulcers are often multiple and the patient usually has evidence of pulmonary or skeletal tuberculosis. Tuberculous ulceration of the calf has been named erythema induratam scrofulosorum or Bazin's disease. Secondary syphilis has become very rare since the introduction of antibiotics, but occasionally a syphilitic gumma may ulcerate, forming a painless, circular punched-out ulcer with a 'wash leather' slough in the base. Yaws may cause similar ulcers.

Other specific infections are leprosy, Guinea worms, caused by the nematode *Dracunculus medinensis*, and anthrax (woolsorter's disease), which rarely occurs on the lower limb. Buruli boil, or Baghdad boil, is caused by *Leishmania tropica* and transmitted by a sand fly. Actinomycosis, epidermophytosis, blastomycosis, moniliasis and mycetoma (Madura foot) are other infections which may cause leg ulceration.

Osteomyelitis

Chronic osteomyelitis of the tibia may discharge to form a sinus which may mimic venous ulceration.

SITE AND APPEARANCE

Osteomyelitis may occur anywhere in the leg but is more likely to be mistaken for venous ulceration when it occurs, as commonly happens, in the lower third of the medial surface of the leg. The appearance of necrotic slough is very hard to distinguish from venous ulceration. Osteomyelitis of the toes may occur in association with ischemic ulceration.

HISTORY AND EXAMINATION

There may be a past history of pulmonary or abdominal tuberculosis or a history of local trauma. Examination is unlikely to show any evidence of venous disorder or ischemia.

INVESTIGATIONS

X-ray examination will normally show bone destruction and sequestrum formation typical of osteomyelitis.

MALIGNANT ULCERS

Squamous cell carcinoma

Squamous cell carcinoma developing in an established venous ulcer is known as Marjolin's ulcer[16] (Plate 8.7). Although this complication of venous ulceration is well described in all standard surgical textbooks and is well known to most medical students, it is in fact remarkably rare. Browse *et al.*[17] have reported seeing only five cases in 25 years. Ryan and Wilkinson[18] reported only three cases of squamous carcinoma in 2000 ulcers. One or two new cases of leg ulcer are referred to the Lewisham Hospital ulcer clinic each week (a total of between 50 and 100 a year). Only two patients have developed Marjolin's squamous cell carcinoma in venous ulcers in the past 12 years and the incidence is therefore similar to that reported by Ryan and Wilkinson.

Squamous cell carcinoma should be suspected if there is any overgrowth of tissue in the base or at the edge of the ulcer. Biopsy and histological examination must then be performed as a matter of urgency.

Squamous cell carcinoma may also develop per primum on the leg and mimic venous ulceration. In the case history in Box 8.6, a number of alternative diagnoses were considered before the correct one was made.

Basal cell carcinoma

Basal cell carcinoma may occasionally occur on the leg. Its appearance is less likely to mimic venous ulceration than squamous cell carcinoma and the diagnosis is established by biopsy. Malignant melanoma is common on the foot and lower leg, but is most unlikely to be confused with venous ulceration.

Box 8.6   Case history: squamous cell carcinoma

A 54-year-old Jamaican woman was referred to the skin clinic with a 4-week history of ulceration on the lateral surface of the left ankle. The appearances were typical of an infected venous ulcer. She was therefore referred to the vascular clinic where examination and Doppler ultrasound examination failed to show any evidence of venous or arterial disorder. It was then found that she had recently returned from a holiday in Jamaica. She said that she had been walking in the country where there were many thorn bushes and she thought she might have been scratched. It therefore seemed likely that the ulcer was a tropical sore. Biopsy of the ulcer edge showed granulation tissue only, with no evidence of malignancy.

X-ray of the leg showed a translucent area in the distal tibia suggestive of osteomyelitis. The diagnosis of tropical sore was abandoned and the patient was referred to an orthopedic surgeon. The apparent sinus was explored. No osteomyelitis was found but further biopsies of the deep tissues showed that the lesion was in fact a squamous cell carcinoma which had invaded bone. The patient was treated by above-knee amputation. Metastatic spread to the inguinal and iliac lymph nodes occurred 8 months later and was treated by block dissection followed by radiotherapy, but in spite of this the patient died after a further 4 months.

Sarcomas and lymphomas

Kaposi's sarcoma may present with skin ulceration. The ulcers are usually small and multiple, similar to vasculitic ulcers. Rare at present, ulcerated Kaposi's sarcoma is likely to become an increasing differential diagnosis with the spread of acquired immune deficiency syndrome (AIDS). Tumours of bone, sarcoma and osteoclastoma may also present with leg ulceration.

Cutaneous B-cell and T-cell lymphomas associated with pyoderma gangrenosum and skin ulcers have been described.[19,20] Pyoderma gangrenosum is also a rare complication of ulcerative colitis or Crohn's disease.

BLOOD DYSCRASIAS

Leg ulceration may occur in conjunction with sickle cell disease, thalassemia, thrombotic thrombocythemia, polycythemia rubra vera and leukemia. These are usually painful and present as small ischemic ulcers. In polycythemia rubra vera, the ischemia may be sufficient to produce small areas of gangrenous skin on the toes.

Cryoglobulinemia and macroglobulinemia cause rouleaux formation of erythrocytes and occlusion of small vessels.

This situation is exacerbated by vasospasm and small ischemic ulcers sometimes result.

NUTRITIONAL ULCERATION

Leg ulceration as a result of malnutrition is most commonly seen in developing countries accompanying such malnutrition states as kwashiorkor, beriberi and scurvy. The situation is likely to be exacerbated by anemia, which results from a combination of malnutrition and hookworm infestation.

Leg ulcers were very common among British servicemen in Japanese prisoner-of-war camps during World War II. These 'tropical sores' are likely to have been due to a combination of malnutrition and local trauma resulting in infection. The condition frequently deteriorated into infected gangrene, requiring amputation.

It should be remembered that malnutrition is not confined to developing countries. The diet of some elderly patients is inadequate, and vitamin C deficiency and anemia must be considered as possible complicating factors in all elderly patients with venous or ischemic ulcers. It used to be thought that zinc deficiency was also important and zinc-containing lotions such as lotio rubra were popular in the treatment of leg ulcers. Dietary zinc is mainly obtained from meat, which may be lacking in the diet of elderly patients on low incomes.

Serum zinc levels were measured in over 30 patients attending the St Thomas's Hospital ulcer clinic in 1973 but no evidence of zinc deficiency was found. Most of these patients were elderly and on low incomes and it was surprising that we were unable to detect any suffering from zinc deficiency. We no longer feel it necessary to check serum zinc levels, except occasionally in elderly patients whose chronic ulcers prove completely resistant to conventional treatment and in whom no other underlying cause can be demonstrated.

IMMUNODEFICIENCY

Leg ulcers with no evidence of venous, ischemic or other etiology are now increasingly being seen in HIV-positive Africans.[21] This must obviously be remembered as AIDS becomes more common.

CONTACT DERMATITIS

Contact dermatitis may result in the failure of existing ulcers to heal or in the development of new ulcers. This condition is the result of sensitivity to medicated bandages or local antibiotics (see Plate 13.1). Steroid applications are particularly likely to produce contact dermatitis. The skin is red and scaly and the ulcers are usually shallow and with a yellow base, and may appear on any surface of the leg or ankle.

Box 8.7 Allergens identified in leg ulcer patients (University Hospital, Leuven, Belgium 1978–90)

Balsam of Peru
Neomycin
Fragrance mix
Wood tars

Benzocaine
Colophony
Cetrimide
Cetyl alcohol
Ammoniated Mercury

The skin of an ulcer-bearing leg is more sensitive than normal skin and contact dermatitis is a common complication of ulcer dressings. For this reason, local steroids, antibiotics and medicated dressings and bandages (particularly zinc) should be scrupulously avoided and replaced by the simple alternatives which are described in Chapter 13.

Cotton compression bandages and stockings are now available and these should be prescribed for patients who are allergic to nylon. Lycra is commonly used in the manufacture of elastic stockings and its use avoids rubber allergies. Allergy to Lycra does occasionally occur, but only very rarely.

Numerous other allergens have been described and those encountered in a Belgian clinic between 1978 and 1990[22] are listed in Box 8.7.

REFERENCES

1. Shami SK, Sarin S, Cheatle TR *et al.* Venous ulcers and the superficial venous system. *J Vasc Surg* 1993; **17**: 487–90.
2. Barwell JR, Davies CE, Deacon J *et al.* Comparison of surgery and compression with compression alone in chronic venous ulceration (ESCHAR study): randomised controlled trial. *Lancet* 2004; **363**: 1854–9.
3. Mackenzie RK, Ludlam CA, Ruckley CV *et al.* The prevalence of thrombophilia in patients with chronic venous leg ulceration. *J Vasc Surg* 2002; **35**: 718–22.
4. Negus D. Calf pain in the post-thrombotic syndrome. *Br Med J* 1968; **2**: 156–8.
5. Callam MJ, Harper DR, Dale JJ, Ruckley CV. Arterial disease in chronic leg ulceration: an underestimated hazard? Lothian and Forth Valley Leg Ulcer Study. *Br Med J* 1987; **294**: 929–31.
6. Moffatt CJ, Franks PJ, Doherty DC *et al.* Prevalence of leg ulceration in a London population. *QJM* 2004; **97**: 431–7.
7. Dodd H, Cockett, FB. *The Pathology and Surgery of the Veins of the Lower Limb*, 2nd edn. Edinburgh: Livingstone, 1956; 254.
8. Klippel M, Trenaunay P. Du noevus variqueux osteo-hypertrophique. *Arch Gen Med (Paris)* 1900; **185**: 641–72.
9. Martorell F. Hypertensive ulcer of the leg. *Angiology* 1950; **1**: 1331–140.
10. Cockett FB. Ulcéré de Martorelle. *Phlébologie* 1983; **36**: 363–72.

11. Meleney FL. *Clinical Aspects and Treatments of Surgical Infections.* London: Saunders, 1949.

12. Henriet JP. Expérience durant trois années de la mousse de polidocanol dans le traitement des varices réticulaires et des varicosités. *Phlebologie* 1999; **52**: 277–82.

13. Tiwari A, Cheng KS, Button M *et al.* Differential diagnosis, investigation, and current treatment of lower limb lymphedema. *Arch Surg* 2003; **138**: 152–61.

14. Landra AD. The tropical ulcer. *Surgery* 1988; **59**: 1402–3.

15. MacGraith B. *Exotic Diseases in Practice.* London: Heinemann, 1965.

16. Marjolin JN. Ulcére. *Dictionaire de Médicine*, Vol. xxx. Paris: Labbé, 1846; 10–31.

17. Browse NL, Burnand KG, Lea Thomas M. *Diseases of the Veins; Pathology, Diagnosis and Treatment.* London: Arnold, 1988; 383.

18. Ryan TJ, Wilkinson DS. Diseases of the veins – venous leg ulcers. In: Rook A, Wilkinson DS, Ebling FJG, eds. *Textbook of Dermatology.* Oxford: Blackwell Scientific Publications, 1985; 1098.

19. Damstra RJ, Toonstra J. Cutaneous B-cell lymphoma mimicking ulcus crus venosum. *Phlebology* 1992; **7**: 82–4.

20. Kitahama A, Roland PY, Kerstein MD. Pyoderma gangrenosum with cutaneous T-cell lymphoma manifested as lower extremity ulcers; case reports. *Angiology* 1991; **42**: 498–503.

21. Bayley AC. Surgical pathology of HIV infection: lessons from Africa. *Br J Surg* 1990; **77**: 863–7.

22. Dooms-Goosens A, Degreef H. Contact allergy of leg ulcer patients. *Phlebol Digest* 1992; **2**: 4–6.

9

Diagnosis: history and examination

DAVID NEGUS

The diagnosis and treatment of the underlying cause of a leg ulcer are as important as the treatment of the ulcer itself. A failure to appreciate this elementary concept is responsible for the majority of recurrent ulcers. Even when this point has been grasped, accurate diagnosis may be hampered by lack of familiarity with methods of investigation. The most frequent error is the failure to recognize that an ulcer is ischemic in origin, and many ischemic ulcers are undoubtedly made much worse by tight compression bandaging, in the mistaken belief that they are venous. As the latter are by far the most common, this is an understandable mistake, but in an aging and cigarette-smoking society, ischemic ulceration is now seen with increasing frequency.

HISTORY

In taking the patient's history, it is important to note the duration of the ulcer, whether there was any precipitating cause, and whether there is any past history of deep vein thrombosis (DVT) or varicose veins. It is also important to enquire whether the patient has experienced symptoms suggestive of ischemia, intermittent claudication or rest pain.

ISCHEMIA

A venous ulcer may be locally painful, but if the patient complains of pain in the toes or forefoot, suspect ischemia. Remember that the history may sometimes be misleading; a history of DVT does not necessarily mean that the ulcer is venous in origin. A typical example is that of a 54-year-old man whose ulcer had been treated for some years by compression bandaging because he had suffered a DVT in the distant past. Examination showed no evidence of deep vein disorder, ankle pulses were absent, and the ulcer was obviously ischemic. Ulcers of mixed venous and arterial origin are not

uncommon, particularly in the elderly, and a history of DVT or varicose veins may coexist with symptoms of intermittent claudication and ischemic rest pain.

PROXIMAL VENOUS OBSTUCTION

Even the symptom of pain on walking, intermittent claudication, may cause diagnostic confusion, as post-thrombotic venous obstruction may also result in severe calf pain on walking, or so-called 'venous claudication'.[1] Venous claudication can be demonstrated by means of a 'stepping test'; patients with significant proximal venous obstruction experience severe calf pain when marking time and are unable to continue this exercise for more than 2.5 min. Proximal venous obstruction can then be confirmed by duplex ultrasound examination or venography, with resting and exercising femoral venous pressure measurements (see Ch. 4, p. 31). Where the history, examination and investigations show no evidence of either venous or arterial cause, other possibilities must be considered. These include rheumatoid arthritis and the hands and other joints should be examined for evidence of arthritis. Diabetic ulcers are usually on the sole of the foot, but may occur elsewhere, and all new patients attending an ulcer clinic must have a routine urine check. Other forms of vasculitis may sometimes present with leg ulcers and these have been considered in Chapter 8. Suspect anemia and vitamin C deficiency in the elderly who live alone and whose diet may be inadequate. The possibility of an ulcer being malignant must always be borne in mind and a biopsy performed if there is any doubt.

EXAMINATION

A full general examination must be carried out and this must include blood pressure measurement and urine testing. Examine the conjunctivae for evidence of anemia. Leg pulses must be palpated in all patients. Ankle pulses are often difficult to feel in the ulcerated and edematous leg and Doppler ultrasound examination must then be used (see p. 78) (Box 9.1).

Careful abdominal examination must be performed to exclude abdominal aortic aneurysm or other abdominal masses. Rectal examination should also be performed, particularly in any patient presenting with a swollen leg. Some textbook accounts still attribute primary varicose veins to compression of venous return by an abdominal tumor. It seems more likely that primary familial varicose veins are the result of an inherited collagen and smooth muscle defect in the vein wall (see Ch. 6, p. 51) and any abdominal mass in such patients is likely to be coincidental. However, leg swelling can certainly occur as a result of iliac vein compression by tumor spread, particularly if this involves perivenous lymph nodes. Carcinoma of the prostate must therefore be excluded in men and uterine and ovarian malignancy in women.

During abdominal examination, the groins must be carefully examined for the presence of dilated collateral veins, the result of iliac venous occlusion. These most often appear as dilated subcutaneous veins rather than true varices. If they are present, or if the patient's history suggests an episode of iliofemoral DVT, calf circumference should be measured to see whether there is any discrepancy. Post-thrombotic iliac vein occlusion, and its attendant physical signs, most often affects the left leg (Plate 9.1).

The colour and temperature of the toes give a good indication of blood flow. Both patients with venous insufficiency and those with ischemia may have cyanosed feet, but cyanosis secondary to venous congestion will show rapid refilling after firm finger pressure to empty the superficial vessels, while an ischemic foot will have a slow refilling time, as long as 4 or 5 s. Following abdominal and pedal pulse examination, careful attention should be paid to the ulcer itself. This must be examined methodically, with particular attention to its site and appearance; appearance is subdivided into base and edge. Venous ulcers most commonly occur in the skin above the malleoli, most usually the medial, the gaiter area of the leg, and often occur in an area of lipodermatosclerosis or pigmentation. Ischemic ulcers are usually on the anterior surface of the leg and dorsum of the foot and diabetic ulcers are most commonly on the sole of the foot. Ulcers are, however, notorious mimics and it is quite common for an ischemic ulcer to occur over the medial malleolus, to all appearances looking exactly like a venous ulcer.

Following general and pedal pulse examination on the examination couch, the patient is asked to stand so that thorough examination of the leg veins can be performed. An 18-cm (7 in) high mounting block is essential to avoid backache in the examiner, and even elderly patients are able to stand on such a low platform with adequate support (Fig. 9.1). A good standard lamp is also essential. Those who design outpatient clinics seem to assume that all examinations are performed with the patient on the couch and usually only provide a wall lamp.

Box 9.1 Case history: overlooked ischemia

A typical example was a young Arab soldier with a 2-year history of ankle ulceration. He had a history of DVT following a comminuted fracture of the left ankle. Examination showed a typical venous ulcer over the medial malleolus and he was treated for several months with bed rest, elevation, dressings and compression bandages. The ulcer failed to heal and he was then referred to the author's clinic. The posterior tibial pulse could not be felt and was therefore checked by Doppler ultrasound examination. This also failed to detect a pulse and subsequent arteriography showed occlusion of the posterior tibial artery, a previously overlooked complication of his fracture. Doppler ultrasound also demonstrated perforating vein incompetence. The ulcer healed following ligation of the incompetent perforating vein and chemical lumbar sympathectomy to improve arterial blood flow to the ankle.

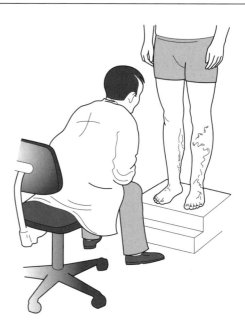

Figure 9.1 *Examination – a suitable platform and good light are essential.*

The leg veins

The lower leg and foot are first inspected for evidence of cyanosis, which may not have been evident in the supine position, particularly if venous in origin. The surroundings of the ulcer are carefully inspected for evidence of lipodermatosclerosis or pigmentation typical of the venous ulcer, and the malleolar skin is equally carefully inspected for the presence or absence of an ankle venous flare (see Plate 3.2 – corona phlebectatica).[2] This fine network of venules is the single most constant indication of calf perforating vein incompetence. A corona phlebectatica is a far more reliable indicator of perforating vein incompetence than 'fascial defects' palpated on the medial surface of the calf. Indentations in the subcutaneous superficial fat can often be felt, but these are more likely to represent superficial varices than defects in the deep fascia, and this is a most unreliable method of examination.

The next step in examining the veins of the lower limb is directed to the saphenous systems, long and short. In patients with varicose veins related to gross venous incompetence, the saphenous veins may be so dilated as to be obvious and no further examination or investigation is then necessary. In cases of doubt, and particularly in the obese patient, a number of simple tests and non-invasive investigations will determine whether these veins are normal or incompetent.

THE PERCUSSION TEST

This useful test was first described by Chevriér in 1908.[3] It is carried out in two steps:

1 *The conventional trapping test*: The watching fingers are placed over the foramen ovale or the popliteal fossa, and the dilated saphenous vein, or a varicose tributary, in the lower leg is tapped briskly with the fingers of the other hand (Fig. 9.2a). The dilated vein transmits the pulse wave thus produced and an impulse can easily be felt by the watching fingers. Strictly speaking, the 'distal tapping, proximal watching' test only indicates a dilated vein, and incompetence should be assessed by the second part of the test.
2 *The reflux tapping test*: the watching fingers and tapping fingers are now reversed (Fig. 9.2b). Tapping in the groin or popliteal fossa will produce a detectable impulse under the distal watching fingers if the vein is incompetent. It is arguable whether this part of the test is really

necessary. While the first test strictly indicates dilatation rather than reflux, it is extremely rare for a competent saphenous vein (e.g. without reflux) to be sufficiently dilated for a tapping impulse to be detected proximally.

The percussion test can more easily be performed in obese patients by the addition of Doppler ultrasound. Instead of the pulse wave being detected by the watching fingers, the Doppler ultrasound probe is placed in the same position and the noise of the pulse wave can easily be heard in an incompetent and dilated vein.

THE TOURNIQUET TEST

This test was described by Trendelenburg in 1891.[4] The patient lies flat and elevates the leg. A tourniquet is applied at upper thigh or below knee level, depending on which saphenous vein is to be examined. Finger occlusion is often quicker. The patient then stands and the leg is inspected to see whether the varices have been controlled. The tourniquet or finger is then suddenly released and the varices rapidly refill (Fig. 9.3).

Like the previous test, this can be enhanced by the use of Doppler ultrasound.[5] With the patient standing, an obvious lower leg varix is marked with a felt-tipped pen. The patient then lies, elevates the leg and the tourniquet is applied as before. The patient stands again and the Doppler probe is placed over the marked point on the lower leg. When the tourniquet is suddenly removed, the rush of blood is detected by Doppler ultrasound and can be heard through its loudspeaker as a roaring noise, like a cascade of water. This modification is very useful in the excessively obese, where distal varices may be difficult to see and feel, and is also a most dramatic demonstration for students.

The author finds the groin cough impulse test of little value and the tourniquet test only useful in the obese or in cases of doubt. The tapping test, with or without help from Doppler ultrasound, remains the mainstay of examination for saphenous incompetence. Like all tests performed in clinical examination, it requires practice, but this is easily attained in a busy varicose vein or ulcer clinic and an experienced examiner can usually detect the termination of the long or short saphenous vein with sufficient accuracy to enable the incision for its ligation to be performed precisely.

Beware 'concealed' or 'straight-through' long saphenous incompetence;[6] ankle edema or ulceration may be related to an incompetent long saphenous vein when is not visible or palpable (usually in the obese) and without any visible varicosities. Doppler ultrasound or duplex scanning must then be used for its diagnosis.

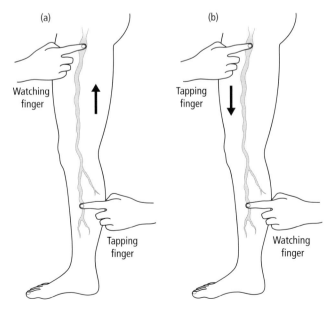

Figure 9.2 *The percussion test for saphenous incompetence: (a) tapping test; (b) reflux tapping test.*

Watching finger

Tapping finger

Tapping finger

Watching finger

(a)

(b)

NON–INVASIVE INVESTIGATIONS IN THE CLINIC

Investigation of the peripheral arteries and veins can be performed by both invasive and non-invasive methods. Invasive

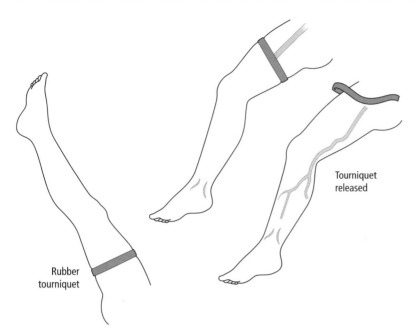

Figure 9.3 *The tourniquet test for saphenous incompetence. Finger pressure can be used as an alternative to the tourniquet.*

investigations include angiography and arterial and venous pressure measurements. Non-invasive methods include photoplethysmography (PPG), Doppler ultrasound, plethysmography (impedance, air or strain gauge) and duplex scanning, in which Doppler ultrasound, flow detection and real-time grey scale ultrasound imaging are combined. Advances in instrument and computer design have resulted in the development of relatively small and portable instruments.

Doppler ultrasound and PPG are two simple, inexpensive and quick investigations which should be available in all vein clinics and used during the clinical examination. The vascular laboratory investigations, Duplex ultrasound and plethysmography are described in Chapters 10A and 11.

Doppler ultrasound examination

Unlike PPG, whose chief value is in distinguishing the edema of calf muscle pump failure from that of non-venous causes, Doppler ultrasound is the single most important instrument in the non-invasive evaluation of the ulcerated limb in the clinic. A simple hand-held instrument is quite adequate, but the more complex instruments with zero crossing circuitry or waveform spectral analysis, and with output to an oscilloscope or LED display, have a number of advantages, particularly in teaching. Two pencil probes are usually used, with operating frequencies of 5 and 8 MHz. The former is suitable for venous investigations, the latter for arterial.

ARTERIAL ASSESSMENT

Doppler ultrasound is invaluable in detecting pedal pulses, particularly in patients with venous edema. Ankle pulses can easily be heard even when they cannot be felt and waveforms can be visualized on the oscilloscope (Fig. 9.4). Ankle pulse

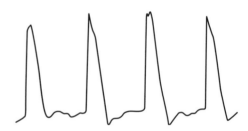

Figure 9.4 *Doppler ultrasound: normal arterial pulsation.*

pressures can be measured by means of a sphygmomanometer cuff applied just above the probe. With the patient horizontal and the sphygmomanometer cuff in position, the flow probe is placed over the posterior tibial or dorsalis pedis artery and the cuff is inflated until the outflow signal ceases. During deflation of the cuff, a return of flow signal indicates the level of the systolic pressure at the ankle. Ankle pressures are compared with brachial systolic pressure measured at the same time and the ankle:brachial pressure index should normally be greater than 1. An ankle systolic pressure of about 80–100 mmHg does not indicate severe reduction in skin blood flow, although such patients usually suffer from intermittent claudication. An ankle pressure of 70 mmHg or less is more usually found in patients whose ulcers are of ischemic origin. A systolic pressure of less than 30 mmHg indicates very severe ischemia which is unlikely to respond to sympathectomy.

A large or tender ulcer may make ankle pulse pressure measurement very difficult, but this problem can be overcome in various ways. The cuff can be placed on the leg above the ulcer, although this is likely to result in an abnormally high pressure being recorded. Alternatively, the ulcer can be covered with a dry dressing held in place with a light cotton bandage and the cuff placed over this. If both these maneuvers are considered impossible, reliance must be placed on the Doppler signal. An experienced operator can get a good idea of pulse pressure simply by listening to the signal and distinguishing the sharp sound of a good systolic pulse wave from the slurred note of a damped wave. With the instrument connected to an oscilloscope or LED display on which the pulse wave can be observed, it is quite easy to tell whether this is suggestive of arterial insufficiency or not by the sharpness of the systolic peaks and the presence or absence of reversed flow. Doppler ultrasound can also be used for evaluating the popliteal pulse; the pulse pressure is measured by inflating a broad thigh cuff.

Evaluation of femoral artery blood flow is more difficult as no cuff can be applied above this point. An audible bruit over the femoral artery indicates stenosis, even if the arteriogram appears normal. As most atherosclerotic plaques in the iliac arteries lie on the posterior wall, an arteriogram film in the anteroposterior plane may well appear normal even in the presence of significant narrowing of the lumen. A crudely quantitative method of evaluating femoral artery blood flow has been described by Gosling et al.[7] This method requires the use of a Doppler ultrasound apparatus which includes the measurement of mean velocity (this can be obtained electronically using the 0.1 Hz upper-frequency cut-off filter of the Hewlett-Packard Biolectric Amplifier, and is included in the Medasonics D10 instrument). Gosling et al. described a parameter called pulsatility index (PI), which is obtained by measuring the peak velocity of forward flow and that of reverse flow and dividing the difference in peak frequencies by the mean frequency. The same measurement is made on the aorta (or, in fat patients, on the brachial artery, on the assumption that there is no stenosis between the suprarenal aorta and the brachial artery), and the ratio of the proximal (brachial) PI to the distal (common femoral) PI is calculated. This is the damping factor (DF). A figure less than 1 indicates some degree of aortic or iliac stenosis. This is a relatively crude investigation, particularly as Skidmore et al.[8] have shown that an abnormal value does not distinguish between inflow stenosis and stenosis of the superficial femoral artery.

VENOUS ASSESSMENT

Venous occlusion

Doppler ultrasound can be used to detect venous occlusion by positioning the probe over the common femoral vein in the groin and squeezing the calf to produce a pulse wave. The patient should be positioned propped up at an angle of 45° with the ankle resting on a pillow so that the calf hangs free (Fig. 9.5). This ensures maximal filling of the capacitance vessels in the calf and therefore a good pulse wave on compression (Fig. 9.6). Patency of the iliac veins is assessed by asking the patient to take deep breaths or to perform a Valsalva manoeuvre; patent veins will transmit the respiratory swings to the common femoral vein where they are detected by the Doppler ultrasound probe. Venous occlusion is not common in the post-thrombotic ulcerated leg and this use of Doppler ultrasound is mainly of value in the early detection of acute DVT.

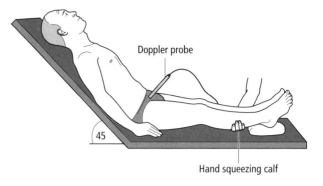

Figure 9.5 *Doppler ultrasound examination for deep venous obstruction: note that the patient's trunk should be elevated to ensure good filling of the calf sinusoids.*

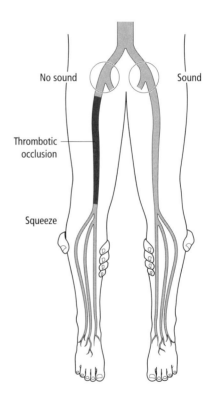

Figure 9.6 *Doppler ultrasound assessment of deep vein patency.*

Venous incompetence

With the patient erect, the Doppler probe can be used to assess competence of each of the important systems: saphenous veins, the direct calf and ankle perforating veins. and the popliteal and femoral veins.

Saphenous veins Examination for great saphenous incompetence by the modified Trendelenburg test using Doppler ultrasound has already been described. Great saphenous incompetence can also be detected by placing the Doppler ultrasound probe over the saphenous vein just below the saphenofemoral junction and listening for reflux after thigh squeezing. Examination for small saphenous reflux is carried out at the same time as examination for popliteal reflux and will be described under that heading.

Direct calf and ankle perforating veins The fascial defects where these veins penetrate the deep fascia may be palpable in a thin leg and sometimes a small varix is visible at this point. Often there is no local varicosity and it is then that Doppler ultrasound is most useful. It is important that the patient is examined in the erect position to ensure maximal filling of the calf venous reservoir. A rough approximation of the site of an incompetent perforating vein can be obtained by observing the anterior and posterior borders of the ankle venous flare (corona phlebectatica) and extending these proximally to the point where the lines cross ('the coastal navigation sign') (Fig. 9.7). The Doppler probe is then placed over this point and the observer's other hand repeatedly squeezes and releases the calf muscles at probe level (or the ankle or foot, distal to the probe) while the probe is moved slowly over the skin surface (Fig. 9.8). A tourniquet is applied above the probe to exclude the effect of saphenous incompetence. Perforating vein incompetence is detected by a characteristic 'in and out' signal which is both audible and can be recorded (Fig. 9.9). It should be emphasized that it is often impossible to carry out this examination satisfactorily in the presence of an infected or painful ulcer. Several weeks of ulcer cleaning and dressing may be necessary before examination is possible.

Femoral, popliteal and small saphenous veins Valvular competence of the superficial femoral, popliteal and short saphenous veins is assessed in similar manner by using the Doppler probe in the popliteal fossa. Maximal arterial pulsation is first found and the probe is then moved a little laterally. The calf is squeezed firmly (Fig. 9.10) and proximal flow can be heard and observed on the oscilloscope or chart recorder. In the presence of normal valves in the popliteal and short saphenous veins, no retrograde flow is heard or observed on release of calf pressure (Fig. 9.11). Valvular incompetence

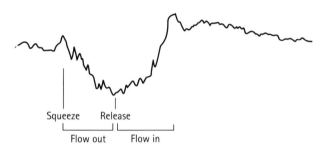

Figure 9.9   *Doppler ultrasound trace showing inflow and outflow through an incompetent perforating vein.*

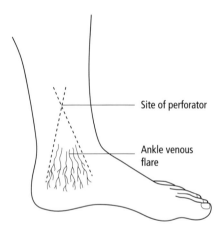

Figure 9.7   *The 'coastal navigation' test for locating an incompetent perforating vein. Extend the anterior and posterior borders of the ankle flare proximally and the perforating vein will be found close to where they cross.*

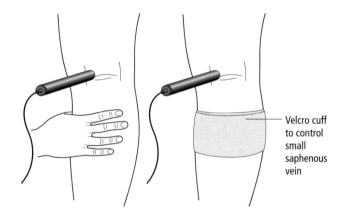

Figure 9.10   *Doppler ultrasound investigation of popliteal and small saphenous incompetence; the cuff is used to occlude an incompetent small saphenous vein.*

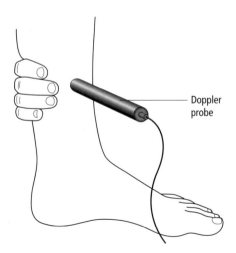

Figure 9.8   *Doppler ultrasound detection of perforating vein incompetence.*

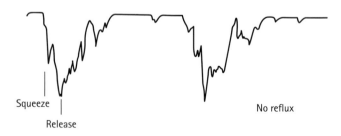

Figure 9.11   *Doppler ultrasound trace demonstrating normal popliteal and small saphenous veins; forward flow only, no reflux.*

7. Gosling RG, Dunbar G, King DH *et al.* The quantitative analysis of occlusive peripheral arterial disease by a non-obstructive ultrasonic technique. *Angiology* 1971; **22**: 52–5.

8. Skidmore R, Woodcock JP, Wells PNT *et al.* Physiological interpretation of Doppler-shift waveforms. III. Clinical results. *Ultrasound Med Biol* 1980; **6**: 227–31.

9. Posnett H, Derodra J. Diagnostic devices in the undergraduate curriculum. *J R Soc Med* 2004; **97**: 310.

10. Flynn WR, Queral LA, Abramowitcz HB *et al.* Photoplethysmography in the assessment of chronic venous insufficiency. In: Nicolaides AN, Yao JST, eds. *Investigation of Vascular Disorders.* New York: Churchill Livingstone, 1981.

11. Zukowski AJ, Nicolaides AN, Szendro G *et al.* Haemodynamic significance of incompetent calf perforating veins. *Br J Surg* 1991; **78**: 625–9.

12. Negus D. The distal long saphenous vein in venous ulceration – a preliminary report. In: Raymond-Martimbeau P, Prescott R, Zummo M, eds. *Phlébologie '92.* Paris: John Libbey Eurotext, 1992; 1291–3.

Anatomical diagnosis: duplex ultrasound

PHILIP D. COLERIDGE SMITH

INTRODUCTION

Duplex ultrasonography has become widely used in the management of varicose veins and leg ulcers. Several papers have been published in which the efficacy of duplex ultrasonography has been reported without comparison to other modalities of investigation.[1–4] Is this investigation essential in all patients with venous disease in the lower limb and are any other tests useful? Plethysmographic tests were commonly used to assess the impairment to venous function but these have been widely abandoned in favor of duplex ultrasonography. These are discussed in more detail in Chapter 11. Vascular surgeons often examine patients with continuous-wave (CW) Doppler ultrasound, since this is a simple investigation which may be accomplished in the clinic. Is this sufficient for some patients or should we always arrange for duplex ultrasonography in addition? Clinical examination is very poor in assessing the source of varices, even when performed by an experienced vascular surgeon.[5]

ASSESSMENT OF PRIMARY VARICOSE VEINS

Considerable reliance is placed on the preoperative assessment of patients in order to obtain a successful outcome following treatment. Most vascular surgeons would be reluctant to use clinical examination alone in the assessment of patients with primary varicose veins before commencing surgery.[6]

Duplex ultrasonography has been compared with clinical assessment and CW (hand-held) Doppler ultrasound.[7–9]

DePalma et al.[7] investigated 40 patients with varicosities in the distribution of the great saphenous vein. They compared clinical examination and CW Doppler with color duplex ultrasonography, which they used as the reference standard. Clinical examination and CW Doppler examination were equally sensitive (48 percent) in detecting great saphenous vein incompetence, missing a startling 26 of 50 incompetent great saphenous veins. In 22 patients who had previously undergone saphenofemoral ligation, the groin recurrence present in nine subjects on duplex was missed by CW Doppler. The CW Doppler examinations in this study were carried out by an experienced vascular surgeon.

In a study carried out by McMullin et al.[8] CW Doppler was compared with duplex ultrasonography in 136 patients presenting with varicose veins. The CW Doppler detected 73 percent of the great saphenous veins found to be incompetent on duplex ultrasonography. Sensitivity in the popliteal fossa for saphenopopliteal incompetence was worse at only 33 percent, and 48 percent for deep vein incompetence. More recently, Mercer et al.[10] re-examined the same question. They found 73 percent sensitivity at the saphenofemoral junction (SFJ), 77 percent at the saphenopopliteal junction (SPJ), and 51 percent for calf perforating veins using CW Doppler in comparison with duplex ultrasound.[10] This led these authors to conclude that duplex ultrasonography is essential before all surgical procedures for the treatment of varicose veins if errors in diagnosis and treatment are to be avoided.

Darke et al.[11] examined patients with primary, uncomplicated varicose veins by both CW Doppler and duplex ultrasonography. For the great saphenous vein, they reported a sensitivity of 95 percent and a specificity of 100 percent in

87 patients shown to have great saphenous vein reflux on duplex ultrasonography. Accuracy at the SPJ was worse: there were five false positives, resulting in a sensitivity of 90 percent and a specificity of 93 percent. They concluded that inappropriate exploration of the SPJ would have been performed in these five cases on the basis of CW Doppler examination alone.

A study in which patients were first examined by a surgeon using clinical examination and CW Doppler to asses the operation has been conducted in 48 patients, 10 of whom were being operated upon for the second time.[9] An operation plan was devised for each patient based on this information. Patients were then examined by colour duplex ultrasonography and the operation plan revised in 18 of 68 limbs. 'Escape points' between the superficial and deep venous systems would have been left intact in 14 limbs had duplex ultrasonography not been performed.

Perforating veins may be assessed by CW Doppler, but doubt has been cast on the reliability of this investigation.[12] Duplex ultrasonography has the ability to asses the size of perforating veins as well as the direction of flow. This has been shown to be a more effective method than phlebography when compared with surgery in one study.[13] A comparison between CW Doppler and duplex ultrasonography shows greater precision for duplex scanning in the detection of calf perforating veins.[14]

Phlebography is no longer widely used for the investigation of primary varicose veins. One series of 68 patients presenting with varicose veins was assessed by colour duplex ultrasonography, phlebography and varicography.[15] Close concordance between the ultrasound and radiological tests was reported for SFJs and SPJs. However, the authors found that ultrasound was insensitive in detecting incompetent perforating veins, demonstrating only 40–63 percent of those shown by phlebography. In a series of patients with deep vein incompetence, duplex ultrasonography was found to be as sensitive as phlebography in the femoral region and detected more cases of popliteal vein incompetence.[16] The difference here is that descending phlebography relies on demonstrating reverse flow in veins into which a hypertonic contrast medium has been injected. This investigation has to be performed at rest. Competent proximal valves may prevent the demonstration of incompetence in the (important) popliteal segment, since contrast medium never descends to this section of the venous system. Duplex ultrasonography relies on the flow of blood in veins, is not restricted by the need for injection of contrast material and is usually carried out with the patient standing, the position in which venous reflux is clinically significant.

The ability of duplex ultrasonography to reveal a wide range of patterns of venous valvular incompetence has led some authors to suggest that varicose vein surgery should be precisely tailored to each patient's needs.[17] Whether this actually improves the results of surgery has not been tested systematically.

In general, CW Doppler examination of the SFJ is reliable enough to be used for clinical purposes in patients with primary varicose veins. However, in the detection of saphenopopliteal or perforating vein incompetence the reliability of this investigation falls. Inappropriate exploration of the popliteal fossa may be undertaken if reliance is placed on this test. Since damage to sural or lateral popliteal nerves may ensue from this, duplex ultrasonography should be used to confirm the exact location of venous reflux or varices arising from the popliteal fossa or from perforating veins.

ASSESSMENT OF PATIENTS WITH RECURRENT VARICOSE VEINS

In patients with recurrent varicose veins, the use of an imaging technique to determine the source of recurrent varices is widely advocated[5] (Plate 10A.1). The most common source of recurrence following surgery of the great saphenous system is the SFJ (Figs 10A.1 and 10A.2).[18–20] However, this only accounts for 40 percent of new varices, and reliable investigation is necessary to determine whether veins fill from other sources. Clinical examination is as unreliable here as it is in other situations. Bradbury et al.[5] studied an unselected series

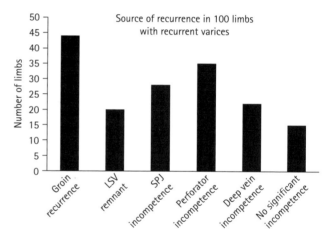

Figure 10A.1 *Sources of recurrent varices in a study by Quigley et al.[19] LSV, long saphenous vein; SPJ, saphenopopliteal junction.*

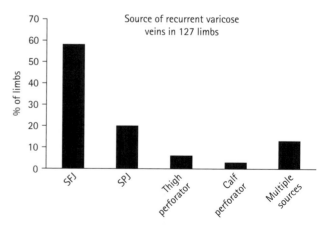

Figure 10A.2 *Sources of recurrent varices in a study by Redwood and Lambert.[20] SFJ, saphenofemoral junction; SPJ, saphenopopliteal junction.*

of 36 patients who has previously undergone ligation of the SFJ. At operation, three-quarters were found to have a patent SFJ. Of 26 cases with an operative diagnosis of a patent SFJ, 17 were identified clinically, and 23 using CW Doppler. However, both these techniques identified further cases where a patent SFJ was not found at operation, resulting in poor specificity for these tests.

A frequently reported problem is persisting reflux in a residual great saphenous vein following earlier saphenofemoral ligation.[19] The anatomy of this and its filling points cannot be reliably determined without an examination that provides imaging information. In fact, incompetence of the great saphenous vein (LSV) trunk may occur in the presence of a competent SFJ, even before surgical intervention, in one-third of patients with primary LSV varices.[21]

Recurrent varices in the popliteal fossa present an especially difficult problem. Using CW Doppler, venous reflux may be audible but may arise from tiny varices. Injudicious exploration of the popliteal fossa may result in damage to important nerves. An exact anatomical map is required before commencing such a procedure. Duplex ultrasonography has been shown to be very reliable when used in this context, giving 100 percent concordance with phlebography in a small series of patients with recurrent SPJ varices.[22] The complexity of recurrence following operations for varices in the popliteal fossa is emphasized by Tong et al.[23] These authors report a series of 70 limbs and define four different patterns of recurrent reflux in this region.

Perforating veins may be an occasional source of recurrent varices. Pierik et al.[24] found that duplex ultrasonography was only about 80 percent sensitive in detecting incompetent calf perforating veins compared with those found at operation in a series of 20 patients undergoing surgical treatment.

In the case of recurrent varicose veins, so diverse are the findings and new sources of venous reflux that use of an imaging technique is easily justified. As with any investigation, interpretation of the findings from duplex ultrasonography requires experience, but basing management on objective data is widely accepted.

PREOPERATIVE VEIN LOCALIZATION

The most common situation in which vein localization is helpful is the popliteal fossa (Plate 10A.2). There is a wide range of anatomical patterns in this region, with the location of the junction of the small saphenous vein to the popliteal vein being very variable. Location of this point using an imaging technique has been widely advocated, but never assessed to determine whether it actually improves the outcome of venous surgery. Such localizations greatly assist the surgical procedure and hopefully reduce the likelihood of neurological injury following popliteal fossa exploration. The marking of perforating veins[25] and residual segments of the great saphenous vein is also reported and greatly facilitates their ligation and removal at surgery.

METHOD OF SCANNING FOR VALVULAR INCOMPETENCE

Patients stand on a low platform elevating them approximately 10–15 cm above the ground and it is useful for them to be provided with a hand-hold in order to steady themselves during examination. Augmentation of venous flow by manually compressing the calf is facilitated if patients take their weight on the opposite limb to that under investigation. The examiner sits, preferably on a chair with adjustable height to assist examination of the entire length of the leg.

Identification of anatomy

Examination starts by imaging the femoral vein in longitudinal section in the groin. From this the SFJ can be easily identified. Examination progresses down the limb to establish the anatomy of the superficial femoral vein and great saphenous vein in the thigh. The trunk of the saphenous vein can be identified readily because it lies in a fascial compartment of its own, resulting in an appearance known as the 'saphenous eye' (Fig. 10A.3). The femoral vein lies deep in the thigh beneath sartorius and adductor muscles. The presence of thigh perforating veins may also be detected. In addition, some patients present with incompetence of the internal pudendal vein and associated thigh varices. These, too, should be sought in the groin. When examination of the great saphenous system and superficial femoral vein in the thigh is completed on both sides, patients should turn away from the examiner to permit examination of the popliteal fossa. The popliteal vein is traced from its upper limit in the popliteal fossa, and the SPJ examined. The small saphenous vein usually enters the popliteal vein from its lateral aspect and may be traced distally to become the most superficial vein in the calf, lying just beneath the facial covering as the transducer passes over the muscles of the calf. This vein also lies within a saphenous eye. In addition, the

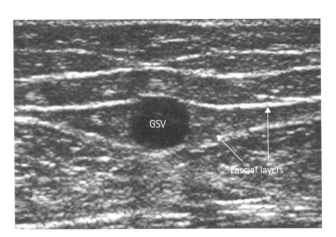

Figure 10A.3 *The major saphenous trunks are encapsulated in a fascial sheath. In transverse section this has the appearance of an 'Egyptian eye' or saphenous eye, seen here in the great saphenous vein.*

popliteal vein also receives tributaries from the gastrocnemius and soleus muscles. These are best traced from the popliteal fossa into the bellies of the medial and lateral gastrocnemius and soleus muscles. Some of these vessels are of large diameter, while others are only a few millimeters (Fig. 10A.4).

Having examined the popliteal fossae comprehensively, patients are then permitted to sit and, through the medial aspect of the calf, the posterior tibial veins can be examined. These are most readily identified just proximal to the ankle where they usually lie within 10–15 mm of the skin surface. Lying more laterally the peroneal veins can often be seen beyond these vessels in their location behind the fibula. Both peroneal veins and posterior tibial veins are usually arranged as a pair of venae comitantes lying beside the accompanying arteries. If the peroneal veins cannot be evaluated from the medial view, they can be imaged easily from a posterolateral approach, their position being identified from the shadow of the fibula. These vessels can be assessed throughout the length of the calf in most patients, and they should be traced up towards the knee. The presence of medial and lateral ankle and calf perforating veins can be determined most readily with a transducer scanning the leg in the transverse section. The anterior tibial vein can also be insonated with patients sitting, although this is rarely the source of significant venous valvular incompetence.

Assessment of venous flow can often be observed using the moving luminal patterns which are seen as the red cells aggregate once patients have been standing for approximately

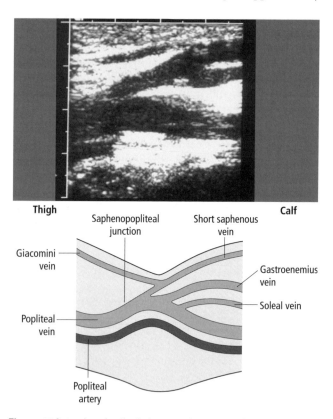

Figure 10A.4 *Longitudinal ultrasound anatomy of the popliteal fossa showing the main groups of deep veins as well as the superficial vein.*

5 min. These are not necessarily the most reliable indicators, but in difficult cases they can give confirmation of the nature of the flow. Venous valves are sometimes visible in the B-mode images when viewed from the correct angle. They are normally much thinner than the current high-resolution imaging systems can resolve (ultrasound resolution, 0.2 mm; valve cusp thickness of 20 μm). The actual functional efficacy of a valve cannot generally be judged from the B-mode appearances.

Duplex ultrasound imaging using the pulsed or colour Doppler modes is the most satisfactory method of determining the direction of flow in veins. Colour flow-mapped duplex ultrasound imaging is more satisfactory than pulsed Doppler alone, permitting several veins to be examined simultaneously, thereby speeding examination. In addition, the presence of small areas of reflux, such as in the region of valves, or regions of scarring with no flow in the lumen as a consequence of previous deep vein thrombosis can be detected.

Colour flow-mapped ultrasound machines differ substantially from manufacturer to manufacturer. I have found it essential in all vascular examinations, both venous and arterial, to use a machine which permits rapid update of the colour image (10–15 times/s) when correctly operated, allowing the dynamic nature of the flow to be assessed.

All deep veins and most superficial veins exhibit forward flow following a calf compression. In this way, each vessel in the anatomical region of the transducer may be examined in turn, and the direction of flow determined before and immediately after relaxation of a manual calf compression. I recommend that calf compression is maintained for 2–3 s before release in order to ensure that it is possible to separate the forward flow and reflux phases. In some veins, during early valve failure, detectable reflux may be confined to the immediate vicinity of the incompetent valve cusp. A careful search may need to be made in order to locate this region when using the pulsed Doppler system. Venous reflux is sometimes seen in patients with normal veins. After examination of substantial numbers of patients with normal veins, I have found that, in the deep and superficial veins, the venous reflux component usually does not exceed 0.5 s in duration following release of calf compression. This observation is in keeping with published evidence from other sources, and the reflux phase must be attributable to the flow required to produce venous valvular closure. Measurement of volumetric flow has been attempted in order to provide a quantitative evaluation of the reverse flow, but this has not become a widely accepted practice. In part, this is due to the need to sum the reverse flow in all veins in order to achieve a final answer. Plethysmographic methods of assessing venous reflux or foot vein pressure measurements may be more appropriate for this purpose.

In the superficial veins, it is sometimes difficult to produce forward flow by manual calf compression, particularly in the great saphenous vein. This is especially true when the veins are normal, and this reflects the fact that the superficial veins do not normally constitute a main axial drainage route. However, in patients with venous reflux there is usually considerable forward as well as reverse flow following calf compression.

PATTERNS OF FLOW IN VENOUS DISEASE – VARICOSE VEINS

Saphenofemoral junction

By far the most common abnormality seen in venous disease is incompetence of the SFJ associated with great saphenous vein reflux. This is usually easy to demonstrate, using the techniques described above. In a substantial proportion of patients, reflux of the SFJ may be absent in the presence of incompetence of the great saphenous vein in the thigh or calf. The incompetent segment may fill from a mid-thigh perforator. More commonly, reflux may arise from forward flow in tributaries of the great saphenous vein. When these reach the main trunk of the saphenous vein below an incompetent valve, antegrade flow in the tributary turns downward towards the feet in the great saphenous vein. This pattern has been observed by other authors and is often the source of varicosities in the calf.

Saphenopopliteal junction

The next most common source is from the SPJ (approximately 20 percent of my patients). Again, this is easily demonstrated by insonating the popliteal junction and SPJ in the popliteal fossa whilst applying and releasing calf compression. It is well known that the site of the SPJ is variable and may lie anywhere from the level of the popliteal skin crease to the mid-thigh region. Sometimes there is no SPJ and the small saphenous vein continues up to the buttock (often referred to as the Giacomini vein in the thigh) to join the ascending inferior gluteal vein, or alternatively passes medially to join a medial branch of the great saphenous vein. Ultrasound imaging is extremely useful in identifying the level of the SPJ. I regularly use it to place marks on the leg preoperatively to facilitate surgical ligation of the SPJ.

Gastrocnemius veins

Gastrocnemius veins (lying within the gastrocnemius muscle) may also be assessed for reflux. These may be the source of varices or liposclerotic skin change. Strictly these are deep veins but have been regarded as superficial veins by a number of authors, and incompetence treated by surgical ligation. Incompetent gastrocnemius veins may be traced into the calf where they join superficial varices by perforating the deep fascia of the leg overlying the gastrocnemius muscles, particularly in the medial calf region.

Calf perforating veins

Enlarged perforating veins of the calf are frequently seen in patients with superficial venous incompetence. Their clinical and functional significance is a matter of debate, and it remains unclear whether or not ligation of these vessels is appropriate. Flow in perforating veins may be either inwards or outwards, even in patients with normal limbs, and it seems that the hallmark of a truly pathological perforator is that both inward and outward flow is observed in the same vessel. Perforating veins are best assessed for inward flow by compressing the limb distally to the perforating vein under investigation either at the ankle or the foot. Outward flow may be elicited by compressing the calf proximal to the level of the perforating vein. Additionally, the size of the veins should be noted since this probably influences surgical management.

RECURRENT VARICOSE VEINS

Recurrence at the SFJ is one of the most common findings in patients with recurrent varicose veins. The site of previous surgical ligation can usually be identified from a bulge on the anterior aspect of the femoral vein. In some patients, a small vessel, 1 or 2 mm in diameter, may be seen coursing between the femoral vein and overlying varices in the groin. My experience of operating on such vessels has been rather unsatisfactory and I now simply manage the associated varices of the lower limb.

Frequently, large communications between superficial varicosities or a persisting great saphenous vein may be identified. Occasionally, the SFJ appears entirely pristine with no previous ligation where presumably the surgeon mistook the anatomy and failed to ligate the SFJ, instead taking a large branch. Patients who have previously had a saphenofemoral ligation, but without great saphenous vein stripping, may have substantial persisting reflux in the remnant of the great saphenous vein, which can be found filling varices in the calf. Less frequently, a mid-thigh perforating vein may be found communicating with a remnant of the great saphenous vein.

In the popliteal fossa, the SPJ may be missed at operation but can easily be identified on ultrasound imaging as the source of recurrent reflux. Following successful ligation of the SPJ, a gastrocnemius vein becomes incompetent and the remnant of the small saphenous vein may communicate with the gastrocnemius, resulting in recurrent varicosities.

Occasionally, calf perforating veins may be associated with recurrent varices and, if there is no other venous abnormality, then it must be assumed that calf perforator ligation is appropriate.

DEEP VENOUS DISEASE

The most common abnormality in the deep venous system is venous reflux alone. This may or may not be accompanied by evidence of previous deep vein thrombosis. Usually the duration of reflux in the deep veins is substantially shorter than that in the superficial veins, although, owing to the diameter of the deep veins, it is quantitatively much more important. It may be difficult to determine whether or not there has been a previous deep vein thrombosis, since deep vein thrombosis proven on venography often cannot subsequently be detected using ultrasound imaging after complete resolution of the thrombus. The signs to look for following a previous deep vein thrombosis are described in detail in the previous section.

Altered patterns of flow may also lead to the suggestion that there has been a previous thrombotic episode in the iliac system. If compression of the calf results in outward flow at the SFJ during the compression phase, then proximal venous obstruction should be suspected. If outward flow in the SFJ during compression is associated with large ascending collateral vessels, particularly those which cross to the contralateral side, it is highly likely that a previous thrombotic episode has resulted in obstruction of the iliac vein. This can be checked by compressing one leg while insonating the SFJ of the other leg. Normally this will result in no alteration of flow at the contralateral SFJ. In the case of proximal iliac obstruction, inward flow can easily be seen on the contralateral side during calf compression. Other sources of collateral flow that should be sought include the great saphenous vein, which often bypasses a scarred or occluded superficial femoral vein, and the small saphenous vein which may carry collateral flow in the event of calf vein obstruction.

CONCLUSIONS

Clinical examination is unreliable in the assessment of venous incompetence of the lower limb and a more reliable form of assessment should be used before embarking on surgical treatment. Continuous-Wave Doppler is effective in assessing the SFJ and LSV where many primary varicose veins arise. However, the popliteal fossa is not reliably assessed by this technique, and when varices are present in this region or venous reflux is detected here on CW Doppler, duplex ultrasonography should be undertaken. In patients who present with recurrent varicose veins, duplex ultrasonography is the investigation of choice in the anatomical assessment of the problem. Where skin changes or ulceration are present, duplex ultrasonography provides essential information required for patient management.

REFERENCES

1. Thibault PK, Lewis WA. Recurrent varicose veins. Part 1: Evaluation utilizing duplex venous imaging. *J Dermatol Surg Oncol* 1992; **18**: 24.
2. Katsamouris AN, Kardoulas DG, Gourtsoyiannis N. The nature of lower extremity venous insufficiency in patients with primary varicose veins. *Eur J Vasc Surg* 1994; **8**: 464–71.
3. Gaitini D, Torem S, Pery M, Kaftori JK. Image directed Doppler ultrasound in the diagnosis of lower limb venous insufficiency. *J Clin Ultrasound* 1994; **22**: 291–7.
4. Quigley FG, Raptis S, Cashman M, Faris IB. Duplex ultrasound mapping of sites of deep to superficial incompetence in primary varicose veins. *Aust NZ J Surg* 1992; **62**: 276–8.
5. Bradbury AW, Stonebridge PA, Callam MJ *et al.* Recurrent varicose veins: assessment of the saphenofemoral junction. *Br J Surg* 1994; **81**: 373–5.
6. Lees TA, Beard JD, Ridler BM, Szymanska T. A survey of the current management of varicose veins by members of the Vascular Surgical Society. *Ann R Coll Surg Engl* 1999; **81**: 407–17.
7. DePalma RG, Hart MT, Zanin L, Massarin EH. Physical examination, Doppler ultrasound and colour flow duplex scanning: guides to therapy for primary varicose veins. *Phlebology* 1993; **8**: 7–11.
8. McMullin GM, Coleridge Smith PD. An evaluation of Doppler ultrasound and photoplethysmography in the investigation of venous insufficiency. *Aust NZ J Surg* 1992; **62**: 270–5.
9. van der Heijden FH, Bruyninckx CM. Preoperative colour coded duplex scanning in varicose veins of the lower extremity. *Eur J Surg* 1993; **159**: 329–33.
10. Mercer KG, Scott DJ, Berridge DC. Preoperative duplex imaging is required before all operations for primary varicose veins. *Br J Surg* 1998; **85**: 1495–7.
11. Darke SG, Vetrivel S, Foy DM *et al.* A comparison of duplex scanning and continuous wave Doppler in the assessment of primary and uncomplicated varicose veins. *Eur J Vasc Endovasc Surg* 1997; **14**: 457–61.
12. O'Donnell TF Jr, Burnand KG, Clemenson G *et al.* Doppler examination vs clinical and phlebographic detection of the location of incompetent perforating veins: a prospective study. *Arch Surg* 1977; **112**: 31–5.
13. Stiegler H, Rotter G, Standl R *et al.* Wertigkeit der Farb Duplex Sonographie in der Diagnose insuffizienter Vv. perforantes. Eine prospektive Untersuchung an 94 Patienten. *Vasa* 1994; **23**: 109–13.
14. Ogi S, Kanaoka Y, Mori T. Diagnosis of incompetent perforators in primary varicose veins by high resolution ultrasonography. *Nippon Geka Gakkai Zasshi* 1994; **95**: 34–9.
15. Phillips GW, Paige J, Molan MP. A comparison of colour duplex ultrasound with venography and varicography in the assessment of varicose veins. *Clin Radiol* 1995; **50**: 20–5.
16. Baker SR, Burnand KG, Sommerville KM *et al.* Comparison of venous reflux assessed by duplex scanning and descending phlebography in chronic venous disease. *Lancet* 1993; **341**: 400–3.
17. Hanrahan LM, Kechejian GJ, Cordts PR *et al.* Patterns of venous insufficiency in patients with varicose veins. *Arch Surg* 1991; **126**: 687–90.
18. Bradbury AW, Stonebridge PA, Ruckley CV, Beggs I. Recurrent varicose veins. correlation between preoperative clinical and hand held Doppler ultrasonographic examination, and anatomical findings at surgery. *Br J Surg* 1993; **80**: 849–51.
19. Quigley FG, Raptis S, Cashman M. Duplex ultrasonography of recurrent varicose veins. *Cardiovasc Surg* 1994; **2**: 775–7.
20. Redwood NF, Lambert D. Patterns of reflux in recurrent varicose veins assessed by duplex. *Br J Surg* 1994; **81**: 1450–1.
21. Abu-Own A, Scurr JH, Coleridge Smith PD. Saphenous vein reflux without incompetence at the saphenofemoral junction. *Br J Surg* 1994; **81**: 1452–4.
22. De Maeseneer MG, De Hert SG, van Schil PE *et al.* Preoperative colour coded duplex examination of the saphenopopliteal junction in recurrent varicosis of the small saphenous vein. *Cardiovasc Surg* 1993; **1**: 686–9.
23. Tong Y, Royle J. Recurrent varicose veins after small saphenous vein surgery: a duplex ultrasound study. *J Cardiovasc Surg* 1996; **4**: 364–7.
24. Pierik EG, Toonder IM, van Urk H, Wittens CH. Validation of duplex ultrasonography in detecting competent and incompetent perforating veins in patients with venous ulceration of the lower leg. *J Vasc Surg* 1997; **26**: 49–52.
25. Hanrahan LM, Araki CT, Fisher JB *et al.* Evaluation of the perforating veins of the lower extremity using high resolution duplex imaging. *J Cardiovasc Surg Torino* 1991; **32**: 87–97.

10B

Anatomical diagnosis: venography of the lower extremity

HUW WALTERS

INTRODUCTION

The introduction of venography into clinical practice was the result of work undertaken by Dos Santos[1] and published in 1938. Within 2 years, Bauer applied the technique to study patients with thromboembolism[2] and then to evaluate the sequelae of deep vein thrombosis in post-thrombotic syndrome.[3]

The clinical diagnosis of deep vein thrombosis is inaccurate, having both low specificity and low sensitivity.[4] The development of venography thus represented a major advance in the ability to examine extremity veins with contrast and to demonstrate acute thrombosis and any subsequent complications of deep vein thrombosis. In the early years, however, the toxicity of contrast media precluded a wide acceptance of the technique. Improvements in contrast agent 'design', with the introduction of the tri-iodobenzates in the 1950s, produced relatively low toxicity compounds. These contrast media were, however, significantly hyperosmolar with respect to plasma.[5] Local endothelial damage may result with their use and this appeared to be largely attributable to their hyperosmolality;[6] on venous injection they may provoke a thrombophlebitis or thrombosis.[7] The introduction of 'low osmolar' contrast media in the early 1980s represented the most significant advance in contrast medium safety and these agents also have a significantly reduced thrombogenic potential.[8]

With these advances in contrast medium chemistry, the safety of venography was substantially improved with greater patient acceptance. The concurrent development through the mid-1980s of non-invasive techniques significantly changed the algorithm of investigation of venous disorders – these have been comprehensively reviewed in earlier chapters. Venography, however, still has an important role, particularly where venous reconstructive surgery is planned and where Duplex ultrasound findings are equivocal.

VENOGRAPHY

Patients presenting with venous ulceration confront the radiologist with an exacting challenge to display the vascular anatomy fully, thus allowing an accurate interpretation of the findings. In its basic form, venography involves the injection of contrast medium into one of the tributaries of the venous system, but requires a variety of special techniques to demonstrate veins in different regions, depending on the clinical presentation. The main variations of technique are in the method of introducing the contrast medium and in the postural and other maneuvers designed to obtain uniform or selective venous filling.

A close clinical liaison with the vascular surgeon is essential so that the appropriate technique can be employed and the investigation tailored to answer the specific question arising from clinical examination, or queries arising from non-invasive vascular laboratory testing. Although there is a degree of overlap, non-invasive methods provide primarily functional information on the state of the veins, while venography provides precise anatomical information. In many clinical situations, non-invasive methods and venography are complementary in providing specific information to enable effective surgical management.

Venographic techniques that may be employed in the investigation of patients presenting with leg ulceration include the basic ascending venogram, a modification of this basic study to demonstrate incompetent communicating veins, varicography, descending venography and iliocaval venography with pressure measurements. The basic equipment required is a radiographic tilting table equipped for fluoroscopy and with a spot-film capability. This system allows the direction of flow of contrast medium to be monitored, and exposures are made only when there is optimal venous filling. Iliocaval venography additionally requires a digital subtraction angiographic facility or, if this is not available, a conventional film angiographic unit.

THE BASIC ASCENDING LEG VENOGRAM

One of the most common indications for the basic ascending venogram in patients with venous ulceration is the demonstration of altered deep venous anatomy in those cases suspected, or shown, to have varying degrees of obstruction on non-invasive testing.

The patient is examined supine with a 20–40° foot-down table tilt. Table hand supports enable patients to maintain position and avoid any weight-bearing on the leg under examination (Fig. 10B.1). The use of tourniquets, together with this semi-upright position, also promotes maximal and uniform filling of veins, thus avoiding flow artifacts.

A self-fastening Velcro tourniquet is applied above the ankle to distend the foot veins. The skin on the dorsum of the foot is

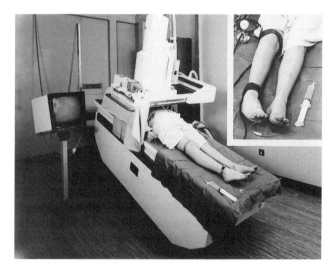

Figure 10B.1 *Fluoroscopy unit with the table in a 30° foot-down tilt. Hand grips provide support for this non-weight-bearing position. The leg under examination (inset) is internally rotated to separate the images of the tibia and fibula.*

cleaned and a 21-gauge butterfly needle is inserted into a distal vein. Although any of these distal veins is acceptable, the medial digital vein of the great toe has the advantage of communicating directly, through the first interosseous space, with the plantar plexus. Injected contrast medium thus passes preferentially into the deep veins. The butterfly needle is secured and the venepuncture checked by injecting saline under direct vision.

A second tourniquet is applied above the knee to delay flow of contrast medium from the calf veins, serving also to promote more uniform filling of the deep distal veins.

The saline syringe is replaced with a syringe containing 60 mL of low osmolar contrast medium. The concentration routinely employed is 250 mg iodine/mL, and is obtained by diluting 50 mL iohexol 300 or iopamidol 300 with 10 mL saline. The volume of contrast medium required varies between patients, reflecting the differing venous capacity of legs. Optimal venous filling is determined by the appearances at fluoroscopy.

With the table at a 20–40° foot-down tilt and the leg under examination internally rotated to separate the images of the tibia and fibula (see Fig. 10B.1, inset), contrast medium is injected by hand under screen control. An injection rate of 0.5–1 mL/s is employed. The venepuncture site is checked to exclude extravasation, and the progress of the contrast medium is followed to ensure that it passes into the tibial veins. The ankle tourniquet pressure may require adjustment at this stage to ensure deep venous filling. The posterior tibial veins are normally the first to fill, followed by the peroneal and anterior tibial veins. The muscular venous arcades of the soleus and gastrocnemius generally fill later than the main stem veins.

Films are exposed in the posteroanterior position when there is uniform filling of the deep veins of the calf. Three exposures are made on a 35 cm × 35 cm radiograph, subdivided into three to include the veins from the ankle to the knee (Fig. 10B.2). Contrast filling of the popliteal venous segment is enhanced by gentle pressure of the deep calf veins just above the ankle. The leg is then externally rotated to obtain lateral views of the deep calf veins, three similar exposures being made to include the veins from the foot to the knee (Fig. 10B.3). These lateral views are important in demonstrating the posterior tibial veins and muscular venous arcades without superimposition of other veins.

The leg is now repositioned to the front and the tourniquets released to allow contrast filling of the superficial and common femoral veins. Two exposures are made of the deep veins in the thigh. The explorator is finally positioned to include the areas of the groin and pelvis. A third exposure is then made following the application of firm pressure to the calf in order to propel contrast medium as a bolus to demonstrate the iliac veins and lower inferior vena cava (Fig. 10B.4).

Following the procedure, and while the radiographs are being processed, the veins are cleared of contrast medium by leg elevation and injecting heparinized saline flush. Once the diagnostic adequacy of the examination is confirmed, the patient is encouraged to walk. Possible thrombotic complications from stasis of the contrast medium are further reduced in this way.

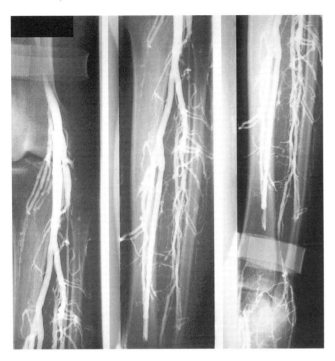

Figure 10B.2 *Uniform filling of the deep calf veins exposed in the posteroanterior position on a divided 35 cm² film. The ankle tourniquet directs contrast into the deep veins; the above-knee tourniquet delays emptying of the calf veins.*

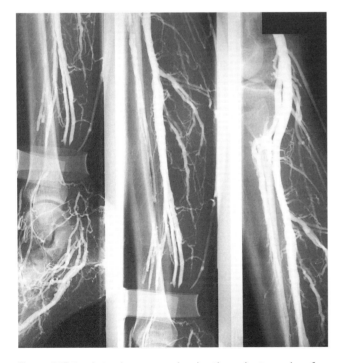

Figure 10B.3 *Lateral exposures showing the main stem veins of the calf with good filling of the calf muscle veins. The plantar veins have been included on the first exposure.*

The appearances of deep vein thrombosis

The post-thrombotic syndrome is a significant cause of venous ulceration, and it is appropriate to briefly describe the venographic appearances of the acute thrombotic event. Practically, in demonstrating the thrombus, the objectives of the standard technique described above are: (i) to show that a filling defect in a vein is persistent and constant in shape on more than one radiograph, thus excluding various artefacts, such as those related to flow; (ii) to fill as many deep veins as possible, including established collaterals around occluded veins; and (iii) to demonstrate the upper extent of the thrombus or occluded vein.

Deep vein thrombosis shows as a filling defect in an opacified vein, and is constant in shape and size on at least two films. The age of the thrombus, as it matures, modifies its appearance. A recent, fresh thrombus typically appears as a translucent defect, separated from the vein wall by a thin white line of contrast medium, producing a 'ground-glass' appearance (Fig. 10B.5). When a thrombus completely occludes a vein, contrast medium may delineate its extent both proximally and distally, and in the adjacent collaterals. These venous collaterals, unlike collateralizing arteries, enlarge almost immediately after obstruction of a venous segment. As the thrombus ages, it retracts and becomes more adherent to one side of the vein wall. The thrombus has a more clearly defined outline and is surrounded by a thicker layer of contrast medium. Finally, recanalization changes take place, the extent of resolution being variable from restoration of a normal venous lumen to the various appearances of the post-thrombotic state described below.

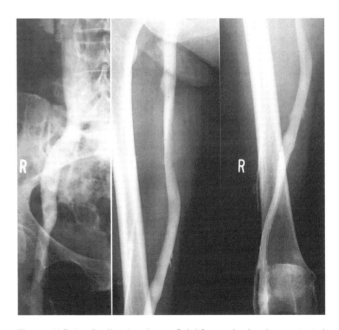

Figure 10B.4 *Popliteal and superficial femoral veins demonstrated after tourniquet release. The final exposure to outline the iliac veins and lower inferior vena cava is made using the bolus technique following calf compression. The profunda femoris vein has not filled in this study.*

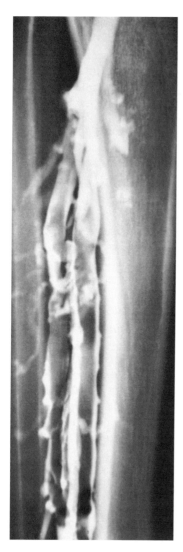

Figure 10B.5 *Recent thrombus in the stem veins of the calf. The thrombus is surrounded by a thin layer of contrast medium.*

Post-thrombotic syndrome

The basic technique will demonstrate the extent of thrombotic occlusion, changes of recanalization, collateral venous pathways and valvular damage or destruction. The resulting impaired function of the calf muscle pump results in the high pressure developed in the deep veins on exercise being transmitted through to the superficial veins via incompetent communicating veins (their localization is described below).

During the procedure, an indication of valvular incompetence secondary to post-thrombotic damage may be made by the performance of a Valsalva maneuver. Venographically, however, descending venography provides a better test of valve function (described below). Using a similar technique, small and great saphenous vein incompetence may be demonstrated when the popliteal and common femoral veins, respectively, are filled – the superficial veins then filling retrogradely. With small saphenous vein incompetence, a tourniquet applied

above its termination will assist its demonstration when the vein fills in a retrograde direction. Radiographs taken in the lateral projection for the termination of the small saphenous vein are important because of the variation of anatomy in this region. Modifications of the basic technique, with exclusion of the ankle tourniquet, may be required to demonstrate the variable termination of the small saphenous vein; alternatively, varicography may be of particular value, especially in patients with recurrent varicose veins. In some patients, this lateral projection will identify other venous tributaries, including incompetent gastrocnemius veins, which join the small saphenous or popliteal vein and may result in calf varices.

MODIFIED BASIC TECHNIQUE TO DEMONSTRATE INCOMPETENT COMMUNICATING VEINS

Incompetent communicating veins play a major role in the etiology of venous ulceration.[9] Precise information on their location is thus essential for effective surgical management.

Modification of the basic technique described above involves the selective delivery of contrast medium into the deep venous system, allowing the identification of the site of these incompetent veins to be seen fluoroscopically as contrast passes through from the deep to the superficial veins. Pneumatic cuffs, as described by Craig,[10] allow more efficient occlusion of the superficial veins at the ankle. The effectiveness of the ankle cuff can be checked on fluoroscopy. An above-knee cuff serves to delay the escape of contrast medium from the tibial veins, and assists in the demonstration of incompetent communicating veins.

The position of the ankle cuff may need to be modified and placed around the forefoot if ulceration is present at ankle level, or if an inframalleolar perforator is suspected. Further calf tourniquets may be required to occlude large incompetent communicating veins, which allow excess filling of varicosities with contrast medium, since this degree of superficial venous filling may obscure more proximal incompetent veins.

The flow of the injected contrast medium is monitored and a radiograph exposed when retrograde flow through the incompetent vein is seen. These early films further aid identification of the precise level of the origin of the incompetent vein from the deep venous system, before excess superficial venous filling occurs. Localization of the level of incompetent perforators can be measured by means of a ruler with 1 cm radio-opaque markers. This allows for magnification and the level is determined by reference to the malleoli (Fig. 10B.6).

The advent of ultrasound as a non-invasive imaging modality has largely replaced contrast venography in the day-to-day laboratory detection of deep vein thrombosis and the investigation of patients presenting with venous insufficiency. However, venography continues to play a role where there are equivocal findings with Duplex ultrasound in the detection of thrombus in calf veins, and proximally in the iliac veins where

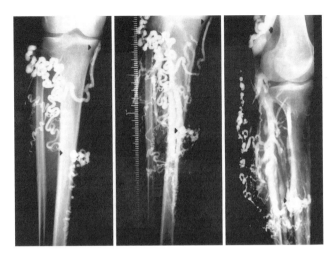

Figure 10B.7 *Left – Varicogram showing complex recurrent varicose network communicating medially with long saphenous varicosities (arrowheads). Centre – Deep venous filling is present, due to perforator (lower arrowhead) at this level. Right – Lateral view showing communication with recurrent short saphenous varicosities (arrow).*

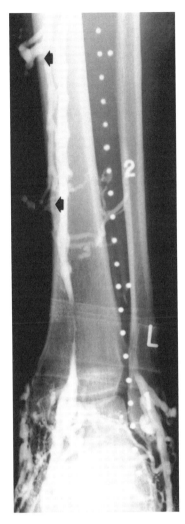

Figure 10B.6 *Ascending venogram with effective ankle tourniquet pressure allowing selective deep venous filling. An early exposure allows identification of incompetent perforating veins (black arrows); their level is determined from the 1 cm radio-opaque markers.*

acoustic access may be difficult. When venous reconstructive surgery is planned, ascending venography is essential in providing precise anatomic detail. The basic ascending venogram and its modifications will demonstrate evidence of thrombus, obstruction and recanalization changes, the presence of any reduplication of deep veins where antireflux procedures are planned, the presence of incompetent perforating veins, the state of the deep venous valves where valve surgery is contemplated and large venous collaterals bypassing an occlusion, which may be misinterpreted for normal anatomy on a Duplex ultrasound.

VARICOGRAPHY

Varicography is the term applied to the technique of direct injection of contrast medium into varicose veins. Although described as a venographic technique nearly 40 years ago,[11]

this method of investigation was not widely practiced. This clinical lack of acceptance was almost certainly due to the high incidence of thrombotic complications which resulted from the injection of high osmolar contrast media into varicosities. The advent of the low osmolar contrast media, with a significantly reduced thrombotic potential,[8] has resulted in a wider application of a valuable technique, particularly in the investigation of recurrent varicose veins.

The patient is first clinically examined in the erect position to display the varicose network of veins optimally. A 21-gauge butterfly needle is introduced into a suitable vein in the symptomatic varicose complex. With the needle secured, the patient lies on the fluoroscopy table in either the prone or supine position, depending on the position of the needle.

The fluoroscopy table is positioned to a 10–20° foot-down tilt, and the flow of contrast medium is monitored to determine the direction of drainage of the varicosities through the perforating veins to the deep venous system. With varicosities in the small saphenous territory, a lower thigh tourniquet, applied above the saphenopopliteal junction, will retard the flow of contrast away from the popliteal vein and enhance the filling of incompetent veins in relation to both the small saphenous and popliteal veins. Lateral projections are essential in this situation to display adequately the variable anatomy which may be found at the saphenopopliteal junction (Figs 10B.7 and 10B.8). The filling of Hunterian and other thigh perforating veins is similarly enhanced with the placement of a tourniquet above the incompetent vein. Lateral views are also helpful with Hunterian perforators to allow accurate localization in two planes. A ruler with opaque distance markers allows for magnification, and the level is determined by reference to the femoral condyles.

In the great saphenous territory, varicose vein recurrences may arise from the groin or more distally through incompetent

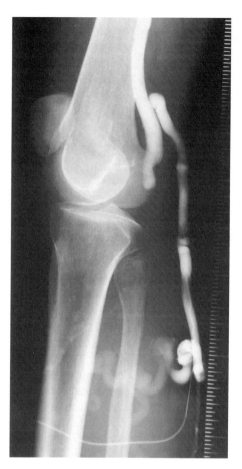

Figure 10B.8 *Varicogram: lateral projection demonstrating termination of short saphenous vein recurrence.*

communicating veins between the deep system and any part of the great saphenous vein not identified at surgery (Fig. 10B.9). It is therefore of considerable importance to determine the site of recurrence to avoid a possible abortive re-exploration in an area distorted by previous surgery. Varicography is initially undertaken with the fluoroscopy table tilted foot-down and, as the contrast injection is continued, the table is moved into a 30–40° head-down position. Table hand supports provide a secure position for the patient. Spot films are made to record the central deep venous communications.

Varicography may, however, fail to demonstrate the full extent of recurrent groin varices, since contrast medium under gravity in the head-down table tilt position will tend to follow the path of least resistance. Descending venography with a Valsalva maneuver will distend the varices and demonstrate their full extent.[12] This technique is described below.

DESCENDING VENOGRAPHY

Descending venography was originally applied in the evaluation of the competence or otherwise of the valves in the deep veins. The procedure involves the placement of a 4 Fr vessel dilator into the common femoral vein under local anesthesia

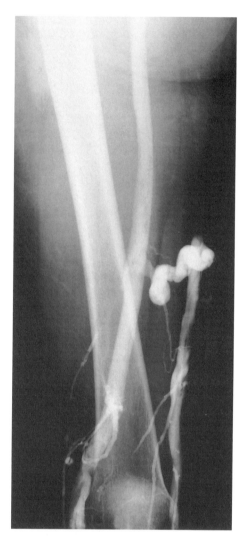

Figure 10B.9 *A large Hunterian incompetent communicating vein not identified at surgery. The long saphenous vein had been ligated just proximal to the incompetent vein.*

and with the tip of the dilator just above the level of the femoral head. The examination is carried out with the patient in the erect or steep semi-erect position. Contrast medium is injected slowly by hand as a 15–20 mL bolus, the initial bolus being to confirm full iliac vein patency. The progress of the contrast is monitored fluoroscopically and spot films are made to record the extent of retrograde flow (Fig. 10B.10). A Valsalva maneuver will assist the retrograde flow of contrast as far as competent valves allow. A 'controlled' Valsalva maneuver may be achieved by having the patient blow into a rubber glove. Valve competency may be graded according to the classification described by Kistner *et al.*[13] Some reflux of contrast medium is normal due to gravity and the density of the medium. Reflux to below-knee level is abnormal, however, and the damaged valves will be apparent. The presence of any deep femoral venous reflux is important to document, as this may affect the result of any planned deep venous reconstruction.

Although Duplex ultrasound with colour flow mapping is the imaging method of choice in diagnosing venous reflux,

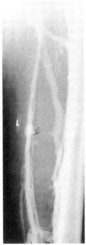

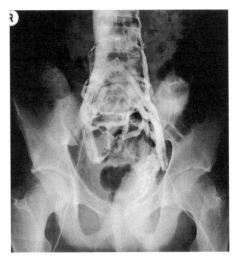

Figure 10B.11 *Left – Post-thrombotic occlusion of the left common iliac vein with established collaterals through the presacral plexus, ascending lumbar vein and developing pudendal collaterals. Right – Ascending venogram also shows post-thrombotic changes in the superficial femoral vein and external iliac vein.*

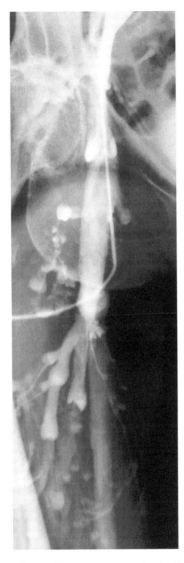

Figure 10B.10 *Descending venogram: contrast reflux down the deep femoral vein – as far as competent valves allow – and down the superficial femoral vein.*

where deep venous reconstruction surgery is contemplated, further precise anatomical information is required from ascending and descending venography. These contrast studies will provide details of any venous obstruction that may coexist with reflux, the presence of incompetent perforating veins, as well as the degree of deep venous reflux. Contrast studies may also allow the etiology of chronic venous insufficiency to be clarified, whether primary in nature or post-thrombotic.

Reference has already been made to the possible application of descending venography in some patients with recurrent groin varices.

ILIOCAVAL VENOGRAPHY

Iliac vein thrombosis frequently fails to recanalize with maturation, and a permanent occlusion may result. When

recanalization does occur, the vein is often narrowed with stenotic segments. Collateral venous pathways then develop and iliac venography will demonstrate these collateral pathways. The development of these venous collaterals may be sufficient to compensate for the iliac vein stenosis or occlusion, so that no functional obstruction results to the venous return from the leg. Pressure measurements are essential to evaluate the functional significance of these occlusions/stenoses, and are an integral part of iliocaval venography.[14] These pressure measurement techniques and interpretation are described in Chapter 4, p. 32.

The patient is examined in the supine position on a fluoroscopy unit which is also equipped for angiography. Two 4 Fr vessel dilators are introduced, one in each common femoral vein, under local anesthesia and with the tips of dilators in the lower external iliac vein. Venepuncture is facilitated by the patient performing a Valsalva maneuver to distend the femoral vein. Test injections of contrast medium confirm correct placement. Low osmolar contrast medium (30 mL) is then simultaneously injected into the common femoral veins by two operators. The injection rate must be such as to deliver the volume in 4–5 s. The exposure sequence is commenced at the same time as the injection.

A single spot film would serve to demonstrate any occlusion but serial exposures allow a better display of the altered anatomy, demonstrating the extent and direction of flow through venous collaterals (Fig. 10B.11). At completion of the procedure, the femoral vein pressures are taken at rest and following exercise.

Where the femoral vein is occluded, the proximal extent of the occlusion can be defined venographically by one of three alternative approaches: retrograde iliac venography, where the contralateral femoral vein is patent; descending

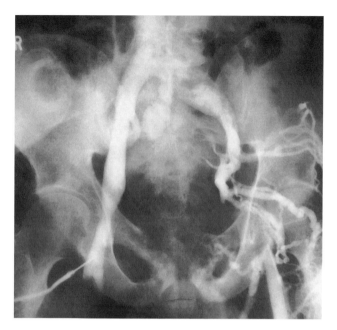

Figure 10B.12 *Pelvic phlebography using a combined approach: a right perfemoral injection and left pertrochanteric intraosseous injection in a patient with an occluded left external iliac vein. The left femoral vein was punctured but the upper extent of the vein could not be defined (history of pelvic surgery followed by radiotherapy).*

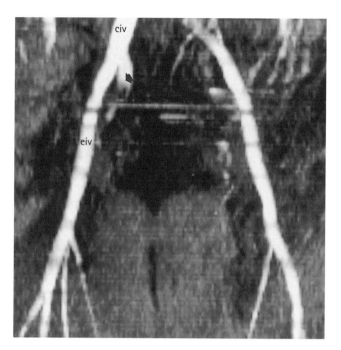

Figure 10B.13 *Anterior coronal magnetic resonance image of pelvic veins with arterial presaturation to suppress arterial signals. Twenty-four-week elderly primigravida with gross perineal/vulval edema due to acute bilateral internal iliac vein thrombosis. Left internal iliac vein totally occluded; right internal iliac vein termination with filling defect due to thrombus (arrow).*

retrograde iliocavography via a catheter introduced from a median antecubital vein; or pertrochanteric intraosseous venography (Fig. 10B.12; with the advent of alternative imaging techniques, this technique is now of mainly historic interest), which requires a general anesthetic.

These techniques are invasive and, in this central venous situation with retrograde catheterization techniques, are limited by the area of opacification because of venous flow pathways away from the site of injection. Duplex Doppler ultrasound may be significantly limited by problems of acoustic access to these areas. The recent introduction of magnetic resonance venography promises to revolutionize the non-invasive evaluation of the major central veins, including the internal iliac veins (Fig. 10B.13).

The percutaneous management of these venous stenoses and occlusions with venoplasty and intravascular stents is described in Chapter 21.

SUMMARY

A number of non-invasive and invasive tests are available to investigate the pathophysiology of chronic venous insufficiency. These investigations should be tailored to the clinical presentation and proceed from non-invasive to invasive testing. Duplex ultrasound has become the cornerstone for

day-to-day evaluation of patients presenting with both deep vein thrombosis and chronic venous insufficiency. However, contrast venography remains the anatomic gold standard and is indicated where reconstructive venous surgery is contemplated.

REFERENCES

1. Dos Santos JC. La phlébographie directe. Conception, technique, premier resultats. *J Int Chir* 1938; **3**: 625–69.
2. Bauer G. A venographic study of thromboembolic patients. *Acta Chir Scand* 1940; **84**(Suppl. 61).
3. Bauer G. A roentgenological and clinical study of the sequels of thrombosis. *Acta Chir Scand* 1942; **86**(Suppl. 74).
4. Leclerc JR, Illescas F, Jarzem P. Diagnosis of deep vein thrombosis. In: Leclerc JR, ed. *Venous Thromboembolic Disorders*. Philadelphia: Lea & Febiger, 1991.
5. Grainger RG. Osmolality of intravascular radiological contrast media. *Br J Radiol* 1980; **53**: 739–46.
6. Raininko R. Role of hyperosmolality: the endothelial injury caused by angiographic contrast media. *Acta Radiol* 1979; **20**: 410–6.
7. Laerum F, Holm HA. Postphlebographic thrombosis. *Radiology* 1981; **140**: 651–4.
8. Walters HL, Clemenson J, Browse NL, Lea Thomas M. ^{125}I-fibrinogen uptake following phlebography of the leg. *Radiology* 1980; **135**: 619–21.

9. Negus D, Friedgood A. The effective management of venous ulceration. *Br J Surg* 1983; **70**: 623–5.

10. Craig JO, In: Saxton HM, Strickland B, eds. *Practical Procedures in Diagnostic Radiology*, 2nd edn. London: HK Lewis, 1972; 250.

11. Dow JD. The venographic diagnosis of the method of recurrence of varicose veins. *Br J Radiol* 1952; **25**: 382.

12. Lea Thomas M, Phillips GW. Recurrent groin varices: an assessment by descending phlebography. *Br J Radiol* 1988; **61**: 294–6.

13. Kistner RL, Ferris EB, Randhawa G *et al.* A method of performing descending venography. *J Vasc Surg* 1986; **4**: 464–6.

14. Negus D, Cockett FB. Femoral vein pressures in post-phlebitic iliac vein obstruction. *Br J Surg* 1967; **54**: 522–5.

11

Functional diagnosis: plethysmography and venous pressure measurement

PHILIP D. COLERIDGE SMITH

INTRODUCTION

Numerous methods of investigation have been used to study the peripheral vascular system. Doppler ultrasound is currently the most widely employed, but several plethysmographic techniques are also currently in use.

METHODS USED TO INVESTIGATE THE PERIPHERAL VASCULAR SYSTEM

Air plethysmography

Air plethysmography is based on volume changes detected by an air-containing compartment or cuff wrapped around part or all of the calf. The cuff is inflated to a low pressure with air, so that fluctuations of calf volume are reflected by a change of pressure within the cuff. This technique has been known for many years,[1–4] but more modern materials have permitted simplification of the equipment.[5] The first descriptions of the equipment, using pneumatic cuffs inflated around short sections of the leg, were devised to assess arterial inflow to the limb. Proximally placed venous occlusion cuffs were used to permit an assessment of volumetric blood flow. Venous function was assessed by quickly tilting the patient from head-up to head-down to determine the rate of venous outflow, in the diagnosis of deep vein thrombosis. The reverse maneuver was used to measure venous reflux.

In the modern air plethysmograph, a plastic sleeve is zipped around the patient's leg and filled with air to a pressure of 6–8 mmHg.[5] This is sufficient to ensure close conformity with the leg, but does not interfere with the venous physiology under study. It is now possible for the device to be calibrated so that absolute volume changes in the limb can be deduced. A commercial source of this device is the APG 1000 (ACI Corporation, San Marcos, CA, USA). It is composed of an air pump that inflates a long tubular air cuff (to a selected pressure of about 6 mmHg), applied to the leg to be measured. A pressure sensor reads the pressure in the cuff, displays the data on a bar graph on the front panel, and sends the pressure signal to a computer. The computer logs the data and assists with measurements from the recorded traces. An example of an APG trace is shown in Figure 11.1. The measurement cuff is applied, inflated and calibrated with the patient lying supine. The patient then stands and the cuff is allowed to fill providing the measurement VV (venous volume). The time taken for 90 percent filling of the calf venous

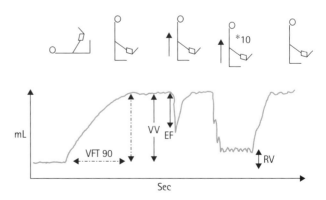

Figure 11.1 *Diagram of traces and measurements made using air plethysmography.*

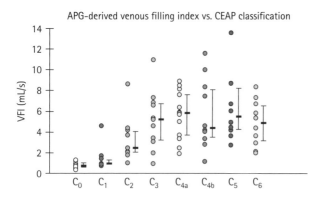

Figure 11.2 *Venous filling index (VFI) measurements made in a series of patients with chronic venous disease and in control subjects. APG, air plethysmograph.*

compartment is the VFT_{90}. The venous filling index (VFI) is calculated as follows:

$$VFI = 90\%VV/VFT_{90}$$

The patient then performs one tiptoe exercise which ejects blood from the calf, which is referred to as ejection volume (EV). From this, the ejection fraction (EF) is calculated as:

$$EF = (EV/VV) \times 100$$

The patient then performs 10 tiptoe movements to empty the venous compartment of the calf more completely. The remaining volume in the calf is referred to as the residual volume (RV) and the residual volume fraction (RVF) is calculated as follows:

$$RVF = (RV/VV) \times 100$$

The VFI is regarded as an index of the severity of venous reflux, whereas the RVF is considered to be analogous to ambulatory venous pressure. These parameters have been shown to correlate with other plethysmographic measures of venous reflux and impairment of calf muscle pump function. McDaniel *et al.*[6] investigated a series of 91 patients with venous ulcers. Where possible, they treated superficial venous reflux and perforating vein reflux by surgical methods. They observed ulcer recurrence in 37 percent of patients at 3 years and 48 percent of patients at 5 years. The VFI measured at the start of the study showed a strong correlation with the likelihood of recurrence.

In a study conducted at the Middlesex Hospital, eight control subjects and 70 patients with venous disease (10 in each of CEAP clinical stages C1, C2, C3, C4a, C4b, C5 and C6) were studied using air plethysmography. The data from VFI measurements is shown in Figure 11.2. This demonstrates that although this parameter increases greatly in the more severe stages of venous disease, it shows considerable spread in each stage making it of little use in predicting the severity of chronic venous disease any one patient would experience.

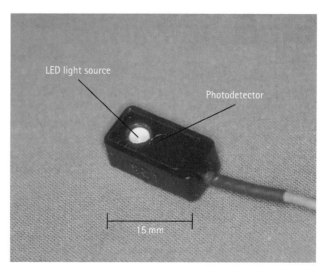

Figure 11.3 *A photoplethysmograph transducer.*

Photoplethysmography

Photoplethysmography, and its more recent development light reflex rheography,[7] have been widely used in the assessment of vascular disease. The photoelectric plethysmograph was first described in the 1930s,[8,9] and was intended for use in the assessment of the arterial system. It was first applied to investigation of the venous system in 1978.[10] The device assesses variation in the light absorption of the skin by hemoglobin in the dermal venous plexuses. When these are full during high venous pressure, the hemoglobin in the red blood cells absorbs light. As venous pressure falls, the venous plexuses become less full and light transmission increases. An example of a photoplethysmography transducer is shown in Figure 11.3.

The photoplethysmograph (PPG) has found wide use in the assessment of the arterial system. It is an effective pulse detector and can be used, with the aid of cuffs, to measure distal pressure in the limbs, including digit pressures. This may be advantageous in patients with diabetes where ankle pressures may be falsely elevated due to heterotopic calcification of the large peripheral arteries.

In order to perform a PPG test of venous reflux in the lower limb, the patient sits with the lower limbs dependent and with the transducers attached 5 cm proximal to the medial malleolus. A stable trace is established. The patient then performs a series of dorsiflexions at the ankle, usually about 10, to activate the calf muscle pump, and then sits at rest. This produces an emptying phase followed by a refilling phase. The time taken for the trace to return to the baseline level is referred to as the PPG refilling time (Fig. 11.4). It has been shown that the refilling time derived by this technique is similar to that obtained by foot vein pressure measurements.[11] Tests can be repeated using tourniquets to compress the superficial veins to establish whether venous reflux lies in

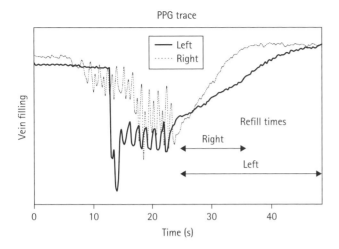

PPG trace

— Left
····· Right

Vein filling

Refill times

Right

Left

0   10   20   30   40

Time (s)

Figure 11.4 *A trace from a photoplethysmograph obtained during a venous refilling test. The venous refilling times are shown on the trace.*

the superficial or deep veins. This is one of the simplest tests to undertake in the investigation of venous reflux.[12]

Light reflex rheography has been shown to detect deep vein thrombosis with 91 percent sensitivity and 93 percent specificity.[13] The subject sits with the foot on the floor and the transducer is applied to the limb 5 cm above the ankle. A series of 10 dorsiflexions of the ankle are performed and the result of venous emptying is recorded on the chart recorder. The calibration possible with this system permits the extent of venous emptying to be assessed, and traces showing failure of sufficient venous emptying are judged to be diagnostic of deep vein thrombosis. The loss of adequate emptying is presumably due to obstruction of the major limb veins which prevent proper functioning of the calf muscle pump.

Strain gauge plethysmography

This method has been used for several years in the assessment of patients with venous disease and is employed to quantify the changes in volume of the calf that occur during exercise or compression of the limb with cuffs. Originally made of mercury in a rubber tube,[14,15] the transducer is now made from a mercury-filled silicone rubber tube. This is stretched around the calf, ankle or foot. The electrical resistance of the tube is dependent on the length of the mercury column and is inversely related to the cross-sectional area of the mercury. As the calf increases in volume, the silicone rubber tube stretches, increasing in length but decreasing in cross-section. This results in an increase in the resistance of the mercury column. The advantage of this system is that the changes in resistance are linearly related to changes in volume, permitting volumetric calibration of the strain gauge system.

The method of strain gauge plethysmography was originally developed to assess arterial inflow into the limbs of patients.[14,15] The strain gauge is placed distally around the limb to monitor the region of interest. More distal regions, such as the hand or foot, where flow is to be disregarded, may be excluded by the application of a cuff inflated above systolic arterial pressure. A proximal venous occlusion cuff is inflated to obstruct venous outflow and the rate of arterial inflow is determined from the upward slope of the plethysmograph trace. Measurements of resting arterial inflow have not proved useful in the management of arterial disease of the lower limb; however, this method is still applicable in situations where quantification of blood flow to a limb is desirable, e.g. as an assessment of the response to treatment.

The strain gauge plethysmograph has been used in the venous system in order to quantify proximal venous obstruction,[16] and to measure the severity of venous reflux.[17] In later modifications the patient was investigated in the standing position, while undertaking tiptoe exercises or walking on a treadmill.[18] Tourniquets are used to differentiate between deep and superficial vein incompetence, in a similar fashion to the photoplethysmograph tests of venous reflux. The technique has been validated against both venography and venous pressure measurements,[19] and results were claimed to be superior to foot volumetry with better separation of the groups, i.e. those with deep and superficial vein incompetence. As with foot volumetry, measures of both the efficiency of venous emptying, from the expelled volume on exercise, and refilling time following exercise are obtained. Both of these parameters have been shown to improve following surgery.[20]

Strain gauge plethysmography has been employed in the diagnosis of deep vein thrombosis. The subject lies supine with the lower limbs elevated by 25–30 cm above the level of the right atrium. Strain gauges are applied at the mid-calf level and thigh cuffs are connected to an inflation system. The cuffs are inflated to 50–60 mmHg for 2 min. During this time, arterial inflow continues but venous outflow is prevented. The calves increase in volume with the retained venous blood. The increase in calf volume, as measured by the strain gauges, is referred to as the 'venous capacitance'. At the end of the inflation period, the cuffs are deflated rapidly, and the rate of blood flowing from the limbs is monitored by the strain gauges. Various measures of the outflow rate have been described, but usually the outflow in the first 1–2 s is converted to flow per minute, expressed as mL%/min. This is the 'venous outflow' (Fig. 11.5). Venous outflow is dependent on the venous capacitance and discriminant tables have been devised to recommend the levels of venous outflow which might be expected for a given venous capacitance. A reduced venous outflow is suggestive of occlusion of one of the main limb veins, and in the absence of another cause for obstruction a diagnosis of deep vein thrombosis may be made. The results of such a diagnosis would usually be confirmed venographically.

Comparison with phlebography[21] and Doppler ultrasound[22] confirms that this investigation has a high degree of

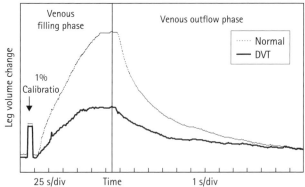

Figure 11.5 *Trace obtained from a strain gauge plethysmography while undertaking a venous outflow test. The first part of the test represents arterial inflow, while the second section is recorded after deflation of the thigh cuffs, resulting in maximum venous outflow.*

sensitivity and specificity in the detection of deep vein thrombosis, detecting 90–95 percent of thromboses with a false-positive rate of 18 percent. The sensitivity falls to 66 percent in isolated calf vein thrombosis,[23] reflecting the dependence of the technique on finding a substantial obstruction to venous flow in the lower limb. The advantage of the system is simplicity compared with venographic or previous plethysmographic methods.

Foot volumetry

Measurements of venous function using foot volumetry were first described by Norgren.[24] In this investigation, the patient stands with each foot in a water bath of known volume (Fig. 11.6). The water bath is then filled to a predetermined level, which permits foot volumes to be established by subsequent volume measurement of the contents of the water bath. Floats or level detectors on the surface of the water bath indicate changes in water level and these can be calibrated to show precise volume changes of the foot. Patients perform a series of 20 knee bends to exercise the calf muscles after which they stand still again. The exercise ejects blood from the foot and the volume change of the foot can be measured precisely. The time taken for half refilling of the venous compartment of the foot is also measured. Combined with a knowledge of the foot volume, fractional measurements of volume change can be calculated. Both expelled volume as a result of exercise and the refilling time were shown to be abnormal in patients with venous disease. These parameters were validated against venous pressure measurements and shown to correlate with decrease in venous pressure and refilling time following exercise.[25] Differentiation of superficial from deep vein incompetence was shown to be possible with the use of tourniquets to occlude the superficial veins.[24] Norgren also showed that

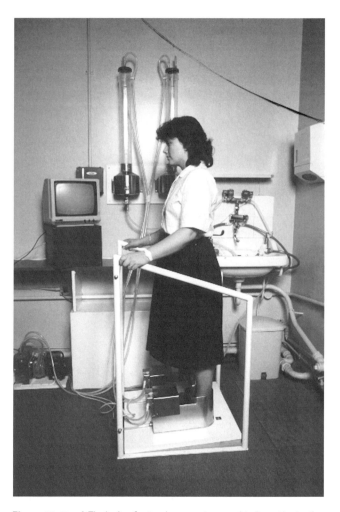

Figure 11.6 *A Thulesius foot volume meter, used to investigate the function of the venous system in the lower limb.*

measurements were normalized following appropriate surgery to correct superficial vein incompetence.[26]

Impedance plethysmography

In this technique four electrodes are applied to the leg with the patient lying supine. Two outer electrodes are used to apply an electrical current to the leg. High-frequency (25–50 kHz) alternating current is used which does not carry the risk of causing cardiac arrhythmias. A current of approximately 0.2–1 mA is passed through the leg. The leg is connected as one 'limb' of an electrical bridge circuit, and an external resistance adjusted so that the bridge is balanced. A chart recorder is used to demonstrate fractional changes in the balance of the bridge in response to arterial inflow and respiration. It is used to measure the rate of venous outflow following a period of venous occlusion,[27,28] in a manner identical to that used in strain gauge plethysmography. Verification of this technique has shown it to be 97 percent specific and 93 percent sensitive for proximal thrombi.[29] Non-occlusive thrombi are more difficult to detect, a sensitivity of 78 percent being reported.

VENOUS PRESSURE MEASUREMENTS

Moritz and Tabora were the first to measure venous pressure directly, in 1910. They cannulated a vein and connected it to a manometer filled with saline and antiseptic, a technique which was subsequently widely used. In 1924, Bedford and Wright[30] cannulated an arm vein and demonstrated that venous pressure was affected by respiration. They also showed that exercise produced a rise in venous pressure. The following year, De Takats et al.[31] reported the results of pressure measurements performed on subjects with varicose veins. They cannulated a vein in the lower leg and connected this to a water manometer, measuring pressure while the subject stood motionless. They concluded that the pressure in varicose veins was higher than normal and attributed the edema and skin changes seen in venous disease to this increased pressure.[31] Using the same apparatus, however, Seiro[32] showed that venous pressure was dependent on posture and was the same in subjects with and without varicose veins. He calculated that venous pressure in the foot, on standing, was equal to the weight of a column of blood from the heart to the foot and therefore only dependent on the height of the heart above the foot. His findings were widely corroborated.

Veal and Hussey,[33] in 1940, cannulated the popliteal vein and performed pressure measurements while the subject performed tiptoe exercises. They confirmed that resting venous pressure measurements were of no use in detecting venous abnormalities. In the face of iliofemoral occlusion by thrombus, they demonstrated that, on exercise, pressure in the popliteal vein rose whereas in a normal limb, although it fluctuated, it remained around the same level.

Smirk[34] first recorded pressure in a vein at the ankle during exercise in 1936 and showed that there was a drop in pressure on walking. He examined only one subject who had no signs of venous disease, but following this, numerous similar studies were performed. Pollack and Wood,[35] in 1949, examined normal subjects, patients with varicose veins and others with a history of deep vein thrombosis. They cannulated the great saphenous vein at the ankle using a no. 17 hypodermic needle through which was passed a polyethylene tube. This was connected to a strain gauge manometer and pressure measurements were recorded on a kymographic camera while the subject walked on a treadmill. They confirmed that pressure in the ankle vein decreased on walking and showed that the decrease in pressure in subjects with varicose veins was less than in normal subjects. Subjects with a history of deep vein thrombosis had a minimal fall in pressure. They also demonstrated that on cessation of exercise, in subjects with venous disease, the pressure returned to the baseline resting pressure much faster than in normal subjects.[36]

Højensgård and Stürup[37] performed a similar study in the same year and reported the same results. They studied patients with varicose veins and those with a history of thrombosis. Again they found that the drop in pressure on walking was greater in the normal subjects and the refilling time faster after cessation of exercise in the post-thrombotic group. In patients with varicose veins, they demonstrated that occlusion of the varicosities by a tourniquet increased the fall in pressure while walking and normalized the venous refilling time. This was also found in a proportion of post-thrombotic limbs. In the remainder of the post-thrombotic limbs, the drop in pressure was not improved by superficial vein occlusion and in some cases this maneuver caused a rise in pressure on walking.

In another study they set out to determine the effect of incompetent perforating veins on pressure measurements. From this study, they concluded that incompetent perforating veins have no effect on ambulatory venous pressure. The ambulatory hypertension seen in venous disease, they concluded, was produced by incompetent superficial and deep veins alone.[38] They showed that raised abdominal pressure, such as produced during a Valsalva maneuver, was transmitted down the deep veins and through incompetent perforating veins to the superficial system. They went on to cannulate the popliteal vein, the posterior tibial vein and the great saphenous vein separately in the same subject. By this means they demonstrated that, in normal limbs, at rest, pressure was the same in the deep and superficial veins. On walking, pressure in the popliteal vein remained the same, but in posterior tibial and saphenous veins it dropped considerably. Increased intra-abdominal pressure was transmitted to the popliteal vein but not to the other veins.[39]

White and Warren[40] used venous pressure measurements to assess the accuracy of the Trendelenberg and Perthes tourniquet tests. They studied limbs with primary varicose veins, those with recurrent varicose veins and limbs with skin changes (post-phlebitic limbs). They found the tourniquet tests unreliable in reaching a diagnosis about the state of the deep veins and showed that, in many cases, 'post-phlebitic' skin changes were due to superficial vein incompetence alone. By application of tourniquets at different levels on the leg while performing the ambulatory pressure measurements, they were able to identify the site of incompetent perforating veins. They concluded that the measurement of venous pressure during exercise was the most accurate method of differentiating superficial varicose veins from those associated with deep vein damage. They recommended, however, that the test was unsuitable for routine use and that in the majority of cases it was unnecessary.

The findings outlined above obtained more than half a century ago have been confirmed by more recent investigation. Ambulatory venous hypertension is a constant pathological feature in venous disease. Nicolaides et al.[41] have shown that the higher the venous pressure during walking, the higher the incidence of ulceration.[41] This hypertension is most commonly due to incompetence of valves resulting in reverse flow of venous blood and ineffective emptying of venous blood from the limb.[42] Outflow obstruction due to thrombosis may also cause ambulatory hypertension.[43] Figure 11.7 shows a patient undergoing venous pressure measurements with pressure transducers attached to needles in both dorsal foot veins.

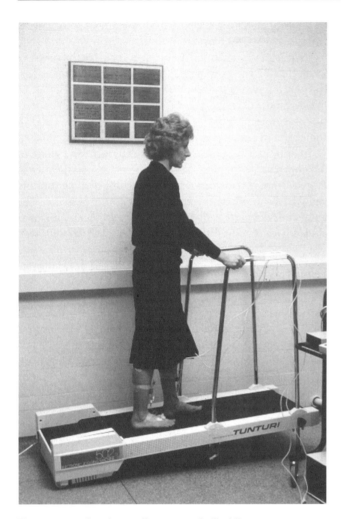

Figure 11.7   *A patient walks on a treadmill whilst venous pressure measurements are made.*

THE ROLE OF FUNCTIONAL VENOUS ASSESSMENT

The tests described above were largely devised before modern duplex ultrasonography came into existence. These tests provided indirect methods of establishing whether venous disease was located in deep or superficial veins and therefore whether surgery could be expected to modify the course of the disease in an individual patient. Much of this information is now obtained from duplex ultrasonography since this technology can rapidly establish whether venous reflux or obstruction is present and which veins are affected. In the management of uncomplicated varicose veins there is little or no advantage in using any of these tests, since only anatomical information is required here.

Patients with leg ulceration present more complex problems, although in general, information concerning which veins are incompetent can be obtained from duplex ultrasonography. Some patients present with combined superficial and deep venous reflux, and in these patients

plethysmographic tests may be used to assess the degree to which venous function might be expected to improve following superficial venous surgery. Deep vein reconstruction is still considered to be experimental surgery and it is highly desirable to monitor the outcome of treatment very closely. This can be done using plethysmographic tests to assess the effects on venous reflux of anti-reflux procedures.

The role of these tests has now greatly reduced with the widespread use of duplex ultrasonography. Some clinical situations remain where these measurements provide useful information.

REFERENCES

1. Mackay IFS, McCarthy G. Measurement of valvular competency in the legs. *J Appl Physiol* 1957; **12**: 329–33.
2. Bygdeman S, Aschberg S, Hindmarsch T. Venous plethysmography in the diagnosis of chronic venous insufficiency. *Acta Chir Scand* 1971; **137**: 423–8.
3. Winsor T, Hyman C. Objective venous studies. *J Cardiovasc Surg* 1961; **2**: 146–52.
4. Sakaguchi S, Tomita T, Endo I, Ishitoba K. Functional segmental plethysmography: a new venous function test. *J Cardiovasc Surg* 1968; **9**: 87–98.
5. Christopoulos D, Nicolaides AN, Szendro G. Venous reflux: quantification and correlation with the clinical severity of chronic venous disease. *Br J Surg* 1988; **75**: 352–6.
6. McDaniel HB, Marston WA, Farber MA *et al.* Recurrence of chronic venous ulcers on the basis of clinical, etiologic, anatomic, and pathophysiologic criteria and air plethysmography. *J Vasc Surg* 2002; **35**: 723–8.
7. Hubner K. Is the light reflection rheography (LRR) suitable as a diagnostic method for the phlebology practice? *Phlebol Proctol* 1986; **15**: 209–12.
8. Cartwright CM. Infrared transmission of the flesh. *J Opt Soc Am* 1930; **20**: 81–4.
9. Hanzlik PJ, Deeds F, Terada B. A simple method of demonstrating changes in blood supply of the ear and effects of some measures. *J Pharmacol Exp Ther* 1936; **56**: 194–204.
10. Barnes RW, Garrett WV, Hummel BA *et al.* Photoplethysmographic assessment of altered cutaneous circulation in the post-phlebitic syndrome. *Arch Surg* 1977; **112**: 1325–30.
11. Abramowitz HB, Queral LA, Flinn WR *et al.* The use of photoplethysmography in the assessment of venous insufficiency: a comparison to venous pressure measurements. *Surgery* 1979; **86**: 434–41.
12. Yao JS T, Flinn WR, McCarthy WJ, Bergan JJ. The role of non-invasive testing in the evaluation of chronic venous problems. *World J Surg* 1986; **10**: 911–8.
13. Thomas PR S, Butler C, Bowman J *et al.* Light reflection rheography: an effective diagnostic test for patients with acute deep vein thrombosis. *Br J Surg* 1990; **77**: 350.
14. Whitney RJ. Measurement of changes in human limb volume by means of a mercury in rubber strain gauge. *J Physiol* 1949; **109**: 5–6P.
15. Whitney RJ. Measurement of volume changes in human limbs. *J Physiol* 1953; **121**: 1–27.

16. Barnes RW, Collicott PE, Mozersky DJ *et al.* Noninvasive quantitation of maximum venous outflow in acute thrombophlebitis. *Surgery* 1972; **72**: 971–9.

17. Barnes RW, Collicott PE, Mozersky DJ *et al.* Noninvasive quantitation of venous reflux in the postphlebitic syndrome. *Surg Gynecol Obstet* 1973; **136**: 769–73.

18. Holm JSE. A simple plethysmographic method for differentiating primary from secondary varicose veins. *Surg Gynecol Obstet* 1976; **143**: 609–12.

19. Mason R, Giron F. Noninvasive evaluation of venous function in chronic venous disease. *Surgery* 1982; **91**: 312–7.

20. Struckmann JR. Assessment of venous muscle pump function by ambulatory calf volume strain gauge plethysmography after surgical treatment of varicose veins. a prospective study of 21 patients. *Surgery* 1987; **101**: 347–53.

21. Hallbook T, Gothlin J. Strain gauge plethysmography in diagnosis of deep venous thrombosis. *Acta Chir Scand* 1971; **137**: 37–52.

22. Barnes RW, Collicot PE, Mozersky DJ *et al.* Non-invasive quantitation of maximum venous outflow in acute thrombophlebitis. *Surgery* 1972; **72**: 971–9.

23. Barnes RW, Hokanson DE, Wu KK, Hoak JC. Detection of deep vein thrombosis with an automatic electrically calibrated strain gauge plethysmograph. *Surgery* 1977; **82**: 219–23.

24. Norgren L. Functional evaluation of chronic venous insufficiency by foot volume try. *Act Chir Scand Supplement* 1974; **444**: 1–48.

25. Lawrence D, Kakkar VV. Post-phlebitic syndrome – a functional assessment. *Br J Surg* 1980; **67**: 686–9.

26. Norgren L. Foot-volume try before and after surgical treatment of patients with varicose veins. *Acta Chir Scand* 1975; **141**: 129–34.

27. Wheeler HB, O'Donnell JA, Anderson FA Jr, Benedict K Jr. Occlusive impedance phlebography: a diagnostic procedure for venous thrombosis and pulmonary embolism. *Prog Cardiovasc Dis* 1974; **17**: 199–205.

28. Wheeler HB, O'Donnell JA, Anderson FA *et al.* Bedside screening for venous thrombosis using occlusive impedance phlebgrophy. *Angiology* 1975; **26**: 199–210.

29. Hull R, van Aken Hirsh J, Gallus AS *et al.* Impedance plethysmography using the occlusive cuff technique in the diagnosis of venous thrombosis. *Circulation* 1976; **53**: 696–700.

30. Bedford DE, Samson Wright. Observations in venous pressure in normal individuals. *Lancet* 1924; **ii**: 106–9.

31. De Takats G, Quint H, Tillotson BI, Crittenden PJ. The impairment of circulation in the varicose extremity. *Arch Surg* 1929; **18**: 672–86.

32. Seiro V. Blutdruck in den krampfadern der unteren extremitaten. *Acta Chir Scand* 1938; **80**: 41–81.

33. Veal JR, Hussey HH. The use of exercise tests in connection with venous pressure measurements for the detection of venous obstruction in the upper and lower extremities. *Am Heart J* 1940; **20**: 308–21.

34. Smirk FH. Observations on the causes of oedema in congestive heart failure. *Clin Sci* 1936; **2**: 318–34.

35. Pollack AA, Wood EH. Venous pressure in the saphenous vein at the ankle in man during exercise and during changes of posture. *J Appl Physiol* 1949; **1**: 649–62.

36. Pollack AA, Taylor BE, Myers TT, Wood EH. The effect of exercise and body position on the venous pressure at the ankle in patients having venous valvular defects. *J Clin Invest* 1949; **28**: 559–63.

37. Højensgård IC, Stürup H. Venous pressure in primary and postthrombotic varicose veins. *Acta Chir Scand* 1949; **99**: 133–53.

38. Stürup H, Højensgård IC. Venous pressure in varicose veins in patients with incompetent communicating veins. *Acta Chir Scand* 1950; **99**: 519–25.

39. Højensgård IC, Stürup H. Static and dynamic pressures in superficial and deep veins of the lower extremity in man. *Acta Physiol Scand* 1952; **27**: 49–67.

40. White EA, Warren R. The walking pressure test as a method of evaluation of varicose veins. *Surgery* 1949; **26**: 987–1002.

41. Nicolaides AN, Zukowski A, Lewis R *et al.* Venous pressure measurements in venous problems. In: Bergan, JJ, Yao, JS T, eds. *Surgery of the Veins.* Orlando: Grune & Stratton Inc, 1985; 111–8.

42. Killewich LA, Martin R, Cramer M *et al.* An objective assessment of the physiologic changes in the post–thrombotic syndrome. *Arch Surg* 1985; **120**: 424–6.

43. Negus D, Cockett FB. Femoral vein pressures in post-phlebitic iliac vein obstruction. *Br J Surg* 1967; **54**: 522–5.

12

Compression therapy in venous leg ulcers

HUGO PARTSCH

INTRODUCTION

Compression therapy is the basic treatment modality in venous leg ulcers. It has been shown to be effective in healing venous ulcers and in preventing their recurrence.[1–5] However, the underlying venous pathology should always be established by investigation of the vascular system. Surgical treatment or sclerotherapy may be indicated to correct superficial or perforating vein incompetence. The reasons for the benefit of leg compression in venous disease have not yet been completely elucidated.[6]

Applying compression bandages skillfully avoids hospital admission and allows patients to continue their work. Therefore this form of treatment is also very cost-effective.

Compression treatment is combined with local dressings, which absorb the exudates and prevent soiling of the compression material.

COMPRESSION DEVICES

Several different devices may be used for compression therapy of venous ulcers (Box 12.1). Table 12.1 shows a categorization of compression devices based on the elastic properties of the material.

Medical compression stockings

For ulcers that are not excessively large (i.e. less than 5 cm^2) and not too long-standing (duration less than 3 months) the use of compression stockings may be considered. Even unskilled patients are able to manage this kind of treatment, which produces a constant degree of pressure and allows the patient

---

Box 12.1 Types of compression devices

- Graduated compression stockings
  - custom made
  - standard size
    - knee length
    - thigh length
    - compression tights
- Bandages
  - inelastic
  - short stretch
  - long stretch
    - single-layer
    - multilayer
- Intermittent pneumatic compression
  - single chamber
  - sequential chambers
    - foot pump
    - lower leg
    - full leg
- Intermittent static pressure
  - 'mercury bath'

---

to change the dressing, clean the ulcer and have a shower. One of the disadvantages is that the exudates may soil the stocking, which then has to be washed frequently, perhaps causing weakening of the stocking fibres.

Light compression stockings may be used for keeping the local ulcer dressing in place. A class 2 compression stocking placed on top will add its pressure to that of the underlying

Table 12.1   *Categories of compression material*

	Inelastic	Short stretch	Long stretch
Stretch	0	<100%	>140%
Application	Trained staff	Trained staff	Every patient
Stays on the leg	Day and night	Day and night	Daytime

Note: Long stretch material changes its elastic property when applied with several layers. Multilayer bandages may therefore also be tolerated during the night.

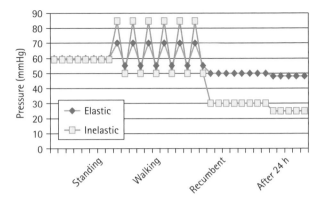

Figure 12.1   *Sub-bandage pressure (mmHg) with elastic and inelastic material both applied with a resting pressure of 60 mmHg at the distal lower leg in the standing position. During walking, the pressure gradient between muscle systole (peak value) and muscle diastole (lowest value) is much higher for the inelastic than for the elastic material. In contrast to the elastic material, the inelastic bandage shows a considerable fall in pressure in the lying position.*

light stocking.[7] In order to facilitate the application of a stocking, some helpful devices have been introduced.

Nylon or silk socks (e.g. Easy slide; Jobst-Beiersdorf, Emmerich, Germany) help to slide the stocking over the foot. Stockings with a zip have also been introduced (Ulcer-care; Jobst-Beiersdorf, Emmerich, Germany).[8] A ready-made tubular device that can be washed and re-used was introduced in some European countries under the name of Tubulcus (Innothera, Arcueil, France).[9]

Usually, below-knee stockings are prescribed. Strong compression stockings exerting a pressure of more than 30 mmHg at ankle level are recommended. To date, only a few randomized controlled trials have reported improved ulcer healing using compression stockings.[7–9]

Inelastic bandages

Zinc paste (Unna boot)[10,11] and rigid gaiters such as Circ-Aid (Circ-Aid Medical Products, San Diego, CA, USA)[12] are examples of inelastic material that can be left on the leg for several days, and even up to 2 weeks. Inelastic compression bandages are difficult to apply and should therefore be used only by trained personnel, exercising great care.

The bandage pressure, which is the most critical parameter for the efficacy of compression treatment, depends on the amount of edema, the walking ability of the patient and the leg circumference. In contrast to bandages containing elastic fibres, this pressure is solely produced by the tension imparted on the bandage during its application. Therefore, the pressure achieved during the application of an inelastic bandage should be much higher than with a bandage made from elastic material.

In a patient with severe edema, the inelastic bandage should be applied to give a pressure of about 60 mmHg to the distal portion of the leg. In keeping with general policies for the use of compression treatment, it is essential to exclude limbs with arterial occlusive disease from bandaging at such high pressures.

An even pressure distribution can be achieved by applying several layers. The applied pressure will decrease from the ankle even when the bandager applies the bandage with the same tension throughout the leg owing to increasing circumference from the ankle to the calf. This is explained by Laplace's Law, which states that the pressure exerted on a cylinder is inversely proportional to its radius.

During walking, sub-bandage pressure peaks reach as much as 80 mmHg with each muscle contraction, followed by a drop to 40–50 mmHg during muscle diastole (Fig. 12.1). The pressure difference between systole and diastole reflects the 'massage effect' of the bandage. The difference between peak pressure and resting pressure, or between muscle systole and muscle diastole,[13,14] correlates with the stiffness of the material.

Several studies have shown the hemodynamic superiority of inelastic bandages compared with elastic material applied with the same resting pressure.[15,16] Venous reflux is moderated by inelastic bandages so that even ambulatory venous hypertension is significantly reduced. Reduced ambulatory venous hypertension was demonstrated following application of inelastic bandages exerting a pressure of more than 50 mmHg on the distal lower leg,[17] but not with elastic compression stockings.[18]

Short stretch bandages

With an extensibility lower than 100 percent (e.g. Rosidal K; Vernon-Carus Ltd, Preston, UK; Comprilan; Jobst-Beiersdorf, Emmerich, Germany) also have to be applied much more strongly than elastic bandages. Usually two 5-m long bandages are used to cover the leg. More important than the details of application in terms of spirals or figures of eight is the high resting pressure on the distal lower leg, which should diminish over the proximal parts in order to create a pressure gradient from distal to proximal.

These bandages are frequently used in continental Europe. They are usually changed once a week, or if there is considerable exudation in the initial phase, they are changed after a few days. The bandages can be washed and re-used. With prolonged use, these bandages lose their elastic properties, which makes them inelastic in character.

Long stretch bandages

Long stretch material is relatively easy to handle and can be usually be applied by patients. In contrast to the inelastic material, these bandages produce an active force by the elastic recoil of their fibres and do not need to be applied with high pressure. The pressure drop after several hours is minimal. Therefore, such bandages may cause pain and discomfort when the patient sits or lies down, especially when they have been applied too tightly. Elastic bandages or compression stockings are therefore applied in the morning, preferably before getting up, and are removed before going to bed at night. During walking, the peak pressure waves are lower than with inelastic material (Fig. 12.1).

New materials with special elastomeric properties (Vari-Stretch system used in ProGuide, Smith & Nephew, Hull, UK) try to overcome the problem of inadequate pressure produced by an inexperienced bandager.[19] The sub-bandage pressure generated by this system remains relatively constant as the tension with which the bandage is applied increases.

In order to provide guidance to the user on the optimal tension and to ensure that two bandage-turns applied with a 50 percent overlap achieve a satisfactory pressure, some bandages with special application aids have been developed (e.g. Surepress; ConvaTec, Uxbridge, UK).[20] Rectangles or ovals of different sizes are knitted into these bandages that change into squares or circles, respectively, when the appropriate level of tension is applied to the fabric.

Several elastic bandages have been supplied with cohesive (self-adhering) or adhesive basic sticky layers in order to prevent slipping down of the bandage. Due to the high friction between several layers, such bandages act like inelastic material. They are also able to maintain prolonged compression.[21]

Multilayer bandages

Applying several layers of bandages not only increases the pressure but also leads to a change of the elastic property of the bandage. The influence of friction on a bandage composed of several layers results in a behavior more similar to an inelastic bandage, with high-pressure peaks during walking and a tolerable pressure drop during rest. Therefore, such multilayer bandages may also remain on the leg for several days.

The so-called four-layer bandage contains four layers of different material: cotton wool, crepe, elastic and self-cohesive. These bandages are relatively easy to apply and have gained widespread use, especially in the UK, where ulcers are treated mainly by nurses.[22,23] In centres that are experienced with applying multilayer short stretch material, no significant superiority of four-layer bandages could be found.[24,25]

Intermittent pneumatic compression

The application of intermittent pneumatic compression in addition to the use of compression bandages is able to accelerate ulcer healing.[26] This adjunctive treatment may be very

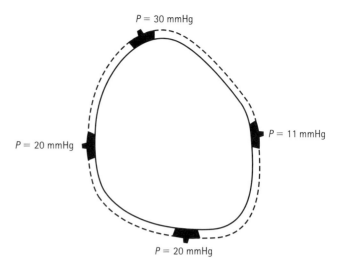

Figure 12.2 *Due to Laplace's Law the local sub-bandage pressure P equals the applied tension divided by the local radius. Over the shin (top of the picture), with its sharp curvature, the pressure will be much higher than over the flat parts of the lower leg, where most venous ulcers are located. In order to increase the pressure over the ulcer area, pads are used which diminish the local radius. The high bandage pressure over the shin can be reduced by applying some cotton wool over the subcutaneous border of the tibia beneath the bandage.*

helpful in those patients who have edema, are unable to walk or who suffer from a stiff ankle, especially when concomitant arterial disease is also present. In such cases, there is often a vicious circle starting with pain and inability to walk, sitting for many hours and progression of edema, which reduces the arterial skin perfusion, which in turn worsens the pain. Bed rest with leg elevation will not be tolerated in such cases. Intermittent pneumatic compression is able to reduce edema and to enhance arterial blood flow.[27–29]

One key advantage of intermittent compression in patients with arterial occlusive disease, as compared with sustained compression with bandages or stockings (which are contraindicated in these patients), is the pressure-free interval between the pressure cycles, in which short periods of reactive hyperemia develop.

Machines developing excessive suprasystolic pressure phases by using mercury-filled cuffs ('mercury bath') have been developed especially for the treatment of patients with lymphedema.[6] Episodic reports also recommend their use in patients with recalcitrant ulcers, specifically of 'mixed' arterial and venous aetiology.

Pads

Venous ulcers frequently occur behind the medial malleolus or on the flat areas of the medial leg. The pressure of a bandage or a stocking will be low in these areas as a result of Laplace's Law, which states that the pressure is inversely proportional to the radius (Fig. 12.2). A local increase of pressure can be achieved by applying rubber foam pads over the ulcer region, thereby decreasing the radius of the leg segment. Care should be taken that the edges of these pads are flattened in order to avoid producing sharp impressions in the skin. The curved prominence of pads (e.g. Komprex; Vernon-Carus Ltd, Preston, UK) should be directed towards the leg.

PREVENTION OF ULCER RECURRENCE

Management of leg-ulcers consists of two phases:

- the healing phase – until complete epithelialization is obtained
- the maintenance phase – after ulcer healing in which the risk of ulcer recurrence should be minimized.

It is often easier to heal a venous ulcer than to keep it healed.

For the healing phase, I prefer zinc paste bandages because of the superior hemodynamic efficacy of inelastic material. Multilayer bandages, which exert similar high levels of compression, may be a good alternative.

To keep the ulcer healed, continuous compression is essential (maintenance phase). Medical compression below-knee stockings, classes 2 and 3 (23–46 mmHg at ankle level) are the preferred method.[2,30,31] Patients who are unable to put on the stockings may use elastic bandages instead. Eradication of superficial venous reflux and perforating vein incompetence by surgery or sclerotherapy should be considered in every patient.

COMPRESSION TECHNIQUES

Many different techniques for compression bandaging have been described. Some general rules are listed below:

- Elastic bandages are easier to handle than inelastic bandages and may also be applied by staff who are not specifically trained and by patients themselves. This is also true for compression stockings.
- Inelastic material, such as zinc paste bandages, should be applied with a much higher resting pressure. The bandage roll is pressed towards the leg, as if moulding clay. It is advisable to cut the zinc bandage when it does not exactly follow the cone shape of the leg during application, in order to obtain a homogeneous pressure distribution without creating constricting bands or folds. A 10 m bandage length is recommended for one leg. After the leg has been covered with the zinc paste bandage, a further 5-m short stretch bandage is added and the patient is encouraged to walk immediately for at least 30 min. The short stretch bandage can be washed and re-used with each change of the bandage.
- After some walking, the pressure drops to around 40 mmHg due to the immediate removal of a considerable amount of edema. In the edematous phase, the bandage will loosen after a few days and should be re-applied or wrapped with a short stretch bandage.

The same is advisable when exudates from the ulceration penetrate the bandage. This may occur especially during the initial treatment phase and the patient should be advised to return for further bandaging if this happens. After the initial phase, the bandage usually changed at weekly intervals.

- Bandaging should cover the foot and go up to the capitulum fibulae. The initial turn may be placed around the ankle or between the heel and the dorsal tendon to fix the bandage. Then the bandage is taken down to the foot as far as the base of the toes. More limited bandaging of the foot is permissible when using short stretch bandages in order to avoid impeding ankle movement. Slight morning edema developing distal to a bandage that only covers half of the foot will disappear soon after starting walking. The ankle joint is always bandaged with maximal dorsiflexion of the foot.
- The bandage is overlapped along the leg in either a spiral fashion or with figures of eight.
- Layers should overlap by between 30 and 50 percent.
- Graduated compression is achieved by exerting higher pressure on the distal leg than on the proximal calf or by using more layers. Pads can increase local pressure over ulcers or firm lipodermatosclerotic areas. Tendons and the shin should always be protected by a layer of cotton wool beneath the bandage.
- The proximal end of the bandage should cover the capitulum fibulae.
- Bandaging of the leg is sufficient for the majority of patients. Only in cases with extensive swelling or phlebitis of the thigh are compression bandages reaching up to the inguinal fold advisable. The flexor tendons at the knee should be protected by cotton wool. Thigh bandages are best applied using adhesive material (e.g. Panelast; Vernon-Carus Ltd, Preston, UK), starting from the proximal calf and going up to the proximal thigh. In order to narrow the veins, the sub-bandage pressure at mid-thigh level should be at least 40 mmHg.
- Highly exudatative ulcers may need frequent dressing changes in the initial phase. However, exudation will subside after several days of firm compression.

Walking exercises are essential to optimize the effect of compression therapy.

HEMODYNAMIC EFFECTS OF COMPRESSION THERAPY

Table 12.2 summarizes haemodynamic parameters that have been measured, and the methodology that has been used.[32,33]

REDUCTION OF EDEMA

Compression is able to reduce the circumference of a swollen leg by several centimetres per week. Walking exercises exert a

Table 12.2 *Effects of compression therapy*[32,33]

Parameter	Investigative method
Edema	Volumetry, isotopes, ultrasound
Venous volume	Phlebography, blood pool scintigraphy, air plethysmography (APG)
Venous velocity	Circulation time (isotopes), duplex ultrasound
Blood shift into central compartments	Blood pool scintigraphy, cardiac output
Venous refluxes	Duplex ultrasound, APG
Venous pump	Foot volumetry, APG, venous pressure
Arterial flow	Duplex ultrasound, xenon-clearance, laser Doppler
Microcirculation	Capillaroscopy, tcPo$_2$, laser Doppler
Lymph drainage	Isotopic and indirect lymphography

kind of massage. By ultrasound B-scans, it can be demonstrated that this diminution of leg volume is caused by a loss of water in the subcutaneous tissue. The reduction of edema is a major cause of the decrease in bandage pressure after 24 h, so that the bandage has to be reapplied. In order to prevent refilling of the leg with edema, permanent compression is essential. Elastic stockings may be able to maintain the edema-free condition but they are less effective at decreasing edema in the massively swollen limb.

SOFTENING OF LIPODERMATOSCLEROSIS

Structural skin changes have been reported after using computed tomograph (CT) and ultrasound.

REDUCTION OF VENOUS VOLUME (NARROWING OF VEINS)

It has been demonstrated by phlebography that firm compression is able to reduce the diameter of superficial and deep veins to the dimension of a thin cord.

By measuring radioactivity in the legs after labelling of red blood cells, it has been shown that blood volume decreases with increasing external pressure up to 40 mmHg in the horizontal position. Blood volume reduction may also be demonstrated by air plethysmography and by duplex ultrasound in the upright position. Non-elastic material applied with the same pressure leads to a greater volume reduction.

ACCELERATION OF VENOUS FLOW

Due to the narrowing of the venous diameter, blood flow velocity increases when the arterial inflow remains unchanged. This may be demonstrated by calculating circulation times after injection of a radioactive tracer into a dorsal foot vein with and without leg compression.

BLOOD SHIFT INTO CENTRAL COMPARTMENTS

Compression of both legs leads to a shift of blood into central vascular compartments, to an increase of the preload of the heart and to an increase of cardiac output. Therefore, compression therapy must be performed with caution in patients with severe cardiac failure. Diuresis may be improved by mobilizing fluid from the extravascular compartment.

REDUCTION OF VENOUS REFLUX

Venous reflux due to valvular incompetence plays a central role in the pathophysiology of chronic venous insufficiency. This may be demonstrated by duplex ultrasound and measured quantitatively by plethysmographic techniques, preferably by air plethysmography.

High levels of compression decrease reflux in the upright position. Again, with the same pressure, inelastic material is more effective than elastic.

Reduction of venous reflux by external compression is also observed in completely avalvular segments and cannot therefore be explained by an approximation of valve leaflets. (Congenital avalvulia is a rare cause for venous ulceration, which develops in late childhood.)

IMPROVEMENT OF VENOUS PUMPING

Foot volumetry can be used to estimate expelled volume, which reflects the amount of venous blood that is pumped up from the foot during standardized knee-bending exercises. This parameter, which is reduced depending on the degree of venous incompetence, shows a steady improvement with increasing external compression pressure.

Simultaneous foot volumetry and peripheral venous pressure measurement showed that a decrease of ambulatory venous hypertension can only be obtained with inelastic, and not with elastic, compression. This fact may be explained by the more intense narrowing of deep veins by inelastic material during walking.

INFLUENCE ON ARTERIAL FLOW

The immediate effect of a firm static compression is a reduction of arterial inflow. In patients with arterial occlusive disease severe skin damage including gangrene may be caused by external compression. However, intermittent pressure waves have been shown to increase blood-flow in the large arteries and in the skin in these patients. Inelastic bandages applied at greatly reduced pressure[34] may exert similar effects when the ankle pump is moved, actively or passively. Reduction of leg swelling by a careful intermittent compression regime may improve peripheral ischaemia, especially when edema impedes the nutrition of the skin in addition to arterial obstruction. These facts are of considerable practical importance, especially in patients with ulcers of mixed arterial and venous etiology, and in edema due to limb dependency.

IMPROVEMENT OF MICROCIRCULATION

Blood flow in the enlarged capillary loops is accelerated, capillary filtration is reduced due to enhanced tissue pressure. Effects on mediators involved in the local inflammatory response may explain both the immediate pain relief that occurs with good compression, and ulcer healing.

IMPROVEMENT OF LYMPH DRAINAGE

Intermittent pneumatic compression enhances extrafascial lymph drainage. Unna boots are able to increase subfascial lymph transport, which is reduced in post-thrombotic syndrome.

Consequent compression leads to a morphological improvement of pathological initial lymphatics in patients with lipodermatosclerosis, which can be demonstrated by indirect X-ray lymphography.

CLINICAL TRIALS

In assessing the outcome of a clinical trial, only the time to complete healing and the healing rate should be considered. The percentage area decrease per unit time is often quoted in such studies but is of secondary importance.

The following conclusions may be derived from several randomized controlled trials and systematic reviews:[1,5]

- Compression increases ulcer healing compared with no compression.
- Multilayer bandages are more effective than single-layer systems.
- High compression is more effective than low compression.
- Differences in efficiency between different types of compression material can mainly be explained by variations in interface pressure that should be measured in future studies.

Compression has been shown to result in faster healing rates of venous ulcers compared with local therapy alone. The augmentation of sustained compression with sequential pneumatic compression promotes ulcer healing.

With adequate compression therapy, 70 percent of venous ulcers should be healed after 12 weeks. Reports with healing rates lower than 50 percent raise the suspicion that the compression technique used in the study was inadequate. This is also true for randomized studies comparing different compression regimes or trying to demonstrate the supplementary effect of drugs. In future studies comparing different materials, it would be desirable to measure the sub-bandage pressure, since this parameter is of crucial importance for the healing of venous ulcers.

With optimal compression therapy, baseline ulcer area and ulcer duration are significant predictors of ulcer healing.[35,36] After the ulcers are healed, venous ulcer recurrence is much more likely in those patients who fail to comply with a regime of wearing compression stockings as a preventive measure.[2]

Recurrence after healing of leg ulcers was shown to be significantly lower if compression stockings with higher pressure were used.

SUMMARY

Compression remains the cornerstone of therapy for patients with venous ulcers. The efficacy of external application of compression depends mainly on the pressure exerted by the bandage or stocking and on the elasticity of the material that is used. Treatment goals include reduction of edema and lipodermatosclerosis, and improvement of venous incompetence in large veins and microcirculation. These effects have been demonstrated experimentally and may explain the healing effects of compression treatment.

During the last few years, several randomized controlled trials have proved the common experience that compression is the most effective, conservative treatment modality for healing venous ulcers. These trials have demonstrated that sustained compression and multilayer bandages provide the best results. No clear conclusions can yet be drawn from experimental work concerning the elastic properties of the material used for a bandage or stocking and its efficacy in healing venous leg ulcers.

Because of the superior hemodynamic efficacy of inelastic materials, I prefer Unna boot or multilayer bandages for the healing phase. To keep the ulcer healed, sustained compression is essential (maintenance phase). For this indication, below-knee medical compression stockings, classes 2 and 3 (23–46 mmHg at ankle level), are the method of choice.

In patients with concomitant arterial occlusive disease, firm compression is contraindicated. However, if applied with the utmost caution, light compression is able to reduce edema, thereby improving arterial flow. Intermittent pneumatic compression and inelastic bandages can be used for this purpose and the resting pressure of the bandage should come close to zero. During walking or passive ankle movement the massage waves with each muscle systole help to squeeze out edema and increase arterial flow.

REFERENCES

1. Cullum N, Nelson EA, Fletcher AW, Sheldon TA. *Compression for Venous Leg Ulcers (Cochrane Review) in the Cochrane Library, Issue 3.* Oxford: Update Software, 2003.
2. Nelson EA, Bell-Syer SE, Cullum NA. Compression for preventing recurrence of venous ulcers. *Cochrane Library. Issue 3.* Oxford, Update Software, 2003.
3. Phillips TJ. Current approaches to venous ulcers and compression. *Dermatol Surg* 2001; **27**: 611–21.
4. Alexander House Group. Consensus paper on venous leg ulcers. *Phlebology* 1992; **7**: 48–58.
5. Fletcher A, Cullum N, Sheldon TA. A systematic review of compression treatment for venous leg ulcers. *Br Med J* 1997; **315**: 576–80.
6. Partsch H, Rabe E, Stemmer R. *Compression Therapy of the Extremities.* Paris: Editions Phlébologiques Francaises, 1999.
7. Horakova MA, Partsch H. Ulcères de jambe d'origine veineuse: Indications pour les bas de compression? *Phlébologie* 1994; **47**: 53–7.

8. Häfner HM, Vollert B, Schlez A, Jünger M. Compression stockings in treatment of ulcus cruris. An efficient alternative to bandages. *Hautarzt* 2000; **51**: 925–30.

9. Jünger M, Partsch H, Ramelet AA, Zuccarelli F. Efficacy of a ready made tubular compression device versus short-stretch compression bandages in the treatment of venous leg ulcers. *Wounds* 2004; **16**: 313–20.

10. Hendricks, WN, Swallow, RT. Management of stasis leg ulcers with Unna's boots versus elastic compression stockings. *J Am Acad Dermatol* 1985; **12**: 90–8.

11. Kikta MJ, Schuler JJ, Meyer JP *et al.* A prospective, randomised trial of Unna's boot versus hydroactive dressing in the treatment of venous stasis ulcers. *J Vasc Surg* 1988; **7**: 478–83.

12. Depalma RG, Kowallek D, Spence RK *et al.* Comparison of costs and healing rates of two forms of compression in treating venous ulcers. *Vasc Surg* 1999; **33**: 683–9.

13. Häfner HM, Piche E, Jünger M. The ratio of working pressure to resting pressure under compression stockings: its significance for the development of venous perfusion in the legs. *Phlebologie* 2001; **30**: 88–93.

14. Stock R, Wegen van der Franken CPM, Neumann HAM. A method for measuring the dynamic behaviour of medical compression hosiery during walking. *Dermatol Surg* 2004; **30**: 721–36.

15. Spence RK, Cahall E. Inelastic versus elastic leg compression in chronic venous insufficiency. A comparison of limb size and venous hemodynamic. *J Vasc Surg* 1996; **24**: 783–7.

16. Partsch H, Menzinger G, Mostbeck A. Inelastic leg compression is more effective to reduce deep venous refluxes than elastic bandages. *Dermatol Surg* 1999; **25**: 695–700.

17. Partsch H Improvement of venous pumping function in chronic venous insufficiency by compression depending on pressure and material. *Vasa* 1984; **13**: 58–64.

18. Mayberry JC, Moneta GL, Taylor LM, Porter JM. Fifteen-year results of ambulatory compression therapy for chronic venous ulcers. *Surgery* 1991; **109**: 575–81.

19. Moffatt CJ on behalf of the EXPECT trial. A multi-centre randomised trial comparing a Vari-stretch compression system with Profore. *13th Conference European Wound Management Association, Pisa.* (Abstract.) Pisa: Felice Editore 2003.

20. Thomas S. High-compression bandages. *J Wound Care* 1996; **5**: 40–3.

21. Travers JP, Dalziel KL, Makin GS. Assessment of a new one-layer adhesive bandaging method in maintaining prolonged limb compression and effects on venous ulcer healing. *Phlebology* 1992; **7**: 59–63.

22. Blair SD, Wright DDI, Backhouse CM *et al.* Sustained compression and healing of chronic venous ulcers. *Br Med J* 1988; **297**: 1159–61.

23. Callam MJ, Harper DR, Dale JJ, Brown D. Lothian and Fourth Valley leg ulcer healing trial, part 1: elastic versus non-elastic bandaging in the treatment of chronic leg ulceration. *Phlebology* 1992; **7**: 136–41.

24. Partsch H, Damstra RJ, Tazelaar DJ *et al.* Multicentre, randomised controlled trial of four-layer bandaging versus short-stretch bandaging in the treatment of venous leg ulcers. *Vasa* 2001; **30**: 2108–13.

25. Meyer FJ, McGuiness CL, Lagattolla NR *et al.* Randomised clinical trial of three-layer paste and four-layer bandages for venous leg ulcers. *Br J Surg* 2003; **90**: 934–8.

26. Coleridge Smith P, Sarin S, Hasty J, Scurr JH. Sequential gradient pneumatic compression enhances venous ulcer healing: a randomised trial. *Surgery* 1990; **108**: 971–5.

27. Eze AR, Comerota AJ, Cisek PL *et al.* Intermittent calf and foot compression increases lower extremity blood flow. *Am J Surg* 1996; **172**: 130–4.

28. Mayrowitz HN, Larsen PB. Effects of compression bandaging on the leg pulsatile blood flow. *Clin Physiol* 1997; **17**: 105–17.

29. Delis KT, Nicolaides AN, Wolfe JHN, Stansby G. Improving walking ability and ankle brachial pressure indices in symptomatic peripheral vascular disease using intermittent pneumatic foot compression: a prospective controlled study with one year follow-up. *J Vasc Surg* 2000; **31**: 650–61.

30. Samson RH, Showalter DP. Stockings and the prevention of recurrent venous ulcers. *Dermatol Surg Oncol* 1996; **22**: 373–6.

31. Harper DR, Ruckley CV, Dale JJ *et al.* Prevention of recurrence of chronic leg ulcer – a randomised trial of different degrees of compression. In: Raymond-Martinbeau P, Prescott R, Zummo M, eds. *Phlebology.* London: John Libbey, 1992; 902–3.

32. Nicolaides AN. Investigation of chronic venous insufficiency. A consensus statement. *Circulation* 2000; **102**: e126–63.

33. Partsch H. Compression therapy of the legs. *Dermatol Surg Oncol* 1991; **17**: 799–805.

34. Stacey M, Falanga V, Marston W *et al.* The use of compression therapy in the treatment of venous leg ulcers: a recommended management pathway. *EWMA J* 2002; **2**: 9–13.

35. Margolis DJ, Berlin JA, Strom BL. Which venous leg ulcers will heal with limb compression bandages? *Am J Med* 2000; **109**: 15–9.

36. Phillips TJ, Machado F, Trout R *et al.* Prognostic indicators in venous ulcers. *J Acad Dermatol* 2000; **43**: 627–30.

13

Primary ulcer healing: dressings and compression

CHRISTINE J. MOFFATT, PETER J. FRANKS

INTRODUCTION

Over the last 20 years there have been rapid developments in the diagnosis of venous disease, and a growing awareness that leg ulceration is often complex, involving several etiological pathways, most commonly related to venous or arterial disorders.[1] Correct assessment of the underlying etiology remains the most important factor in evidence-based leg ulcer practice. Moreover, treatment cannot be considered in isolation, but must also be considered in relation to the systems of care delivery. In some countries, it is the physician who treats patients with ulceration. In others, it may be the surgeon, whilst in the UK, for example, by far the greatest proportion of patients (>80 percent) are treated by nurses in the community. There has been a proliferation in the number of integrated leg ulcer services, where hospital support is available to all community patients who are treated within community leg ulcer clinics.[2]

Clearly, the infrastructure which supports care will lead to differences in emphasis on the management of venous ulceration wherever and by whomever it is being delivered. Each system of care, and the clinical area within each system, will place a different emphasis on the care that is being delivered, be it surgical interventions, tissue engineering, pharmaceuticals, compression or novel adjunctive therapies. In addition, it is likely that different patient populations may exist in different clinical areas. It is important that these are taken into consideration when reviewing the evidence in terms of the practical aspects of the interventions, and the potential benefits that are likely to come from a particular patient group. It is also important to appreciate the changes which are occurring in medicine and health care, most importantly the rapidly changing health systems throughout the world and the development of guidelines based on systematic literature reviews. These synthesize the evidence whilst providing recommendations for care based on this evidence.[3]

PRIORITIES IN ULCER MANAGEMENT

The first priority of leg ulcer management is to correct the underlying cause of the ulcer, where possible. It has been suggested that up to 40 percent of patients with leg ulceration have a correctable vascular abnormality, although robust evidence for this statement is lacking.[1] There is also evidence that an increasing number of elderly patients suffer from complex ulceration involving a number of etiological factors.[4] Other management priorities are: to create the optimum local wound healing environment; improve the factors which may delay wound healing; prevent avoidable complications such as exogenous dermatitis, wound infection or tissue damage due to overtight bandaging; and maintain skin integrity when healed.[5]

Wound bed preparation

Falanaga's[6] aims for wound bed preparation and management are:

- restoration of bacterial balance
- management of necrosis
- control of exudate
- correction of cellular dysfunction
- restoration of biochemical balance.

There has been a resurgence of interest in the potential role that bacteria may play in the wound healing process.[7]

Debate has centered around the difficulties of assessing the bacterial load within ulceration and the possible effects of heavy colonization of bacteria on ability of the wound to heal. This subject is further considered in Chapter 6.

Severely infected ulcers should be treated with a 2-week course of an appropriate oral antibiotic. Local antibiotic powders should be avoided, as allergic reactions are common. Anaerobic bacteria are usually present and metronidazole should be included in the prescribed antibiotics.

Debridement, which involves the removal of devitalized tissue and cellular exudate at the outer surface, is an integral part of the wound cleansing process. The accumulation of these products in the wound is generally thought to prevent or delay granulation and epithelialization. Debridement is therefore thought to facilitate healing.[8]

Debridement should aim to remove foreign bodies; minimize clinical infection; remove dead and devitalized tissue, slough and pus; protect peri-ulcer skin integrity by prevention of maceration and further tissue breakdown; and protect granulating tissue. It can be achieved by a number of methods. Mechanical methods such as surgical debridement can be used, although products containing enzymes which lyse the debris within the wound are also popular, e.g. Debrisan (Pharmacia) and Varidase (Lederle).

Biosurgical techniques using sterile maggots have proved useful in certain clinical situations. The choice of dressings may also aid debridement by creating a moist wound environment promoting autolytic debridement, although this process may be slower than other methods. A number of dressing types are promoted as aiding the debridement process. At present, however, there is insubstantial evidence on which debridement method should be used. Patients with uncomplicated venous ulceration rarely require debridement, provided that optimum compression is being used, since compression creates the correct microenvironment for healing.

Compression therapy

Compression therapy is the deliberate application of pressure in order to produce a desired clinical effect.[9] This is usually achieved by appropriate bandaging or with elastic stockings. Graduated compression bandaging applies external pressure to the limb and, as a result:

- reduces the distension of superficial veins by counteracting high venous pressure[10]
- encourages and enhances blood flow velocity in the deep veins[11]
- partially restores venous valve function and reduces deep vein reflux[12,13]
- enhances lymphatic circulation both at skin level and within the deep, subfascial system[14,15]
- reduces edema by reducing the pressure difference between the capillaries and the tissues[16]
- may play a role in preventing neutrophil activation and the dissolution of fibrin cuffs[17,18]

- improves the condition of skin[19]
- provides comfort by reducing symptoms of venous disease, such as aching limbs and pain from the ulcer.[20]

Graduated compression therapy applied from toe to knee has been shown to heal between 40 and 80 percent of venous leg ulcers within 12 weeks.[21,22] The compression is graduated to apply higher pressure at the ankle and lower pressure below the knee in order to significantly increase venous return. The optimum pressure required to heal venous ulcers is still a matter of debate, but it is generally agreed that to promote ulcer healing a pressure of 30–40 mmHg compression should be applied at the ankle, reducing to 15–20 mmHg at the calf.[23] Ankle pressures of 40 mmHg have been shown to produce healing rates of 74 percent in 12 weeks.[24]

There are a number of principles which govern the application of graduated external compression to a limb. Compression should:

- be applied only after significant arterial disease has been ruled out and following an ankle brachial pressure index assessment
- always start at the distal end of the extremity and then continue proximally (towards the heart) (Fig. 13.1)
- be correctly applied to protect the limb from pressure damage
- stay in place until a dressing requires removal
- be used to treat uncomplicated venous ulcers and prevent ulcer recurrence.

The pressure exerted by a bandage depends on how much it has been stretched (the tension), the shape and size of the leg, and the number of layers applied. According to Laplace's

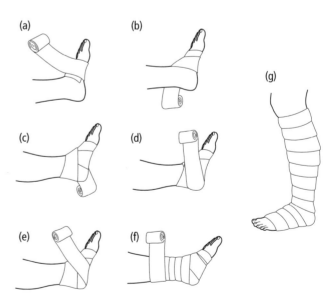

Figure 13.1 *The standard bandaging technique. Two important points: (1) enclose the heel; (2) each turn overlaps the previous turn by half its width.*

law, sub-bandage pressure is proportional to bandage tension and inversely proportional to the radius of the limb, i.e.:

Pressure = (tension × number of layers × constant)/(circumference of limbs × bandage width)

Considering each of these factors:

- Tension – bandage tension depends on the elasticity of the bandage; the tension is produced according to the stretch is applied on bandage application
- Layers of bandage – the more layers applied, the higher the sub-bandage pressure
- Limb radius – given a constant tension and number of layers along the leg, a bandage will produce a higher pressure on a small limb than on a large limb
- Bandage width – a narrow bandage applied at a constant tension with 50 percent overlap will produce a high pressure, as more layers are applied with a narrow bandage; generally a 10 cm bandage should be used on the lower limb.

BANDAGING

Classification of bandages

One of the major difficulties in describing compression systems relates to the classification systems in use.[25] Bandages are classified according to their response to stretching. At present, bandages are classified as highly extensible, minimally extensible or inextensible. Highly extensible bandages are those containing elastomeric fibres and are capable of exerting medium to very high pressure on the limb. Minimally extensible bandages are made of twisted fibres and are also known as inelastic or short stretch bandages. Inextensible bandages are made of woven fibres and are also known as non-elastic or inelastic bandages (Box 13.1). However, with the advent of multilayer systems, this classification system is inadequate to capture the combination

---

Box 13.1   Bandage classification.

Type 1 – conforming stretch, retention bandages
Type 2 – provide light support
Type 3 – compression bandages further differentiated according to the amount of ankle pressure they produce.
   – 3a: light compression, 14–17 mmHg ankle pressure
   – 3b: moderate compression, 18–24 mmHg ankle pressure
   – 3c: high compression, 25–35 mmHg ankle pressure
   – 3d: extra high compression, up to 60 mmHg ankle pressure

---

of bandages currently in use. For instance, the Charing Cross system of bandaging known as the four-layer system (Fig. 13.2) is described as an elastic system, although it contains bandages that are both highly extensible (layer 3) and minimally extensible (layer 4). In addition, the current classification does not adequately describe bandages with either a cohesive or adhesive property. Bandages are also divided into passive and active systems based on their properties. Active compression uses minimally extensible bandages which, when applied, produce a cuff around the lower limb. During exercise, a steep rise in sub-bandage pressure occurs, with low pressure when the patient is at rest. The term 'active' implies the ability of the bandage to work in conjunction with the patient to enhance effect. Passive compression involves the application of bandages with elastomeric fibres that sustain a more constant level of pressure irrespective of the patient's position or activity level.

The poor performance characteristics of type 1 bandages means that they provide no compression and are ineffective in the management of venous ulcers.[21] Table 13.1 identifies the range of bandages commonly used in the management of venous ulcers.

Multilayer bandage systems are used in various combinations in order to provide high compression. These include:

- two-layer regimen – consisting of a base layer of absorbent padding, and a compression layer (class 3c bandage, applied in a spiral)
- three-layer regimen – consisting of a first layer of absorbent padding, a second layer of class 3c bandage and a third layer of a tubular retaining bandage
- four-layer regimen – made up of a first layer of padding, a second layer of crepe bandage to smooth the first layer, a third layer of class 3a bandage applied in a figure of eight and a fourth layer of cohesive bandage applied in a spiral.

INELASTIC/SHORT STRETCH BANDAGES

These are inextensible bandages, which can be used to apply graduated compression. These systems are particularly popular in mainland Europe and are used in the treatment of venous and lymphatic disorders. They are made of cotton and applied to the limb at between 90 and 100 percent extension. Short stretch bandages form a firm 'skin' over the leg, and when the calf muscle contracts, the bandage cannot yield and the pressure under the bandage will increase. These bandages require the patient to be mobile and may be therapeutic by enhancing the action of the calf pump. They are frequently used as part of a two-layer bandage regimen. Short stretch bandages rapidly lose their pressure on application and with a reduction in edema will require regular re-application in the early stages of treatment. Examples of short stretch bandages include Comprilan and Rosidal K. These bandages have the advantage of being re-usable. Some inelastic bandages have the additional benefit of having a cohesive layer, preventing the problem of slippage, which is common with such products. An example of this type of product is Actico (Activa Health Care, Burton-on-Trent, UK).

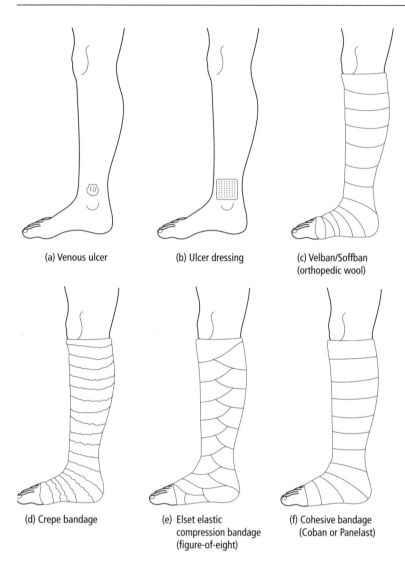

(a) Venous ulcer

(b) Ulcer dressing

(c) Velban/Soffban
(orthopedic wool)

(d) Crepe bandage

(e) Elset elastic
compression bandage
(figure-of-eight)

(f) Cohesive bandage
(Coban or Panelast)

Figure 13.2   *Four-layer bandaging.*

Table 13.1   *Bandages used in the management of venous ulcers*

Classification	Examples	Indication	Comments
Type 2: light support minimal stretch bandages	Elastocrepe Crepe K Lite	Prevention of edema Support in the management of sprains or strains	Support tissue without applying compression Rapid fall in pressure over first few hours of wear make them ineffective in venous ulcer management Can be used as part of a multilayer high compression system
Type 3a: light compression bandage (used in multilayer bandage systems)	K- Plus Elset Litepress	Treatment of mild varices, varices associated with pregnancy Leg ulcer prevention Mild-to-moderate edema management	Can be used alone or as part of a multilayer compression bandage system Application is in spiral or figure of eight
Type 3c: high-compression bandages	Tensopress Surepress	Treatment of severe varices Management and prevention of venous leg ulcers Treatment of post-thrombotic syndrome and gross edema	Sustained compression Can be washed and re-used Can be worn continuously for up to 1 week

COHESIVE BANDAGES

These are minimally extensible bandages which can be used to prevent bandage slippage when used over non-adhesive bandages. They are single-use bandages which sustain compression well and are used as part of a two-, three- or four-layer bandage system. Examples include Co-plus (Smith & Nephew Healthcare, Hull, UK) Coban (3M, Bracknell, UK) and Actico.

Bandage choice

High compression is more effective than low compression in healing venous ulcers. Low-compression bandages such as crepe lose between 40 and 60 percent of their tension within 20 min of application.[26] Dale et al.[27] showed that 30 min after application of an Elastocrepe bandage, pressure at the ankle fell from 44 to 36 mmHg. If the bandage was washed, the fall-off increased, dropping to 29 mmHg after 30 min, rendering it ineffective.

In a randomized controlled trial, Callam et al.[28] compared three-layer high-compression bandaging using Tensopress with inelastic compression using Elastocrepe in 132 patients with venous ulcers. Complete healing was achieved in 54 percent of the high-compression group at 12 weeks compared with 28 percent in the inelastic compression group. Duby et al.[22] also found that higher compression with either four-layer or short stretch bandaging resulted in higher healing rates. Forty-four percent of venous ulcers healed at 3 months compared with 23 percent of ulcers in the paste, elastocrepe and tubigrip group which provided lower compression.

Several types of high-compression systems are available. Two small trials compared the four-layer system with a single-layer compression bandage. No significant difference was found in healing between four-layer and the single adhesive layer.[29,30] However, in a larger trial, the four-layer system was shown to increase the healing rate of ulcers at 12 and 24 weeks, respectively, when compared with a single-layer compression bandage.[31,32] In a meta-analysis, healing rate using a four-layer system was more than twice that of a single-layer bandage.[33]

In another large randomized controlled trial, two four-layer bandage regimens were compared for their effectiveness in the healing of venous ulcers. The study compared the original 'Charing Cross' four-layer system with the newer Profore (Smith & Nephew) four-layer kit system.[34] After 12 weeks of treatment 65 percent of ulcers were healed using the original system compared with 79 percent using the Profore system. After completion at 24 weeks the difference had reduced to 82 percent using the original and 84 percent using the Profore system. The difference did not achieve statistical significance.

The most effective intervention for the treatment of venous ulcers is the provision of appropriate high-compression regimens. The evidence from randomized controlled trials suggests that systems using cotton crepe bandages alone are less effective than four-layer, short stretch and elastomeric three-layer systems. Multilayer systems appear to be more effective than single-layer systems, and there is little evidence

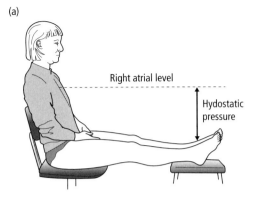

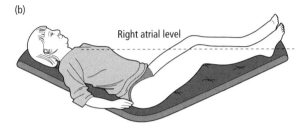

Figure 13.3   *Leg elevation: (a) the wrong way; (b) the right way.*

to recommend one high-compression regimen over another. Research has also highlighted that bandage application is often poor. Training in the correct use of compression is essential if these systems are to reach their full potential in clinical practice. The success of bandage systems such as the four-layer system has partly been due to their use in well organized services with adequate nurse supervision and access to specialist expertise.

Leg elevation

Patients being treated for venous ulceration by dressings and compression bandaging must be firmly advised to avoid prolonged standing and to rest with the leg well elevated as much as possible. Simply elevating the leg on a stool or chair (Fig. 13.3a) while sitting upright is both uncomfortable and ineffectual. The leg must be elevated to heart level by lying back on a sofa or bed so that the foot and ankle are at or above the level of the right atrium. The best designed piece of furniture for this purpose is a garden lounger (Fig. 13.3b). Patients' and nurses' cooperation can easily be achieved by a simple description of the hydrostatic pressures involved in venous return to the heart. Elevation and dressings can usually be carried out in the patient's home; admission to hospital is only necessary for the most severe ulcers or in unacceptable social conditions.

ULCER CLEANING AND DRESSING

Cleaning

The length of time between changes of dressings depends on the amount of exudate. The ulcer and surrounding skin should be cleaned before a new dressing is applied. Scaly surrounding skin, which may harbor bacteria, is gently cleaned away with a little light vegetable oil and the ulcer surface is gently cleaned. Care must be taken not to damage the delicate healing epithelium and strong antiseptic solutions must be avoided. In rabbit ear experiments, Leaper and Brennan[35] demonstrated that all antiseptics are toxic to fibroblasts and that hypochlorite solution causes capillary shutdown. Therefore, only sterile water or saline is used to clean the ulcer itself.

Dressings

There are a number of physiological and pathophysiological factors which inhibit wound healing, including:

- dry wound bed
- presence of devitalized tissue/slough
- presence of clinical infection
- poor blood supply
- poor nutrition
- venous hypertension.

Wound dressings are designed to keep the wound clean, free from contamination and to promote healing. Dressings are classified according to their properties and mode of action. The range of products available has increased in recent years, with a wide choice available in both hospital and community services.

Absorbent dressings
These dressings tend to have a drying effect, as they will absorb exudate from the wound. They should not be used directly on the surface of a moist wound as they will adhere to the wound, causing damage and pain on removal, [e.g. gauze, Surgipad (Johnson & Johnson Medical, Ascot, UK)].

Alginate dressings
Alginates are derived from seaweed. They react with exudate or blood to produce a strong viscous gel. Owing to their absorbent properties they are suitable for exuding wounds [e.g. Kaltostat (Convatec, Ickenhom, UK), Algisite M (Smith & Nephew)].

Antiseptic dressings
These include Inadine (J & J), which is a knitted viscose fabric impregnated with 10 percent povidine iodine. Iodine is rapidly inactivated in the presence of pus and serum exudate, therefore, medicinal effect of the iodine may be exhausted well before the dressing is changed.

Bead dressings
Examples are Iodosorb or Iodaflex (Smith & Nephew). These are cadexomer iodine dressings which have the advantage of reducing the number of organisms present in the wound. The iodine is absorbed systemically and should be used with care on patients with a history of thyroid disorders.

Charcoal and silver dressings
These dressings contain activated charcoal, which acts like a filter, absorbing odoriferous chemicals liberated from the wound before they pass to the air. Examples are Kaltocarb (Convatec) and Lyofoam C (SSL, London, UK). Actisorb Plus (Johnson & Johnson) also contains silver and is an adsorbent dressing (unsuitable as a primary wound contact layer), which can be used in addition to the primary dressing. A number of new products containing silver are now marketed, e.g. Acticoat (Smith & Nephew). It is believed that silver will reduce the bacterial burden within the wound and promote healing.

Foam dressings
These are hydrophilic, semi-occlusive dressings which provide a warm and moist environment. They are able to absorb significant volumes of exudate in some cases. Examples include Allevyn (Smith & Nephew) and Lyofoam Extra (SSL).

Hydrocolloid dressings
These occlusive dressings contain a hydrocolloid matrix. On contact with wound exudate, the hydrocolloid matrix absorbs water, swells and liquefies to form a moist gel [e.g. Granuflex, Duoderm, Combiderm (Convatec), and Comfeel (Coloplast, Peterborough, UK)].

Hydrogels
These consist of a starch polymer, such as carboxymethylcellulose, and up to 80 percent water. They have the ability to absorb wound exudate or rehydrate a wound depending on whether the wound is exuding heavily or dry and necrotic [e.g. Granugel (Convatec), Intrasite (Smith & Nephew)].

Low adherent
Several dressings fall into this category, including knitted viscose, wound contact layer [e.g. Tricotex (Smith & Nephew) or NA dressing (Johnson & Johnson)] (Fig. 13.4). These

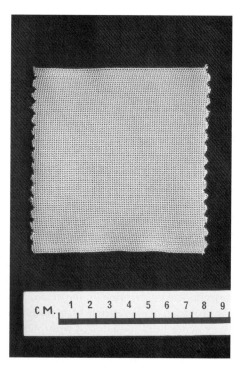

Figure 13.4 *Non-adhesive dry dressing (NA dressing) (sterile knitted viscose primary dressing, BP; Johnson & Johnson, Ascot, UK).*

dressings must be covered with an absorbent dressing (cotton gauze) to absorb exudate. Some low-adherent dressings are impregnated with silicone, e.g. NA ultra (Johnson & Johnson) and Mepitel (Mölnlycke, Dunstable, UK), which have superior non-adherent properties preventing wound trauma and pain.

Impregnated dressings

Made from cotton or cotton and viscose woven fabric, these have been impregnated with white soft paraffin [e.g. Jelonet (Smith & Nephew) or Paratulle (SSL)]. Although described as low adherent, they frequently become firmly attached to the wound surface. Epidermal cells and capillary loops can grow into the dressing, resulting in tissue damage, pain and interference with healing. A number of tulles containing antiseptics and antibiotics are available but are not recommended for use in treating venous ulceration.

Semi-permeable film dressings

These are transparent, vapour-permeable film dressings [e.g. Opsite Flexigrid (Smith & Nephew), Tegaderm (3M)]. They are useful for superficial wounds and are not generally used in the management of leg ulcers.

Zinc impregnated dressings

These are open weave bandages with medicated paste which act as a buffer between fragile inflamed skin and a compression bandage [e.g. Steripaste (Medloch Medical, Oldham, UK), Zipzoc and Viscopaste PB7 (Smith & Nephew)]. Patients may become sensitive to some of the constituents, e.g. parabens and lanolin (Plate 13.1). These constituents have been removed from both Steripaste and Zipzoc in order to reduce sensitivity reactions. This type can be useful for mild dermatitis and lichenification. Other types of paste bandage incorporate other medicaments, such as ichthammol and calamine, which are now used infrequently.

EVIDENCE ON THE USE OF DRESSINGS IN VENOUS ULCERATION

Alginates

Stacey et al.[36] carried out a randomized controlled trial which included 113 patients with venous ulcers. Patients received either zinc paste bandage and alginate or zinc stockinette and alginate. The groups received similar compression systems in the form of two elastocrepe bandages and a layer of tubigrip. They reported 20 percent more ulcer healing under paste bandage than with the alginate. Alginate against zinc stockinette found no difference in the proportion of ulcers healed over the trial period. However, the choice of compression in this trial is less than optimal to achieve healing. Moffatt et al.[37] also evaluated an alginate (Tegagel; 3M) in a randomized controlled trial involving 60 patients compared with a low-adherent dressing (NA dressing; Johnson & Johnson) as the control. All patients received the standard four-layer high-compression bandage, and only patients with ulcers less than 10 cm^2 were included in this study. No significant difference in healing rates was observed; it was equally high in both groups: 80 percent complete healing at 12 weeks in the NA dressing group and 87 percent complete healing at 12 weeks in the Tegagel dressing group.

Foam dressings

In one trial, Pessenhoffer and Stangl[38] compared a foam dressing with traditional sterile gauze compress in 48 patients with venous ulcers. They reported a reduction in wound area with the foam dressing compared with an increase in the mean wound size under the sterile gauze compress. Callam et al.[21] evaluated the effectiveness of a foam dressing (Allevyn) compared with a low-adherent dressing (Tricotex) in 113 patients with venous ulcers. At the end of 12 weeks, 47 percent of ulcers in the Allevyn group were completely healed compared with 35 percent in the Tricotex group. The difference, however, did not reach statistical significance.

Zinc impregnated dressings

In the study described above, Stacey et al.[36] compared a zinc oxide stockinette with a zinc oxide cotton gauze bandage. Patients receiving the paste bandage fared significantly better than those receiving the stockinette. Complete healing was achieved in 60 percent of patients at 3 months, compared with 50 percent of the stockinette group. The reason for the difference in these results is likely to be due to the effect of the paste bandage, which is able to offer a degree of compression compared with the stockinette.

Hydrogels

Gibson[39] made a comparison of two hydrogels (Granugel and Intrasite) in a study of 62 patients with leg ulcers. Outcome measures were a reduction in wound area and a reduction in slough area. The trial found no statistical difference between the two groups after 3 weeks.

Hydrocolloid dressings

Each hydrocolloid differs in composition and construction. Their performance can vary according to the structure. They are generally regarded as impermeable to gases, including water vapour. The pH of wounds have been found to be more acidic under a hydrocolloid, which may have an inhibiting effect on the growth of some bacteria. The pectin present within some hydrocolloids is thought to have a fibrinolytic effect to reduce the diffusion barrier to O_2 and nutrients in patients presenting with lipodermatosclerosis. Amery et al.[40] found that hydrocolloids induce the growth of new blood vessels (angiogenesis). The effectiveness of hydrocolloid dressings versus several other therapies for venous leg ulcer management has been examined in several randomized controlled trials.[41–44] Whilst there was some evidence of benefit of hydrocolloids over simple dressings, only one trial achieved statistical significance,[42] although this could be explained by substantial differences in ulcer size between the groups at baseline.

At present there is little evidence that dressings enhance the healing of venous ulceration, provided that compression is applied. However, the wrong selection of dressing may significantly delay healing if factors such as exudate are not appropriately managed. Patient factors such as wound pain may also be significantly reduced by choosing a product that creates a moist wound environment. Comparisons between hydrocolloids, alginates, hydrogels, foams and low-adherent dressings have failed to show that any product is more effective than the rest. In one trial, which compared a zinc paste bandage with an alginate, the zinc bandage was more effective at ulcer healing.[37] This result may be more attributable to the greater level of compression beneath the paste bandage, reiterating the greater therapeutic role of compression in ulcer healing. Many of the studies providing evidence on the effectiveness of treatment lacked methodological rigour. Sample sizes were too small to detect significance and, in some cases, baseline comparability of groups was poor, leading to bias. A standardized objective end-point would aid comparison as well as a complete description of concurrent treatment regimes, which was lacking in some cases.

ADJUNCTIVE THERAPIES

Whilst bandages and dressings offer the main source of treatment for venous ulceration, there are a number of other therapies which have been advocated for use in conjunction with these.

Ultrasound

Ultrasound has received little attention as an adjunct to compression therapy in venous ulceration. A randomized controlled trial of 24 patients treated with ultrasound found greater percentage reductions in area in the treated group compared with the controls (55.4 vs. 16.5 percent, $P < 0.007$), both groups receiving elastic compression.[45] A similar study of 38 patients showed similar reductions in area after 8 weeks (41 vs. 11 percent, $P < 0.05$)[46]. It would appear that ultrasound may be beneficial to patients with venous ulceration, although the cost-effectiveness of this procedure has still to be evaluated.

Intermittent pneumatic therapy

The use of intermittent pneumatic therapy is attractive, since it attempts to mimic the calf muscle pump performance by applying external compression to the affected limb. One possible limitation is the requirement for long periods of intermittent pneumatic compression (IPC). In a trial of 21 patients treated 4 h/day, 10 (42 percent) healed completely, compared with just 1/24 (4 percent) in the control group.[47] A further study has examined the use of IPC 3 h/day over 6 months, and demonstrated higher healing rates (76 vs. 64 percent) than with the Unna boot.[48] However, both of these studies are small, and require more extensive research to demonstrate clinical effectiveness in terms of ulcer healing and the necessary protocol for the treatment regimen.

Hyperbaric oxygen

The value of hyperbaric oxygen in chronic wounds including venous ulceration has been considered for decades, although there is a dearth of objective randomized trials in this area. Whilst there is some evidence of benefit in patients with diabetic foot ulceration, the information on patients with chronic venous ulceration is largely limited to case studies.

Laser therapy

The Cochrane Review of laser therapy in venous ulcer healing identified four randomized controlled trials in relation to complete healing of the ulceration.[49] Two trials compared laser with a sham,[50,51] one with ultraviolet therapy[52] and one with unpolarized red light.[53] The results suggested that there was no evidence of a significant effect of laser therapy on venous ulcer healing.

Other therapies

In recent years there have been a number of other adjunct therapies for use in wound healing. Vacuum-assisted closure and warming therapy may offer benefits in terms of accelerated closure of venous ulcers, but these techniques have not been subjected to randomized clinical trials.

Adjunctive therapies may benefit patients in accelerating healing beyond that experienced using high-compression therapy alone. Again the frequency of therapy usage must be balanced within a cost-effectiveness assessment to ensure that quality care is given for an appropriate benefit.

DISCUSSION

The treatment of venous ulceration should not be seen in isolation, but as part of the holistic approach to patient assessment, diagnosis and care of all patients with chronic leg ulceration. It is outside the remit of this chapter to describe the overall management of patients with leg ulceration, although a number of issues must be addressed to ensure the appropriate treatment of patients. It is recommended that the patient's care should be incorporated into appropriate guidelines. There are a number of guidelines available on the management of patients with leg ulceration, such as those produced by the Royal College of Nursing in the UK.[3] However, the production of guidelines will not improve practice in itself. Recent work has demonstrated that the availability of guidelines and clinical nurse education do not in themselves produce tangible improvements in patient outcomes. The issue of implementation of evidence-based guidelines will be the major challenge over the next decade, as we strive to improve patient care whilst providing cost-effective treatment, and improve patients' quality of life.

REFERENCES

1. Nelzen O, Bergqvist D, Lindhagen A. Leg ulcer etiology – a cross sectional population study. *J Vascular Surg* 1991; **14**: 557–64.
2. Moffatt CJ, Franks PJ, Oldroyd M *et al.* Community clinics for leg ulcers and impact on healing. *Br Med J* 1992; **305**: 1389–92.
3. Clinical Practice Guidelines. *The Management of Patients with Venous Ulcers.* London: Royal College of Nursing, 1998.
4. Moffatt CJ, Doherty DC. Franks. Community based leg ulcer classification and its relationship to healing. *Int Angiol* 2001; **20**(Suppl. 1): 291.
5. Morison M, Moffatt CJ. *A Colour Guide to the Assessment and Management of Leg Ulcers*, 2nd edn. London: Mosby, 1994.
6. Falanga V. Classifications for wound bed preparation and stimulation of chronic wounds. *Wound Repair Regen* 2000; **8**: 347–52.
7. Krasner DL. How to prepare the wound bed. *Ostomy Wound Manage* 2001; **47**: 59–61.
8. Bergstrom N, Bennett MA, Carlson CE *et al. Treatment of Pressure Ulcers. Clinical Practice Guideline, No. 15.* Rockville, MD: US Department of Health and Human Services. Public Health Service, Agency for Health Care Policy and Research, 1994.
9. Thomas S. Bandages and bandaging the science behind the art. *Care Sci Prac* 1990; **8**: 56–60.
10. Sigg K. Compression with compression bandages and elastic stockings for prophylaxis and therapy of venous disorders of the leg. *Fortchrifthiche Med* 1963; **15**: 601–6.
11. Sigel B, Edelstein AL, Savitch L *et al.* Types of compression for reducing venous stasis. *Arch Surg* 1975; **110**: 171–5.
12. Sarin S, Scurr JH, Coleridge-Smith PD. *Mechanisms of Action of External Compression in Venous Disease.* In: Raymond Martinbeau P, Prescott R, Zummond M, eds. *Phlebology.* Paris: John Libbey, 1992.
13. Partsch H. *Kontrolle Therapeutischer Effekte im Bereich der Venosan Stranbahn Mittels Doppler-Ultrashalll.* In: Hild H, Spanng, eds. *Therapiekontrolle in der Angiologie.* Baden-Baden: Wirtzstock, 1979; 437–41.
14. Bollinger A, Junger M, Jager K. Fluorescence video microscopy techniques for the evaluation of human skin microcirculatin. *Prog Appl Microcirc* 1986; **11**: 77–9.
15. Partsch H, Lofferer O, Mostbeck A. Zur Beurteilung der Lymph und Venenzirkulation am bein mit und ohme Kompression. In: Zeitler E, ed. *Diagnostik Mit Isotopen bei Arteriellen und Venosan, Durchblutung-Sstorungen der Extremitaten. Akt Probl Angiol 19.* Wien: Huber, 1973.
16. Fentem PH. Defining the compression provided by hosiery and bandages. *Care Sci Prac* 1990; **8**: 53–5.
17. Coleridge-Smith PD. The role of leucocytes in venous ulceration. In: Negus D, Jantet G, Coleridge Smith PD eds. *Phlebology, Suppl. 1*, 1995; 125–7.
18. Burnand K, Clemenson G, Morland M. Venous lipodermatosclerosis: treatment by fibrinolytic enhancement and elastic compression. *Br Med J* 1980; **280**: 7–11.
19. Vin F. The physiology of compression: clinical consequences, precautions and contra-indications. In: Negus D, Janet G, Coleridge-Smith PD, eds. *Phlebology '95. Proceedings of the XII World Congress Union Internationale de Phlebologie 2.* Berlin: Springer Verlag, 1995; 1134–7.
20. Moffatt CJ, Harper P. *Access to Clinical Education: Leg Ulcers.* London: Churchill Livingstone, 1997.
21. Callam MJ, Dale JJ, Ruckley CV, Harper DR. Lothian and Forth Valley leg ulcer healing trial-part 2: knitted viscose dressing versus a hydrocolloid dressing in the treatment of chronic leg ulceration. *Phlebology* 1992; **7**: 142–5.
22. Duby T, Cherry G, Hoffman D *et al.* A randomised trial in the treatment of venous leg ulcers comparing short stretch bandages, four-layer bandage system, and a long stretch paste bandage system. *Wounds: A Compendium of Clinical Research and Practice* 1993; **5**: 276–9.
23. Stemmer R. Ambulatory elasto-compressive treatment of the lower extremeties particularly with compression stockings. *Kassenartz* 1969; **9**: 1–8.
24. Blair SD, Wright DDI, Backhouse CM *et al.* Sustained compression and healing of chronic venous ulcers. *Br Med J* 1988; **297**: 1159–61.
25. Thomas SL, Wilde G, Loveless P. Performance profiles of extensible bandages *Phlebology* 1986; **226**: 667–70.
26. Tennant W, Park K, Ruckley CV. Testing compression bandages. *Phlebology* 1988; **3**: 55–61.
27. Dale J, Callam M, Ruckley CV. How efficient is a compression bandage? *Nurs Times* 1983; **79**: 49–51.
28. Callam MJ, Harper DR, Dale JJ *et al.* Lothian & Forth Valley Leg Ulcer healing Trial, Part 1. Elastic versus non-elastic bandaging in the treatment of chronic leg ulceration. *Phlebology* 1992; **7**: 136–41.
29. Kralj B, Kosicek M. A randomised comparative trial of single layer and multi layer bandages in the treatment of venous ulcers. In: Cherry GW, Gottrup F, Lawrence JC *et al. Proceedings of the Conference of the European Wound Management Association.* London: Macmillan Magazines, 1996; 158–60.
30. Travers J, Dalziel K, Makin G. Assessment of a new one layer adhesive bandaging method in maintaining prolonged limb compression and effects on ulcer healing. *Phlebology* 1992; **7**: 59–63.
31. Nelson E, Harper D, Ruckley C *et al.* A randomised trial of single layer and multi-layer bandages in the treatment of chronic venous ulceration. *Phlebology* 1996(Suppl. 1); **1**: 915–6.
32. Colgan M, Teevan M, McBride C *et al.* Cost comparisons in the management of venous ulceration. In: Cherry GW, Gottrup F, Lawrence JC *et al. Proceedings of the 5th European Conference on Advances in Wound Management.* London: Macmillan Magazines, 1996; 8.
33. Fletcher A, Cullum N, Sheldon T. A systematic review of compression therapy for venous ulcers. *Br Med J* 1997; **315**: 576–80.
34. Moffatt CJ, Simon DA, Franks PJ *et al.* Randomised trial comparing two four layer bandage systems in the management of chronic leg ulceration. *Phlebology* 1999; **14**: 139–42.
35. Leaper DJ, Brennan SS. *Let's Have a Rethink About the Use of Antiseptics for Venous Ulcers.* In: Negus D, Jantet G, eds. Phlebology '85. London: Libbey, 1986; 580–3.
36. Stacey MC, Jopp-McKay AG, Rashid P *et al.* The influence of dressings on venous ulcer healing. In: Cherry GW, Gottrup F, Lawrence JC *et al. Proceedings of the 1st European Conference on Advances in Wound Management. Cardiff, UK.* London: Macmillan Magazines, 1992; 145–6.
37. Moffatt CJ, Oldroyd MI, Franks PJ. Assessing a calcium alginate dressing for venous ulcers of the leg. *J Wound Care* 1992; **1**: 22–4.
38. Pessenhofer H, Stangl M. The effect of a two-layered polyurethane foam wound dressing on the healing of venous leg ulcers. *J Tissue Viability* 1992; **2**: 57–61.

39. Gibson B. A cost effectiveness comparison of two gels in the treatment of sloughy leg ulcers. *Advanced Wound Care Symposium, San Diego, USA*. King of Prussia: Health Management Publications, 1995.

40. Amery M, Ryan T, Cherry G. Successful treatment of venous ulcers with a new hydrocolloid dressing – passive or active in wound healing. *Phlebology*. London: Libbey, 1986.

41. Backhouse CM, Blair SD, Savage AP *et al*. Controlled trial of occlusive dressings in healing in chronic venous. *Br J Surg* 1987; **47**: 626–7.

42. Meredith K, Gray E. Dressed to heal. *J Distr Nurs* 1988; **7**: 8–10.

43. Moffatt CJ, Oldroyd MI, Dickson D. A trial of hydrocolloid dressing in the management of indolent ulceration. *J Wound Care* 1992; **1**: 20–2.

44. Bowszyc J, Silny W, Bowszyc-Dmochowska M *et al*. A randomised controlled comparative clinical trial of Lyofoam versus Granuflex in the treatment of venous leg ulcers. In: Harding KG, Dealey C, Cherry G, Gottrup F, eds. *Proceedings of the 3rd European Conference on Advances in Wound Management*. London: Macmillan Magazines, 1994. 34–7.

45. Peschen M, Weichenthal M, Schopf E, Vanscheidt W. Low frequency ultrasound treatment of chronic venous leg ulcers in an outpatient therapy. *Acta Dermatol Venereol (Stockh)* 1997; **77**: 311–4.

46. Weichenthal M, Mohr P, Stegmann W, Breitbart EW. Low frequency ultrasound treatment of chronic venous ulcers. *Wound Repair Regen* 1997; **5**: 18–22.

47. Colerdge Smith P, Sarin S, Hasty J, Scurr JH. Sequential gradient pneumatic compression enhances venous ulcer healing: a randomised controlled trial. *Surgery* 1990; **108**: 971–5.

48. Schuler JJ, Maibenco T, Megerman J *et al*. Treatment of chronic venous ulcers using sequential gradient intermittent pneumatic compression. *Phlebology* 1996; **11**: 111–4.

49. Flemming KA, Cullum NA, Nelson EA. A systematic review of laser therapy for venous leg ulcers. *J Wound Care* 1999; **8**: 111–4.

50. Lundeberg T, Malm M. Low power HeNe laser treatment of venous leg ulcers. *Ann Plastic Surg* 1991; **27**: 537–9.

51. Malm M, Lundeberg T. Effect of low power gallium arsenide laser on healing of venous ulcers. *Scand J Plastic Reconstr Surg Hand Surgery* 1991; **25**: 249–51.

52. Crous L, Malherbe C. Laser and ultraviolet light irradiation in the treatment of chronic ulcers. *Physiotherapy* 1988; **44**: 73–7.

53. Bihari I, Mester AR. The biostimulative effect of low level laser therapy of long standing crural ulcers using helium neon laser, helium neon plus infrared lasers and non coherent light: preliminary report of a randomised double blind comparative study. *Laser Ther* 1989; **1**: 97–8.

14

Skin grafting of venous ulcers

PHILIP D. COLERIDGE SMITH

INTRODUCTION

In the majority of cases, venous ulcers can be managed by complete investigation, surgical intervention to treat incompetent superficial veins and perforating veins where appropriate, and compression bandaging. In a number of cases, these measures may fail to heal the ulcer or ulcer healing may be very slow. There are a number of reasons for this. Patients with very large or long-standing ulcers are the most difficult to heal and, with the progression of time, increasing age and immobility may prove resistant to conventional treatment. In patients with coexisting venous and arterial disease, it may not be possible to use the highest levels of compression because of the risk of causing skin necrosis of bony prominences. In these cases, skin grafting or vascular flaps may be considered. This subject has been recently reviewed in the Cochrane Database.[1]

A number of techniques are available to achieve complete cover of the ulcer with new skin. The most frequently used method is to take an autograft such as a pinch graft, split-thickness skin graft, full-thickness skin graft, a pedicle graft or free vascular graft. Cultured autologous keratinocytes have also been used. Allografts of cultured keratinocytes or cultured epidermal fibroblasts avoid the need to harvest the graft from the patient, offering much greater convenience for both surgeon and patient. Xenografts, usually of porcine origin, have been employed.

More recently, artificial skin such as Apligraf (see p. 128) has been used. This comprises bovine collagen and contains human keratinocytes and fibroblasts obtained from donor skin. This graft is cultured in the laboratory so that the keratinocytes form a surface layer equivalent to the epidermis.[2]

METHODS OF SKIN GRAFTING

Pinch grafting

This type of graft is formed by lifting the donor site with a needle and cutting a 3–5 mm diameter disk of skin with a scalpel blade (Fig. 14.1). The donor site heals in 1 or 2 weeks, or can be excised and sutured. Usually several grafts are taken in order to cover a substantial proportion of the ulcer base. Healing takes place from the islands that these form within the base of the ulcer. Poskitt *et al.*[3] have used this technique in a clinical trial to compare the healing rate of leg ulcers treated

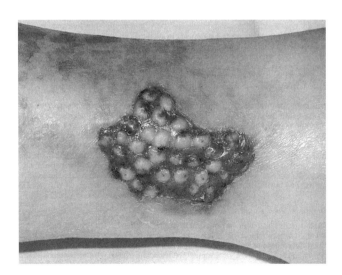

Figure 14.1 *Skin grafting: pinch grafts on a leg ulcer 3 weeks postoperatively.*

by pinch grafting with that obtained by grafting with a porcine xenograft. They randomized 25 ulcers to pinch graft treatment and 28 to treatment with the xenograft. The healing rate in the pinch graft group was 15 cm^2 per week and in the xenograft group was 3.5 cm^2 per week. By 12 weeks 74 percent of ulcers were healing in the pinch graft group compared with 46 percent in the porcine group.

Split-skin grafting

In this technique, donor skin is cut with a grafting knife which removes a thin layer comprising the epidermis and upper layers of the dermis. The donor area heals from the epidermis remaining in the skin adnexae (sweat glands and hair follicles) over a period of about 2 weeks. The harvested skin is very thin but contains a layer of healthy epidermis. It may be meshed to expand its area of coverage and to permit wound exudate to escape from beneath the graft. The ulcer should be clean and granulating before the application of the graft. An alternative strategy is to excise the ulcer, removing liposclerotic skin before applying the graft.

Warburg used skin grafting in addition to excision of the ulcer and perforating vein ligation in a study which contained a control group that received neither surgery nor skin grafting. He found that split-skin grafting achieved more rapid healing than was obtained in the control group. Perforating vein ligation achieved no further benefit after a 12-month follow-up period.

Schmeller et al.[4] reported a variation of this treatment commonly used in German-speaking countries, referred to as 'shave therapy'. The treatment involves resecting the ulcer and all diseased tissue using a skin grafting knife repeatedly to remove the tissue in layers until healthy tissue is exposed. Meshed split-skin graft is then applied to the resected area. The advantage of this method is that the resulting wound is more aesthetically contoured than would be the case if the ulcer was simply excised with a scalpel. Schmeller et al. reported an 88 percent long-term healing rate after a follow-up of 2.7 years. They have subsequently reported normalization of the magnetic resonance imaging appearance of muscle and fascia of the calf in patients treated in this way,[5] implying that if the diseased tissue can be removed and healing achieved, the edema and other inflammatory processes subside.

Free tissue transfer

A more radical approach to replacing the skin in patients with leg ulceration is to use a free tissue transfer technique. The donor skin is derived from an anatomical location where muscle, fat and skin can be obtained with a vascular pedicle that can be attached to the posterior tibial or other crural vessels. Most frequently, a latissimus dorsi or rectus abdominis flap has been used for this purpose. The donor tissue is carefully harvested whilst preserving its vascular pedicle. Meanwhile, the ulcer and all liposclerotic tissue are excised.

The donor flap vessels are anastomosed to the leg vessels using an end-to-side anastomosis. This technique is reserved for young patients troubled by extensive ulceration which is resistant to conventional treatment. A number of clinical series have been reported.[6–8] The most recently published paper records the outcome in 22 patients receiving 25 free flap procedures with a mean area of 237 cm^2 after excision of the diseased skin.[8] Twenty-one patients had been followed up for 5 years and no ulcer had occurred in the region of the flap. Three patients had new ulcers in the treated leg. The transferred skin appears to be protected against venous ulceration, at least for the first 5 years. This method has proven useful in cases where other forms of skin grafting have failed and the ulcer is causing considerable morbidity.

Allografts

The outcome of a clinical trial using 'Apligraf' (Organogenesis Inc., Canton, MA, USA) is a synthetic 'skin' which contains both the cellular elements of the epidermis and dermis. Falanga et al.[2] has used this in a randomized trial comparing patients treated with Apligraf with those treated with standard dressings. He entered 309 patients and evaluated 275 for efficacy of the treatment. In the active treatment group, 92/146 patients healed their ulcer, compared with 63/129 in the control group. In essence, a healing rate of 40 percent was improved to 60 percent by the use of this treatment, representing a modest influence on wound healing.

In other studies, cryopreserved or fresh keratinocytes have been applied to the ulcer in order to achieve healing.[9–11] These trials included relatively few patients (a total of 92 patients over all three studies) and found no evidence of any influence on wound healing.

THE ROLE OF SKIN GRAFTING

The evidence from many studies shows that when managed appropriately using well-established techniques, including standard wound management, dressings and compression, leg ulcers will heal in the majority of patients within 4–6 months. A substantial proportion of patients have incompetent superficial and perforating veins which may benefit from superficial venous surgery. The ESCHAR study has demonstrated that treatment of superficial venous reflux does not lead to an acceleration in wound healing, but does prevent recurrence once ulcers have healed.[12] Sustained healing of ulcers may also be achieved where patients can be persuaded to wear medical compression stockings following ulcer healing.

In a proportion of patients, leg ulcers are resistant to these standard measures and skin grafting can be considered as a method of increasing the likelihood of obtaining healing. This is most likely to occur in large or long-standing ulcers. However, some patients seem especially resistant to conventional compression treatment and their ulcers remain unhealed.

Skin grafting may help considerably in speeding the resolution of the ulcer in these patients. The most simple measure is to undertake pinch grafting. This may be achieved simply in the outpatient clinic under local anesthesia. A few grafts carefully placed and secured in the ulcer base may act as foci of healing.

The use of tissue-engineered skin is an alternative to using pinch grafts. These materials avoid the need to make further incisions in the patient's skin remote from the region of ulceration. However, the costs of these grafts is considerable and the current generation of grafts have to be stored in a frozen state until used. Hence, handling the grafts requires additional facilities in leg ulcer clinics. A modest acceleration in wound healing can be expected following this treatment.

The combination of ulcer excision and split-skin grafting usually requires general or regional anesthesia but may be more effective than simple skin grafting. Excision of liposclerotic skin may seem a rather radical step to take, but in a clinical series this has been found effective in achieving healing. The cosmetic results of this are likely to be inelegant but many patients will be grateful for relief of pain and other symptoms attributable to their ulcer. The 'shave' type excision using a skin grafting knife as reported by Schmeller et al.[4] may offer a slightly more aesthetic outcome whilst maintaining clinical efficacy. However, no clinical trials have been conducted with sufficient rigor to confirm the efficacy of these techniques compared with control treatment.

A small group of patients are especially troubled by their ulcers. Usually of a younger age group with ulcers that fail to heal despite all interventions, this group may benefit from free tissue transfer. The surgical procedures to achieve a successful outcome are complex and protracted, usually being carried out by a plastic surgical team. There is a risk of failure of the graft because of the need to create a vascular anastomosis between the graft and native vessels. Postoperative monitoring and care of the transferred tissue require special skills from the staff of a plastic surgery department. Elderly patients would probably not benefit from such treatment to the same extent as younger patients. The long-term outcome from successful grafting of this type seems to be good. The transferred tissue usually remains free from lipodermatosclerosis and is not usually the site of recurrent ulceration. The cosmetic result of these operations is likely to be imperfect, but in a young patient this is likely to be preferable to the consequences of an open ulcer.

In conclusion, a number of skin grafting techniques are available and can be used to achieve healing of leg ulcers where conventional measures have failed.

REFERENCES

1. Jones JE, Nelson EA. Skin grafting for venous leg ulcers (Cochrane Review). In: *The Cochrane Library, Issue 3*. Chichester: John Wiley, 2004.
2. Falanga V, Margolis D, Alvarez O *et al*. Rapid healing of venous ulcers and lack of clinical rejection with an allogeneic cultured human skin equivalent. *Arch Dermatol* 1998; **134**: 293–300.
3. Poskitt K, James A, Lloyd-Davies E *et al*. Pinch skin grafting or porcine dermis in venous ulcers: a randomised clinical trial. *Br Med J* 1987; **294**: 674–6.
4. Schmeller W, Gaber Y, Gehl HB. Shave therapy is a simple, effective treatment of persistent venous leg ulcers. *J Am Acad Dermatol* 1998; **39**: 232–8.
5. Gaber Y, Gehl HB, Schmeller W. Changes of fascia and muscles before and 12 months after successful treatment of recalcitrant venous leg ulcers by shave therapy. *Vasa* 2003; **32**: 205–8.
6. Dunn RM, Fudem GM, Walton RL *et al*. Free flap valvular transplantation for refractory venous ulceration. *J Vasc Surg* 1994; **19**: 525–31.
7. Weinzweig N, Schuler J. Free tissue transfer in treatment of the recalcitrant chronic venous ulcer. *Ann Plast Surg* 1997; **38**: 611–9.
8. Kumins NH, Weinzweig N, Schuler JJ. Free tissue transfer provides durable treatment for large nonhealing venous ulcers. *J Vasc Surg* 2000; **32**: 848–54.
9. Duhra P, Blight A, Mountford E *et al*. A randomized controlled trial of cultured keratinocyte allografts for chronic venous ulcers. *J Dermatol Treatment* 1992; **3**: 189–91.
10. Lindgren C, Marcusson J, Toftgard R. Treatment of venous leg ulcers with cryopreserved cultured allogeneic keratinocytes: a prospective open controlled study. *Br J Dermatol* 1998; **139**: 271–5.
11. Teepe R, Roseeuw D, Hermans J *et al*. Randomized trial comparing cryopreserved cultured epidermal allografts with hydrocolloid dressings in healing chronic venous ulcers. *J Am Acad Dermatol* 1993; **29**: 982–8.
12. Barwell JR, Davies CE, Deacon J *et al*. Comparison of surgery and compression with compression alone in chronic venous ulceration (ESCHAR study): randomised controlled trial. *Lancet* 2004; **363**: 1854–9.

15

Surgical treatment of superficial venous incompetence: surgery of the saphenous veins

PHILIPP A. STALDER, DAVID C. BERRIDGE

DEFINITION AND CLASSIFICATION

Although varicose veins are easily recognizable, there are a number of different definitions. Arnoldi[1] defined varicose veins as any dilated, elongated or tortuous vein, irrespective of size. The World Health Organisation (WHO) classification defines varicose veins as a 'saccular dilatation of the veins which are often tortuous'.[2] The 1978 Basle Study, an epidemiological study on 4529 healthy employees of pharmaceutical companies, separated varicose veins into trunk varicosities (dilated tortuous trunks of the long or small saphenous vein and/or their tributaries), reticular veins (dilated tortuous subcutaneous veins, not belonging to the main trunk or tributaries) and hyphenwebs (intradermal vein ectasias).[3] The CEAP classification (see Box 6.1, p. 46) was an attempt to classify chronic venous disease, based on clinical, etiologic, anatomic, and pathophysiologic data.[4,5] Whilst it may have a number of flaws, it is nevertheless a useful comparative guide for venous interventions and outcomes.

INCIDENCE

Varicose veins are common. The Edinburgh Vein Study[6] examined 1566 randomly selected men and women aged 18–64 years. Forty percent of the men and 32 percent of the women had trunk varices, whereas more than 80 percent had mild hyphenwebs and reticular varices.

The Basle Study[3] also found varicose veins to be more common in men than in women: 4529 chemical workers were examined, and 5.2 percent of the men and 3.2 percent of the women had severe varicose veins. It was shown that 10 percent of the population between 25 and 34 years had varicose veins, while 50 percent of those between 64 and 75 years had varices.

Beaglehole et al.[7] examined the Maori population in New Zealand in 1976: he found an incidence of 21.5 percent in men and 40.4 percent in women. A survey in Finland, examining 8000 people aged 30 years and over, found 25 percent of women and 7 percent of men having varicose veins diagnosed by a physician.[8] National Surveys in the past in the USA, UK, Denmark and Canada reported incidences of varicose veins of around 2.25 percent, with more women affected than men.[9–12] However, these were carried out by untrained personnel by questionnaire and probably underestimate the prevalence. The San Valentino Vascular Screening Project in Italy screened 30 000 subjects in a real whole-population study with clinical assessment and duplex scanning. The global prevalence was 7 percent.[13] A survey of schoolchildren aged 10–12 years in Germany found 12 percent saphenofemoral junction (SFJ) incompetence, but no associated varicose veins. Eight to 10 years later, aged 20 years, 20 percent had reflux and 8 percent had varicose veins.[14,15]

ETIOLOGY

There are two main theories: first, that varicose veins are caused by incompetent valves; and second, that the walls of the veins are defective, leading to a secondary widening and incompetence of the valves. Traditionally, it was thought that a major proximal valve, e.g. the SFJ, became incompetent, which would then subject the more distal valves in succession from proximal to distal to become incompetent. However, increasingly we have become aware that varicose veins can occur in association with great saphenous segmental reflux with no actual SFJ incompetence. Biochemical abnormalities might contribute to the weakening of the wall. Similarly, an inherited collagen/smooth muscle defect may be the initiating event.

The end-point is an incompetence from deep to superficial venous system. Clinically, the most important sites of reflux are SFJ (53–82 percent),[16–18] the saphenopopliteal junction (20–29 percent),[17,19,20] incompetent perforating veins (35 percent)[17] and non-saphenofemoral reflux (i.e. reflux in veins that are not part of the saphenous veins, e.g. from the pelvis and abdominal wall) in about 10 percent.[21–23]

SYMPTOMS

The most common symptoms include heaviness, aching and swelling, but these are non-specific and are also found in subjects without varicose veins. In an international survey by Kurz et al.,[24] 85.8 percent of patients with varicose veins reported at least one of these symptoms, but 76.1 percent also complained of this in the control group. Of the patients with varicose veins, 34.8 percent had varicose veins alone, whereas 65.2 percent of patients had concomitant venous disease: 11.9 percent had varicose veins with edema, 40.9 percent had varicose veins with skin changes, 9.5 percent had a healed ulcer and 2.9 percent had an active ulcer.

When quality of life was assessed in these patients, an impairment in physical quality of life was associated with concomitant disease, rather than the presence of varicose veins per se.[24]

Other authors, who included patients with varicose veins without ulcers, demonstrated that varicose veins per se significantly affect patients' quality of life.[25] Overall symptoms improved significantly after an operation when assessed pre- and postoperatively with a health assessment questionnaire.[26]

TREATMENT

Treatment should aim to reduce symptoms, provide a good cosmetic result, prevent complications, such as skin changes, edema, venous ulcerations, superficial thrombophlebitis and external bleeding, and minimize recurrence. Options for treatment include compression therapy, sclerotherapy and surgical treatment, which will be discussed here. Newer methods of potential surgical treatment, including transilluminated powered phlebectomy (TriVex), endovenous heat ablation (VNUS-closure) and laser great saphenous vein (GSV) occlusion will be discussed in subsequent Chapters 16.

The decision whether to operate or treat conservatively is made after a thorough history and clinical examination using hand-held Doppler. Our unit routinely performs venous duplex imaging on all patients before undertaking saphenous vein surgery. For patients with saphenopopliteal incompetence, incompetent mid-thigh perforators and/or residual GSV in patients with recurrence, a preoperative duplex marking scan is also performed.

A small number of patients are referred to the vascular clinic without any symptoms. If the clinical examination fails to demonstrate any complications, such as skin changes, edema or superficial phlebitis, and the patient does not wish to undergo any treatment, no further investigations are performed. If the varicose veins are symptomatic, a whole-leg duplex scan is obtained and the patient is reviewed in the clinic again with the results. If the duplex scan shows any incompetence along the long or small saphenous vein (SSV), and if there are no contraindications for surgery, we generally recommend operative treatment. Trials looking at the quality of life after surgery for varicose veins showed that surgery led to an improvement in disease-specific quality of life in 87 percent at 2 years.[27]

If the symptoms with which the patient presents are not clearly attributable to the varicose veins, we will review the patient after a trial of compression stockings for 3–6 months. If the patient is not well enough or does not want an operation, class 2 compression stockings are prescribed, after major peripheral vascular disease is excluded by measuring the ankle brachial pressure index (ABPI >0.8). Stockings are a valuable alternative to operative treatment, as they have been shown to improve venous function.[28,29] They have also been shown to improve skin changes in trials where elastic stockings were used.[30,31]

It is still not universally accepted that all patients undergoing varicose vein surgery need duplex examination. However, several studies have shown that duplex scanning is important to plan the appropriate operation: in our own unit, a comparison between clinical examination together with hand-held Doppler and duplex imaging was performed which clearly showed that surgery planned on the basis of hand-held Doppler examination would have left 24 percent of reflux sites untreated (sensitivity of hand-held Doppler is only about 75 percent for the SFJ and saphenopopliteal junction (SPJ) and only 50 percent for the thigh perforators).[17] Jutley et al.[19] scanned 223 limbs with varicose veins; 19 percent had saphenopopliteal reflux, of which 67 percent was clinically unsuspected.[19] In contrast, another study from Inverness showed that saphenopopliteal incompetence was only demonstrated in 42 percent of cases where reflux in the popliteal region was suspected by hand-held Doppler, thus avoiding a potentially harmful operation.[16] Furthermore, duplex scan also allows the location and marking of incompetent perforators as well as a double saphenous vein.

If the patient meets the criteria for day-case surgery <35, no severe or untreated concomitant disease [body mass index (BMI)], we aim to perform even bilateral varicose vein surgery as a day case. Preoperative blood tests include electrolytes, creatinine and a full blood count. If there is a history of previous deep vein thrombosis or thrombophlebitis, an additional thrombophilia screen is also performed.

Low-molecular-weight heparin injections are given to all patients for deep vein thrombosis prophylaxis. Stopping the oral contraceptive pill routinely is probably not justified,[32] but we do discuss the options with patients who are on it. If they wish to do so, they are offered an operation date 4–6 weeks following stopping the oral contraceptive pill, using an alternative contraception method in the interval. The vast majority of patients take up this option. We do not stop hormone replacement therapy (HRT), although there does seem to be an up to fourfold increase in risk of deep vein thrombosis when using HRT.[33–35]

Patients on oral contraceptives or HRT, or with a history of previous deep vein thrombosis, are given a 5-day course of low-molecular-weight heparin (Clexane 20 mg s.c. o.d.).

Patients with a past history of deep vein thrombosis are re-imaged by duplex ultrasound at 1 week.

Great saphenous vein

The concept of ligation of the great saphenous vein was introduced 1891 by Trendelenburg,[36] whilst the concept of flush ligation with the femoral vein in the groin was first described in 1916 by Homans.[37] Flush ligation prevents reflux in any of the tributaries which join the femoral and great saphenous vein in the groin and therefore reduces the incidence of recurrence. Stripping the great saphenous vein was introduced by Mayo[38] and further developed by Babcock[39] and Myers and Cooley.[40] The great saphenous vein was stripped in toto from the ankle to the groin. Several studies, however, have now shown that stripping the GSV from the SFJ down to or just below the knee carries significantly less risk of saphenous nerve injury, with the same long-term result.[41] Randomized prospective studies comparing total versus partial stripping of the GSV from the groin to just below the knee demonstrated that outcome was no different 3 months postoperatively in both groups, apart from a significantly higher percentage of saphenous nerve injury in the group with total stripping (39 vs. 7 percent, $P < 0.001$). Three years later, 29 percent of patients who had had total stripping of the GSV had permanent lesions of the saphenous nerve, whereas only 5 percent with partial stripping had persistent lesions ($P < 0.01$). There was no difference in recurrence rate (10 percent in both groups).[42–44]

In a 1992 study comparing GSV ligation with ligation and stripping to the upper calf, Sarin et al.[45] reviewed patients 3 months after surgery: There were significantly fewer persisting incompetent GSVs in the calf when the GSV was stripped than after saphenofemoral ligation alone ($P < 0.01$). Stripping the GSV to the upper calf did not result in a higher incidence of injury to the saphenous nerve.[45]

Dwerryhouse et al.[46] compared patients treated by ligation only versus ligation and stripping of the great saphenous vein in the thigh. Five years after surgery, patients with stripping required significant fewer re-operations than patients

with ligation only (21 vs. 6 percent, $P < 0.02$). Despite this significant difference in re-operations required, recurrent visible varicosities were not different in either group (34 vs. 40 percent). Duplex imaging revealed that 71 percent of patients with ligation only had incompetence in the remaining GSV compared with 29 percent when the GSV was stripped ($P < 0.0001$). Recurrence was thought to arise mainly from neovascularization, connecting to the non-stripped GSV.[46] These results were similar to an earlier study by Sarin et al.: 17 percent of patients who had had a saphenofemoral ligation alone were recurrence-free after a median of 21 months following surgery. If partial stripping of the GSV was added, 65 percent were recurrence free ($P < 0.001$). The reduced recurrence rate was thought to be due to disconnection of thigh perforators. Patient satisfaction was also significantly better in the group that had the saphenous vein stripped compared with saphenofemoral ligation alone (65 vs. 37 percent, $P < 0.05$).[47]

A study published in 2002 by MacKenzie et al.[48] compared complete GSV stripping to incomplete GSV stripping in terms of quality of life. After adjustment in terms of recurrent versus primary disease, there was a significant difference between these groups. Successful stripping was associated with a significant reduction in reflux in the below-knee GSV, whereas popliteal vein reflux actually worsened in the incompletely stripped group. Although complete stripping was attempted in all patients, this was successfully achieved in only 32 percent. Quality of life improved in both groups, but more so when complete stripping was achieved.[48] Reasons for incomplete stripping may have been the presence of a duplicated saphenous vein, which is present in 49 percent of venograms performed for bypass surgery. Approximately 40 percent of these extended from the thigh to the calf.[49]

In an assessment of high ligation without stripping of the GSV, it could be shown by duplex scanning that, in 24 of the 52 legs scanned, there was postoperatively persistent reflux down the GSV. In only two of these could this be attributed to mid-thigh perforating veins.[50] Another study showed that 80 percent of patients with varicose veins had one incompetent thigh perforator on ascending deep to superficial venography and 20 percent had more than one incompetent thigh perforator. In this study, 92 percent of the limbs studied had concomitant incompetent calf perforator.[51]

The clinical significance of perforating veins, however, is far from clear. Stuart et al.[52,53] demonstrated that, in the absence of main-stem venous reflux, incompetent perforators were rarely observed (only in about 2 percent), and if main-stem reflux is eradicated, the majority of incompetent perforating veins return to a calibre and functional state similar to normal values. Another small study randomized 38 legs having surgery for uncomplicated varicose veins to additional ligation of incompetent perforators or follow-up: the results of plethysmography were not different in either group.[54] If the deep venous system is incompetent, however, saphenous surgery alone is less reliable in normalizing perforating veins in the calf. The Edinburgh group could demonstrate that 80 percent of perforating veins were competent after venous reflux in the saphenous system was abolished in the absence of deep venous reflux. If deep venous reflux was present or surgery failed to eradicate main-stem reflux completely, only 28 percent of perforating veins were competent postoperatively $(P < 0.01)$.[53]

As vein is universally accepted as the best available material for infrainguinal bypass and coronary artery bypass surgery, it has been suggested that the GSV should remain *in situ* and only flush ligation should be performed. But even with stripping of the GSV, Rutherford *et al.*[55] still found enough residual vein to perform bypass surgery. They scanned residual lengths of saphenous veins segments after either previous stripping or harvesting for visceral, peripheral or coronary bypass. Combining residual GSV and SSV segments of usable calibre, 100 percent of high ligation only, 93 percent of partial distal removal and 74 percent of partial proximal removal had more than 60 cm in total length, and most total removal had more than 40 cm usable SSV in the ipsilateral vein.[55] Even with previous total removal of the GSV, infrainguinal bypass should therefore often still be possible with vein harvested from the ipsilateral leg. The contralateral limb or arm veins were not included in this study. Furthermore, the frequency of patients with previous surgery to the saphenous vein presenting for bypass procedures is not that high in clinical practice. Of the 117 patients scanned by Rutherford *et al.*, only five needed vein harvesting for bypass. This was also demonstrated by Hammarsten *et al.*[56]

We routinely perform a flush ligation and stripping of the GSV in all patients. We also strip the GSV in patients who on Duplex examinations only have reflux in the GSV, and no confirmed reflux at the SFJ, as we believe this to be a disease in progress. This is supported by Schultz-Ehrenburg *et al.*,[14,15] who investigated children in secondary schools. Ten- to 12-year-old children had evidence of venous reflux, but none had visible varicose veins. Eight years later, 20 percent had developed reflux and 8 percent had varicose veins.

OPERATION FOR GSV

The varicosities are marked by the operating surgeon with an indelible pen, with two parallel lines along the vein, to avoid an incision through the marking, which anecdotally can result in tattooing (Fig. 15.1). We tend not to do any stab avulsions below the ankle as any paresthesia in this region may prejudice the comfort of wearing shoes. Groin and legs are shaved immediately before surgery. We generally perform the operation under general anesthesia, as this allows patients to walk around as soon as they are awake, further minimizing the risk of deep vein thrombosis. It also shortens time spent on the day-case unit with earlier discharge. Regional anesthesia is a valuable alternative (most often spinal anesthesia). Flush ligation of the GSV can be done under local anesthesia, but as we nearly always strip the GSV we rarely perform it. Stab avulsions alone can also be done under local anesthesia, but as they tend to be numerous if

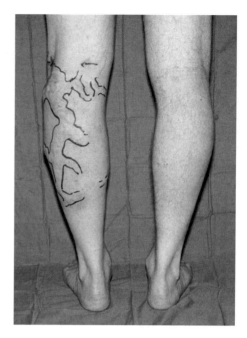

Figure 15.1 *Preoperative marking of varicose veins with an indelible pen. Note the arrow marking the site of the saphenopopliteal junction.*

surgery is intended, general or regional anesthesia is preferred.

The patient is positioned supine on the operating table, legs abducted, in a 25° Trendelenburg position, to reduce haemorrhage. It is routine hospital practice to administer a single-shot antibiotic prophylaxis (cefuroxime 1.5 g i.v.). A 3–4 cm oblique skin incision is made in the skin crease of the groin. Alternatively, the incision can be made just above the crease, but we have found the incision in the skin crease cosmetically more satisfactory.

The SFJ has to be identified beyond any doubt (Fig. 15.2). No longitudinal vessel should be ligated before the SFJ and the femoral vein 1 cm proximally and distally to it have been identified. All tributaries should be dissected and ligated. Careful dissection of the medial as well as the lateral wall of the femoral vein is necessary, in order to identify and ligate medial and, more rarely, lateral branches leading directly into the femoral vein. These might be responsible for non-saphenofemoral reflux in the groin, as found by Jiang *et al.*[22] in 9.9 percent of 1022 limbs prospectively examined with duplex scanning and air plethysmography. Although the reflux was mild, it was more often found in recurrent varices, suggesting a possible role in recurrence if not ligated.

A landmark is the external pudendal artery, originating from the femoral artery, crossing the GSV, most often dorsally, just distal to the SFJ. In a small number, however, it crosses the GSV anteriorly. It is advisable not to injure this small artery, as it bleeds profusely, obscuring vision. If it bleeds or prevents access, it should be ligated. If possible, it should be preserved, as there is a possible association with postsurgical erectile dysfunction following ligation of external pudendal arteries and aberrant arterial supply.[57]

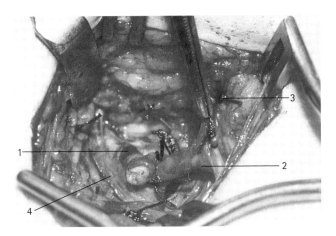

Figure 15.2 *Intraoperative finding: saphenofemoral junction. 1, femoral vein; 2, great saphenous vein; 3, ligated tributary; 4, cribriform fascia. The black ties (Silk 2/0) represent smaller, ligated and dissected tributaries.*

The GSV is double-ligated flush to the femoral vein. We use 2-0 silk (Ethicon Ltd, Edinburgh, UK), but 2-0 Vicryl (Ethicon) can also be used. The GSV then is dissected some 5–10 cm further down, as there is quite often a medial tributary, which should be ligated before the GSV is stripped to prevent the development of a large hematoma. The Oesch perforating-invagination (PIN) stripper (Credenhill Ltd, Ilkeston, UK) is then inserted into the GSV and guided down the GSV just below the knee joint. A straight clip attached to the proximal end allows guidance of the bent tip. Once the stripper is passed down, the tip is pressed into the skin, and a stab incision is made on top of the stripper (Fig. 15.3). A number 2 silk tie is then tied to the proximal end of the stripper and about 4 cm away from it to the vein, allowing an invaginating stripping (Fig. 15.4). The PIN stripper (Fig. 15.5), developed by Oesch,[58] is a modified invaginating method, said to be less traumatic, causing less hematoma, less injury to saphenous nerve and less postoperative pain. Lacroix et al.[59] examined 30 patients with bilateral GSV stripping: on one side with invaginating and on the other limb with conventional stripping. The size of the hematoma, the pain score, and incidence of saphenous nerve injury (13 vs. 17 percent) were all statistically insignificant. There seemed to be a tendency that 1 month following surgery, the leg treated by invagination stripping was less painful (33 percent claimed standard stripping was more painful, 23 percent said invaginating was more painful). Durkin et al.[60] prospectively compared 80 patients' quality of life measures after PIN-stripping vs. conventional stripping: Whilst overall quality of health improved in the conventional group, this appeared to be to a lesser extent than in the PIN group. The cosmetic outcome seems to be better using the PIN stripper, as the exit wound is significantly smaller compared with the wound when using the conventional stripper. There seems to be no clinically significant difference in the formation of haematoma 1 and 6 weeks postoperatively.[61] However, another study looked into hematoma formation using radioisotope red blood cell labelling and reported a

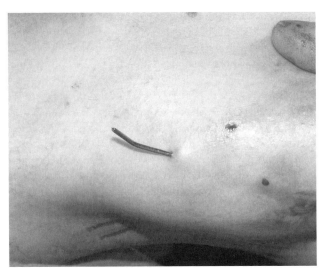

Figure 15.3 *Distal end of the perforating-invagination (PIN) stripper. The bent tip facilitates navigating the stripper down the saphenous vein. Note the size of the incision for the exit of the PIN stripper as well as the incisions for the two stab avulsions on the right side in comparison with the surgeon's thumb.*

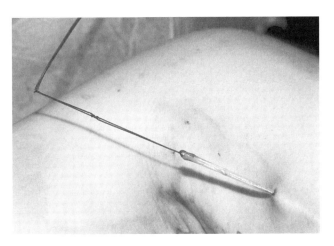

Figure 15.4 *Perforating-invagination (PIN) stripping at the level of the knee, exit wound, demonstrating eversion. The distal great saphenous vein has already been removed by separate stab avulsions.*

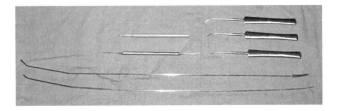

Figure 15.5 *Instruments for varicose vein operation. Top to bottom, right side: Oesch hooks in three different sizes. Top to bottom, left side: Microknife used for the small, 1–2 mm wide incisions for stab avulsions, Varady hook. Bottom: Retrieval device, perforating-invagination (PIN) stripper.*

significant reduction in thigh hematoma in the track of the GSV if the PIN stripper was used.[62]

We always aim to strip the GSV to the level of the knee, to disconnect any possible deep to superficial perforators, especially in the adductor canal. If the GSV ruptures whilst stripping, the retrieval stripper (Fig. 15.5) (Credenhill) is tied to the proximal end of the PIN stripper, to extract the remaining vein.

Once the GSV is stripped, we routinely close the cribriform fascia with 2-0 Vicryl, aiming to reduce neovascularization. In a study where 210 limbs had a silicon sheet sutured to the saphenous stump and the cribriform fascia closed on top, neovascularization was only found in 6 percent, compared with 17 percent in the 212 limbs without a silicon sheet 12 months postoperatively ($P < 0.05$).[63] Small stab incisions are then placed at the markings, using the Micro-Knife (Fig. 15.5) (Micro-Knife 30°; Medtronic UK Ltd, Watford, UK) and the varicosities removed with Oesch phlebectomy hooks (Figs 15.5–15.7) (Credenhill). The Varady hook (Fig. 15.5) (B. Braun Medical Ltd, Sheffield, UK) is similar to Oesch hooks and is preferred by some surgeons. Care is taken to remove only the varicosities and to avoid avulsion of the nerves, lymphatics or

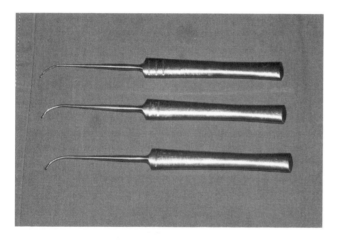

Figure 15.6 *Oesch hooks, different sizes.*

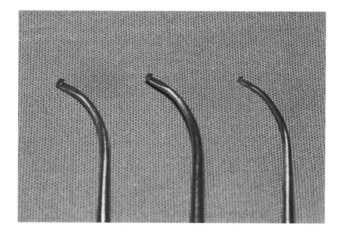

Figure 15.7 *Oesch hooks, detail. Left to right: size one, used for large varicose veins (usually thigh); size two, our preferred size; size three (the smallest one), helpful in small varicosities, such as venules in the skin.*

connective tissue. Special care is taken at the head of the fibula to preserve the lateral popliteal and common peroneal nerve, the tibial nerve at the medial malleolus, the sural nerve at the median line of the posterior calf and the saphenous nerve over the medial calf. Extraction of fatty tissue should be avoided, as this can leave unsightly depressed scars.

We do not routinely use tourniquets. Several small studies have suggested that using tourniquets might decrease blood loss and hematoma, as well as operating time, and would give a better cosmetic result.[64–67] A Cochrane review in 2002 by Rigby *et al.*[68] only found three prospective randomized studies, and due to different methods of collecting data, meta-analysis was not possible. It was concluded that the use of a tourniquet would appear to reduce blood loss, but there was no difference in complications or morbidity. Problems such as nerve damage and burns have been associated with the use of a tourniquet in skin contact. The stab avulsions are closed with adhesive tapes (3M Steri-Strip Skin Closures; 3M Health Care Ltd, Leicestershire, UK). This is a fast and cheap method, with a good cosmetic result. We close the incision in the groin with subcuticular 3/0 Monocryl after evacuating the hematoma from the saphenous channel. Firm compression bandages from foot to proximal thigh are applied – we use an adhesive bandage (Panelast; Lohmann + Rauscher International GmbH & Co, Rengsdorf, Germany) as we believe these maintain compression better than crepe bandages, which tend to slip. As all bandages tend to slip down and become uncomfortable, as well as inhibiting movement of the knee, we usually change the bandages on the first postoperative day when an inpatient or in the next few days when an outpatient. We use class I above-knee compression stockings (TED Stockings; Tyco Healthcare UK Ltd, Hampshire, UK) for a total of 6 weeks during the day. This is nevertheless contentious.

Low-compression stockings may have as good results as high-compression stockings (15 vs. 40 mmHg).[69] Compression bandages are thought to reduce hematoma formation,[70] but Raraty *et al.*[71] could not demonstrate any clinical benefit after compression bandages following varicose vein surgery. One prospective study randomized 69 patients to above-knee stockings class II vs. no stockings. Interestingly, of the patients wearing stockings only 6 percent had recurrence 12 months postoperatively, compared with 71 percent of patients wearing no stocking. However, 39 percent of the patients wearing stockings were lost to follow-up, and 11 percent declined to wear them.[72] A rare complication is the compartment syndrome, and patients as well as nurses should be made aware of it and remove compression bandages if there is any doubt.[73]

We routinely follow up each patient clinically once 6–8 weeks postoperative, although other authors have debated whether this is essential.[74,75]

Small saphenous vein

In 44–60 percent of patients, the SSV joins the popliteal vein at or just above the popliteal fossa. In about one-third, the SPJ is higher, and in about 10 percent it is lower.[76,77] The small saphenous vein is usually considered to join the popliteal on its posterior surface and occasionally on the medial or lateral surface of the popliteal vein However, in our own study, the majority of SSVs joined the popliteal vein laterally (47 percent). In 23.7 percent, the SSV joined the popliteal vein posteriorly, in 10.5 percent posteromedially, in 6.6 percent posterolaterally, in 9.2 percent medially and in 2.6 percent it did not join the popliteal vein but the gastrocnemius vein

Table 15.1 *Termination of short saphenous vein by duplex. (After Bhasin et al.[78])*

	n	%
Laterally	36	47.3
Medially	7	9.2
Posterolaterally	5	6.6
Posterior	18	23.7
Posteromedially	8	10.5
From medial gastrocnemius	2	2.6

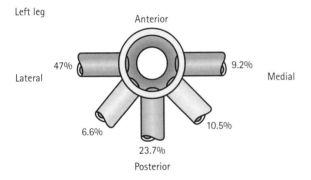

Figure 15.8 *Termination of short saphenous vein. (After Bhasin et al.[78])*

(Table 15.1, Fig. 15.8).[78] In addition to localizing the exact height of the SPJ, we have found the Duplex report helpful in localizing the junction precisely due to these anatomical variations. The vertical position, the coronal insertion and its depth all contribute to accurate localization (Fig. 15.9).

In order to be able to do a flush ligation of the SSV, the SPJ needs to be visualized. The exact localization of the SPJ should be carried out by either intraoperative phlebography[76,77] or preoperative marking with duplex imaging. Simple hand-held Doppler was not found to reliably localize the SPJ compared with duplex imaging.[79]

OPERATION FOR THE SSV

The patient lies prone in a Trendelenburg position. A transverse skin incision is performed approximately 2 cm below the site of the marked SPJ.[80] The fascia is divided transversally, and bipolar diathermy is used. The short saphenous vein is readily identified

The SPJ is carefully dissected, identifying the proximal and distal popliteal vein prior to ligation. Occasionally the medial gastrocnemius vein will join the SSV immediately prior to the short SPJ itself. In contrast to the operation in the groin, we tend to avoid self-retaining retractors, but prefer four Langenbecks retractors in order to minimize the chance of injuring the sural or tibial/peroneal nerves. Care must be taken not to injure the median popliteal nerve, which gives off the sural nerve and lies very close to the popliteal vein and SSV. Localizing the SSV by duplex imaging can also be helpful to accurately identify the SPJ itself. All tributaries must be carefully dissected and ligated, especially the vein of Giacomini, which was first described in 1893.[81] This is an anastomotic branch between the long and small saphenous veins which can transmit reflux from the GSV or thigh perforators into the SSV, or transmits reflux from the SPJ to the

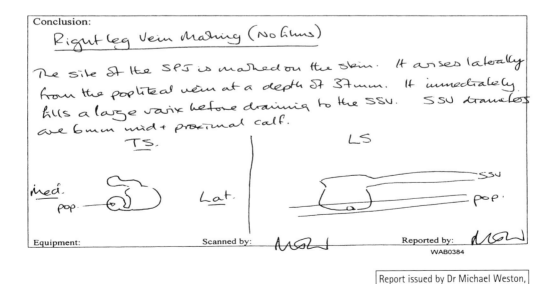

Figure 15.9 *Preoperative duplex marking and report prior to short saphenopopliteal junction ligation.*

GSV or thigh varicose veins and can cause recurrence if missed. In Giacomini's anatomical dissections, this anastomosis was present in 72 percent of limbs. A more recent series of dissections found the intersaphenous anastomosis present in 56 percent.[82] However, with duplex scanning, this kind of anastomosis was present in only 6.2 percent.[83]

After the junction is carefully dissected out, the SSV is double-ligated with 3-0 silk, dissected, if possible, down distally a further 5–10 cm and resected after ligation. We do not strip the SSV. There are no level 1 data to suggest that stripping the SSV reduces recurrence. Proponents of stripping mention communicating veins which drain into the SSV, while opponents are concerned about possible sural nerve injury.

Results after operation for SSV incompetence are scarce in the literature. We reviewed a small number of patients after they underwent surgery for duplex-confirmed saphenopopliteal reflux. The operation was performed by an experienced vascular consultant after localizing the SPJ. In 57 percent there was no persistent small saphenous reflux. Forty-three percent had persistent SSV reflux, the main reason being formation of new collaterals (38 percent). In 6.7 percent the SPJ was missed, although the SPJ was localized by duplex in every patient. There were no major postoperative complications.[79] In another study by Rashid et al.[84] in 2002, the SPJ was missed in 36 percent when reviewing 59 patients retrospectively. In this series, there were two deep vein thromboses, one popliteal vein injury and one sural nerve palsy.[84] In a retrospective study by Lucertini et al.,[85] two out of 104 patients who had SSV surgery had a foot-drop due to an injury to the trunk of the common peroneal nerve, which had completely recovered 1 year later. They also observed hypoesthesia and/or dysesthesia in 14 percent.[85]

Recurrent varicose veins: incidence and etiology

Recurrence after surgery for varicose veins is common. Five years after surgery, recurrence rates from 10–40 percent are reported.[43,46] A follow-up 35 years after SFJ ligation with stripping of the whole GSV with excision of side branches demonstrated a recurrence rate of 60 percent, and 21.6 percent required re-operation.[86] In clinical practice, about 20 percent of varicose vein surgery is for recurrent varicose veins.[16,87] The majority of recurrence arises in the groin with SFJ incompetence. As in primary varicose veins, only about 20 percent of patients have saphenopopliteal incompetence, but this percentage rises to about 55 percent if an additional ulcer is present.[16] Whether recurrence is due to insufficient surgery at the time of the first operation or due to neovascularization is not clear. In 1992, in Edinburgh, Bradbury et al.[88] found that of 118 patients operated on for recurrence, only 28 percent had a tied SFJ, 44 percent had an intact major tributary and 73 percent had an intact GSV. In addition, of the 45 legs with saphenopopliteal reflux, only four previously had saphenopopliteal ligation, saphenopopliteal reflux either missed at the first operation or reflux arisen after surgery. Darke[87] operated on 95 patients for recurrence and found a recurrence pattern suggesting incomplete surgery at the first procedure. Forty-eight percent had saphenofemoral incompetence and 10.5 percent had saphenopopliteal reflux, of which 94 percent had previous great saphenous surgery. However, in over half of the patients with saphenofemoral reflux, recurrence was caused by reconstitution of the junction by neovascularization. Other studies found neovascularization to be the main reason in up to 77 percent of saphenofemoral recurrence.[16,89]

In a clinicopathological study, evidence of neovascularization was present in histological sections in 27 out of 28 groins. In 19 legs (68 percent) it was the sole identified cause of recurrent saphenofemoral incompetence, while in eight it coexisted with veins missed at the original operation.[90] Another possibility is that recurrence is not only due to inappropriate/inadequate surgery or neovascularization, but also to altered venous hemodynamics. Nine out of 46 patients (19.5 percent) in a small study had new sites of reflux 6 weeks after the operation, as demonstrated by duplex. Re-imaging 12 months postoperatively showed that this reflux had disappeared in five patients, but remained in four. Of the 37 patients without reflux at the 6-week postoperative scan, three were found to have new reflux (one new incompetent SPJ, one incompetent medial thigh vein and one neovascularization at the SPJ). Twelve months postoperatively, therefore, 7/46 (15.2 percent) had reflux or a site of incompetence, none of them due to inappropriate surgery, and only in two (4.3 percent) was it due to neovascularization.[91] The diagnosis and treatment of recurrent varicose veins is described in Chapter 24, page 219.

REFERENCES

1. Arnoldi CC. The aetiology of primary varicose veins. *Dan Med Bull* 1957; **4**: 102–7.
2. Prerovsky I. Diseases of the veins. World Health Organisation, internal communication. MHO-PA 10964.
3. Widmer LK. *Peripheral Venous Disorders. Prevalence and Socio-medical Importance. Observations in 4529 Apparently Healthy Persons. Basle 111 Study.* Bern: Hans Huber, 1978.
4. Kistner RL, Eklof B, Masuda EM. Diagnosis of venous disease of the lower extremities. The CEAP classification. *Mayo Clin Proc* 1996; **71**: 338–45.
5. *Ad hoc* Committee, American Venous Forum. Classification and grading of chronic venous disease in the lower limb. A consensus statement. *J Cardiovasc Surg (Torino)* 1997; **38**: 437–45.
6. Evans CJ, Fowkes FG R, Ruckley CV, Lee AJ. Prevalence of varicose veins and chronic venous insufficiency in men and women in the general population: Edinburgh Vein Study. *J Epidemiol Community Health* 1999; **53**: 149–53.
7. Beaglehole R, Salmond CE, Prior IAM. Varicose veins in New Zealand. Prevalence and severity. *NZ Med J* 1976; **84**: 396–9.
8. Sisto T, Reunanen A, Laurikka J *et al.* Prevalence and risk factors of varicose veins in lower extremities: mini-Finland health survey. *Eur J Surg* 1995; **161**: 405–14.
9. US Department of Health Education and Welfare. *National Health Survey.* Washington, DC: USDHEW 1938; 1935–6.

10. Logan WPD, Brooke EM, eds. *Studies on Medical and Population Subjects. Number 12. The Survey of Sickness 1943–52.* London: General Register Office, 1957.

11. The Sickness Survey of Denmark. The committee on the Danish National Morbidity Survey. Copenhagen: 1960.

12. Department of National Health and Welfare and the Dominion Bureau of Statistics. Illness and health care in Canada. *Canadian Sickness Survey 1950–51.* Ottawa: Department of National Health and Welfare and the Dominion Bureau of Statistics, 1960.

13. Cesarone MR, Belcaro G, Nicolaides AN et al. 'Real' epidemiology of varicose veins and chronic venous diseases: the San Valentino Vascular Screening Project. *Angiology* 2002; 119–30.

14. Schultz-Ehrenburg U, Weindorf N, Vonuslar D, Hiche H. Prospective epidemiologische Studie ueber die Entstehungsweise der Krampfadern bei Kindern und Jugendlichen (Bochumer Studie I und II). *Phlebol Proktol* 1989; **18**: 3–11.

15. Schultz-Ehrenburg U, Weindorf N, Matthes U, Hirche H. [An epidemiologic study of the pathogenesis of varices. The Bochum Study I–III.] *Phlébologie* 1992; **45**: 497–500.

16. Wong JK, Duncan JL, Nichols DM. Whole-leg duplex mapping for varicose veins: observations on patterns of reflux in recurrent and primary legs, with clinical correlation. *Eur J Vasc Endovasc Surg* 2003; **25**: 267–75.

17. Mercer KG, Scott DJ, Berridge DC. Preoperative duplex imaging is required before all operations for primary varicose veins. *Br J Surg* 1999; **86**: 570.

18. Sakurai T, Gupta PC, Matsushita M, Nishikimi N, Nimura Y. Correlation of the anatomical distribution of venous reflux with clinical symptoms and venous haemodynamics in primary varicose veins. *Br J Surg* 1998; **85**: 213–6.

19. Jutley RS, Cadle I, Cross KS. Preoperative assessment of primary varicose veins: a duplex study of venous incompetence. *Eur J Vasc Endovasc Surg* 2001; **21**: 370–3.

20. Quigley FG, Raptis S, Cashman M, Faris IB. Douplex ultrasound mapping of sites of deep to superficial incompetence in primary varicose veins. *Aust NZ J Surg* 1992; **62**: 276–8.

21. Myers KA, Zeng GH, Ziegenbein RW, Matthews PG. Duplex ultrasound scanning for chronic venous disease: recurrent varicose veins in the thigh after surgery to the great saphenous vein. *Phlebology* 1996; **11**: 125–31.

22. Jiang P, van Rij AM, Christie RA et al. Non-sapheno-femoral venous reflux in the groin in patients with varicose veins. *Eur J Vasc Endovasc Surg* 2001; **21**: 550–7.

23. Labropoulos N, Tiongson J, Pryor L et al. Nonsaphenous superficial vein reflux. *J Vasc Surg* 2001; **34**: 872–7.

24. Kurz X, Lamping DL, Kahn SR et al. Do varicose veins affect quality of life? Results of an international population-based study. *J Vasc Surg* 2001; **34**: 641–8.

25. Smith JJ, Garatt AM, Guest M et al. Evaluating and improving health-related quality of life in patients with varicose veins. *J Vasc Surg* 1999; **30**: 710–9.

26. Baker DM, Turnbull NB, Pearson JC, Makin GS. How successful is varicose vein surgery? A patient outcome study following varicose vein surgery using the SF-36 Health Assessment Questionnaire. *Eur J Vasc Endovasc Surg* 1995; **9**: 299–304.

27. MacKenzie RK, Paisley A, Allen PL et al. The effect of great saphenous vein stripping on quality of life. *J Vasc Surg* 2002; 6.

28. Sjoberg T, Einarsson E, Norgren L. Functional evaluation of four different compression stockings in venous insufficiency. *Phlebology* 1987; **2**: 53–8.

29. Struckmann J. Compression stokings and their effect on the venous pump – a comparative study. *Phlebology* 1986; **1**: 37–45.

30. Burnand KG, Powell S, Bishop C, Stacey M et al. Effect of Paroven on skin oxigenation in patients with varicose veins. *Phlebology* 1989; **4**: 15–22.

31. Belcaro G, Marelli C. Treatment of venous lipodermatosclerosis and ulceration in venous hypertension by elastic compression and fibrinolytic anhancement with defibritide. *Phlebology* 1989; **4**: 91–106.

32. Throboembolic Risk Factors (THRIFT) Consensus Group. Risk of and prophylaxis for venous thromboebolism in hospital patients. *Br Med J* 1992; **305**: 567–74.

33. Daley E, Vessey MP, Hawkins MM. Risk of venous thromboembolism in users of hormone replacement therapy. *Lancet* 1996; **348**: 977–80.

34. Jick H, Derby LE, Myers MW. Risk of hospital admissions for idiopathic venous thromboembolism among users of postmenopausal oestrogen. *Lancet* 1966; **348**: 981–3.

35. Grodstein F, Stampfer MJ, Goldhaber SZ. Prospective study of exogenous hormones and pulmonary embolism in women. *Lancet* 1996; **348**: 983–7.

36. Trendelenburg F. Ueber die Unterbindung der Vena saphena magna bei Unterschenkelvarizen. *Beitr Klein Chir* 1891; **7**: 195–210.

37. Homans J. Operative treatment of varicose veins and ulcers. *Surg Gynaecol Obstet* 1916; **22**: 143–58.

38. Mayo Ch. Treatment of varicose veins. *Surg Gynecol Obstet* 1906; **2**: 385–8.

39. Babcock WW. A new operation for the exstirpation of varicose veins of the legs. *NY Med J* 1907; **86**: 153–6.

40. Myers TT, Cooley JC. Varicose vein surgery in the management of the post-phlebitic limb. *Surg Gynecol Obstet* 1954; **99**: 733–44.

41. Negus D, Nichols RWT. Is it necessary to strip the incompetent saphenous vein to the ankle? In: Negus D, Jantet G (eds). *Phlebology '85.* London: Libbey, 1986: 148–50.

42. Holme JB, Skajaaa K, Holme K. Incidence of lesions of the saphenous nerve after partial or complete stripping of the great saphenous vein. *Acta Chir Scand* 1990; **156**: 145–8.

43. Holme K, Matzen M, Bomberg AJ et al. Partial or total stripping of the great saphenous vein. 5-year recurrence frequency and 3-year frequency of neural complications after partial and total stripping of the great saphenous vein. *Ugeskr Laeger* 1996; **158**: 405–8.

44. Irace L, Siani A, Laurito A et al. Indication for short stripping of the great saphenous vein. Results and indications. *Minerva Cardioangiol* 2001; **49**: 383–7.

45. Sarin S, Scurr JH, Coleridge-Smith P. Assessment of stripping the great saphenous vein in the treatment of primary varicose veins. *Br J Surg* 1992; **79**: 889–93.

46. Dwerryhouse S, Davies B, Harradine K, Earnshaw J. Stripping the great saphenous vein reduces the rate of reoperation for recurrent varicose veins: five year results of a randomized trial. *J Vasc Surg* 1999; **29**: 589–92.

47. Sarin S, Scurr JH, Coleridge-Smith PD. Stripping of the great saphenous vein in the treatment of primary varicose veins. *Br J Surg* 1994; **81**: 1455–8.

48. MacKenzie RK, Lee AJ, Paisley A et al. Patient, operative, and surgeon factors that influence the effect of superficial venous surgery on disease-specific quality of life. *J Vasc Surg* 2002; **36**: 896–902.

49. Corrales NE, Irvine A, McGuiness CL et al. Incidence and pattern of great saphenous vein duplication and its possible implications for recurrence after varicose vein surgery. *Br J Surg* 2002; **89**: 323–6.

50. McMullin GM, Coleridge Smith PD, Scurr JH. Objective assessment of high ligation without stripping the great saphenous vein. *Br J Surg* 1991; **78**: 1139–42.

51. Papadakis K, Christodoulou C, Christopoulos D *et al.* Number and anatomical distribution of incompetent thigh perforating veins. *Br J Surg* 1989; **76**: 581–4.

52. Stuart PS, Lee AJ, Allan PL *et al.* Most incompetent calf perforating veins are found in association with superficial venous reflux. *J Vasc Surg* 2001; **34**: 774–8.

53. Stuart WP, Adam DJ, Allan PL *et al.* Saphenous surgery does not correct perforator incompetence in the presence of deep venous reflux. *J Vasc Surg* 1998; **28**: 834–8.

54. Fitridge RA, Dunlop C, Raptis S *et al.* A prospective randomised trial evaluating haemodynamic role of incompetent calf perforating veins. *Aust NZ J Surg* 1999; **69**: 214–6.

55. Rutherford RB, Sawyer JD, Jones DN. The fate of residual saphenous vein after partial removal or ligation. *J Vasc Surg* 1990; **12**: 422–8.

56. Hammarsten J, Pedersen P, Cederlund CF, Companello M. Long saphenous vein-saving surgery for varicose veins. A long term follow-up. *Eur J Vasc Surg* 1990; **4**: 361–4.

57. Henriet JP. Sexual complications from superficial venous surgery. *Phlébologie* 1993; **46**: 569–75.

58. Oesch A. PIN stripping a novel method of atraumatic stripping. *Phlebology* 1993; **8**: 171–3.

59. Lacroix H, Nevelsteen A, Suy R. Invaginating versus classic stripping of the great saphenous vein. A randomized prospective study. *Acta Chir Belg* 1999; **99**: 22–5.

60. Durkin MT, Turton EP, Scott DJ, Berridge DC. A prospective trial of PIN versus conventional stripping in varicose vein surgery. *Ann R Coll Surg Engl* 1999; **81**: 171–4.

61. Durkin MT, Turton EP, Wijesinghe LD *et al.* Long saphenous vein stripping and quality of life-a randomised trial. *Eur J Vasc Endovasc Surg* 2001; **21**: 545–9.

62. Kent PJ, Maughan J, Burniston M *et al.* Perforation-invagination stripping of the great saphenous vein reduces thigh haematoma formation in varicose vein surgery. *Phlebology* 1999; **14**: 43–7.

63. De Maeseneer MG, Giuliani DR, Van Schil PE, De Hert SG. Can interposition of a silicone implant after sapheno-femoral ligation prevent recurrent varicose veins? *Eur J Vasc Endovasc Surg* 2002; **24**(5): 445–9.

64. Robinson J, Macierewicz J, Beard JD. Using the Boazul cuff to reduce blood loss in varicose vein surgery. *Eur J Vasc Endovasc Surg* 2000; **20**: 390–3.

65. Sykes TC, Brookes P, Hickey NC. A prospective randomised trial of tourniquet in varicose vein surgery. *Ann R Coll Surg Engl* 2000; **82**: 280–2.

66. Thompson JF, Royle GT, Farrands PA *et al.* Varicose vein surgery using a pneumatic tourniquet: reduced blood loss and improved cosmesis. *Ann R Coll Surg Engl* 1990; **72**: 119–21.

67. Corbett R, Jayakumar KN. Clean up varicose vein surgery – use a tourniquet. *Ann R Coll Surg Engl* 1989; **71**: 57–8.

68. Rigby KA, Palfreyman SJ, Beverley C, Michaels JA. Surgery for varicose veins: use of tourniquet. *Cochrane Database Syst Rev* 2002; **4**: CD001486.

69. Shouler PJ, Runchman PC. Varicose veins. optimum compression after surgery and sclerotherapy. *Ann R Coll Surg Engl* 1989; **71**: 402–4.

70. Travers JP, Rhodes JE, Hardy JG, Makin GS. Postoperative limb compression in reduction of haemorrhage after varicose vein surgery. *Ann R Coll Surg Engl* 1993; **75**: 119–22.

71. Raraty MG, Greavey MG, Blair SD. There is no benefit from 6 weeks of compression after varicose vein surgery: a prospective randomised trial. *Br J Surg* 1997; **84**: A575.

72. Travers JP, Markin GS. Reduction of varicose vein recurrence by use of post-operative compression stockings. *Phlebology* 1994; **9**: 104–7.

73. Widmer MK, Hakki H, Reber PU, Kniemeyer HW. Rare, but severe complication of varicose vein surgery. *Zentralbl Chir* 2000; **125**: 543–6.

74. Bailey J, Roland M, Roberts C. Is follow up by specialists routinely needed after elective surgery? A controlled trial. *J Epidemiol Community Health* 1999; **53**: 118–24.

75. Wedderburn AW, Dodds SR, Morris GE. A survey of post-operative care after day case surgery. *Ann R Coll Surg Engl* 1996 March; **78**(2 Suppl.): 70–1.

76. Hobbs JT. Peroperative venography to ensure accurate sapheno-popliteal ligation. *Br Med J* 1980; **2**: 1578–9.

77. Corcos L, Peruzzi GP, Romeo V, Fiori C. Consideration of the anatomical variations in the venous system of the lower limbs in varicose disease. *Phlebology* 1989; **4**: 259–70.

78. Bhasin N, Lee MH, Weston MJ *et al.* Quality assurance following saphenopopliteal junction ligation for varicose veins.

79. Vrouenraets BC, Keeman JN. [Physical diagnostics–duplex scanning is necessary only for selected patients with varicose veins]. *Ned Tijdschr Geneeskd* 2001; **18**(145): 1613–4.

80. Pittanthankal AA, Adamson M, Richards T *et al.* Duplex-defined anatomy of the saphenopopliteal junction. *Submitted for publication* 2005.

81. Giacomini C. Osservazione anatomiche per servire allo studio della circolazione venosa delle estremita inferiori. *Giornale della R Accademia di Medicina di Torino* 1873; **13**: 109–215.

82. Hoffman HM, Staubesand J. Die venoesen Abflussverhaeltnisse des Musculus triceps surae. *Phlebologie* 1991; **20**: 164–8.

83. Georgiev M, Myers KA, Belcaro G. The high extension of the lesser saphenous vein: from Gaciomini's observations to ultrasound scan imaging. *J Vasc Surg Surg* 2003; **37**: 558–63.

84. Rashid HI, Ajeel A, Tyrell MR. Persistent popliteal fossa reflux following saphenopoliteal disconnection. *Br J Surg* 2002; **89**: 748–51.

85. Lucertini G, Viacava A, Grana A, Belardi P. Injury to the common peroneal nerve during surgery of the lesser saphenous vein. *Phlebology* 1999; **14**: 26–8.

86. Fischer R, Linde N, Duff C *et al.* Late recurrent sapheno-femoral junction reflux after ligation and stripping of the greater saphenous vein. *J Vasc Surg* 2001; **34**: 236–40.

87. Darke SG. The morphology of recurrent varicose veins. *Eur J Vasc Endovasc Surg* 1992; **6**: 512–7.

88. Bradbury AW, Stonebridge PA, Ruckley CV, Beggs I. Recurrent varicose veins. correlation between preoperative clinical and hand-held Doppler ultrasonographic examination, and anatomical findings at surgery. *Br J Surg* 1993; **80**: 849–51.

89. Jones L, Braithwaite BD, Selwyn D *et al.* Neovascularisation is the principal cause of varicose vein recurrence: results of a randomized trial of stripping the great saphenous vein. *Eur J Vasc Endovasc Surg* 1996; **12**: 442–5.

90. Nyamekye I, Shephard NA, Davies B *et al.* Clinicopathological evidence that neovascularisation is a cause of recurrent varicose veins. *Eur J Vasc Endovasc Surg* 1998; **15**: 412–5.

91. Turton EPL, Scott DJA, Richards SP *et al.* Duplex-derived evidence of reflux after varicose vein surgery: neoreflux or neovascularisation? *Eur J Vasc Endovasc Surg* 1998; **17**: 230–3.

16

Surgical treatment of superficial venous incompetence: recent advances

JOHN J. BERGAN

INTRODUCTION

Treatment of superficial venous incompetence at the turn of the twenty-first century was marked by an increasing use of minimally invasive techniques, outpatient treatment, and an influx of physicians from non-surgical specialties into the treatment arena. Obliterating the greater saphenous vein, thus preventing venous reflux rather than physically removing the vein from the thigh, became possible through use of radiofrequency (RF) energy and laser light applied via catheters placed in the lumen of the saphenous vein. Mechanical phlebectomy became an option to replace stab avulsion. Catheter-based ablation of the saphenous vein could be practiced by non-surgeons, but mechanical phlebectomy kept that part of superficial venous surgery in the operating room.

ATTEMPTS AT SAPHENOUS ABLATION

Recognizing that removing the saphenous vein from the circulation is essential to ensuring good long-term results, methods other than surgery have been explored. Attempts to destroy the venous wall by coagulation have a long history. Initial attempts involved creation of a thrombus within the vessel lumen. This was done by applying direct current to the outside of the vessel wall.[1] In theory, the negative charge on platelets would be attracted to the positive charge on the electrode on the vessel wall and platelet aggregation would initiate the coagulation cascade. This theory was supported by studies which

demonstrated that the amount of thrombus formed by direct-current application was less in volume in thrombocytopenic animals.[2] Direct-current application to the adventitia of vessels produced occlusion, but only after several hours of stimulation. It was logical, therefore, to apply direct current to the lumen of the vessel.[3] At the same time, a change to the use of alternating current to destroy the vessel was made.[4] As a result of these modifications, thrombotic occlusion time was reduced to a matter of 10–20 s.

In general, direct and alternating current produce vessel occlusion in different ways. Direct current causes localized thrombosis by prolonged electrolysis. In contrast, high-frequency alternating current causes a rapid thermal electro-coagulation of the soft tissues of vein wall and valves.

MODERN SAPHENOUS ABLATION

Prolonged exposure to high-frequency alternating current, RF energy results in total loss of vessel wall architecture, disintegration, and carbonization.[5–7] Application of this knowledge has allowed treatment of the greater saphenous vein by intraluminal techniques.[8] Preliminary results obtained in 389 patients treated with RF energy were complicated by third-degree burns of the skin, saphenous nerve injury, periphlebitis, peroneal nerve injury and wound infection. However, this complication was totally prevented when high-volume local anesthesia is introduced around the saphenous vein.

Now, elimination of saphenous vein reflux is done using RF heating.[8] The VNUS vein treatment system utilizing the

Closure catheter (Fig. 16.1) (VNUS Medical Technologies, Sunnyvale, CA, USA) is the most used system in the USA and in Western Europe. This system uses electrodes specifically designed for treatment of the saphenous vein and includes monitoring of electrical and thermal effects of the catheter (Fig. 16.2). Clinically, the device produces precise tissue destruction with minimal formation of thrombus. Bipolar electrodes are used to heat the vein wall. The net effect is venous spasm and collagen shrinkage, which produces maximal physical contraction.

The catheter is introduced into the great saphenous vein in the region of the knee by ultrasound-guided puncture or by cut-down onto the vessel. It is then passed proximally to the saphenofemoral junction under ultrasound guidance. Elimination of venous blood from the saphenous vein is

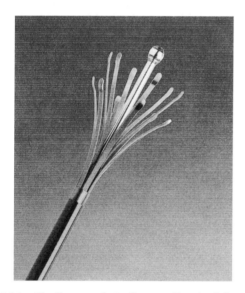

Figure 16.1   *The Closure catheter illustrated here is 8F diameter and delivers radiofrequency energy to the vein wall while monitoring temperature and delivering this information to the control unit.*

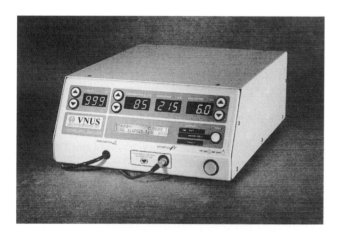

Figure 16.2   *VNUS Technologies has produced a radiofrequency (RF) generator which delivers energy and provides information to the operator. From left to right: Total time of RF delivery (s), temperature (degrees Celsius), impedance (ohms), and power (watts).*

necessary to allow vein wall heating and prevention of superficial thrombophlebitis. This is accomplished by Esmarch bandaging and proximal saphenofemoral junction compression. Alternatively, large amounts of dilute local anesthetic solution will accomplish the same thing. Saphenous vein ablation has been performed using intravenous sedation and tumescent anesthesia alone[9] and with general anesthesia,[10] with and without proximal saphenofemoral ligation.[11] Anesthesia is required because the heating process produces significant pain, and superficial varices may be removed by hook phlebectomy at the same procedure. Starting at the saphenofemoral junction, the saphenous vein is heated and the catheter is withdrawn slowly, ensuring that all parts of the vein are heated sufficiently to produce ablation of the vein. Postoperatively the patient wears a compression stocking for 10–14 days. Postoperative bruising and discomfort are greatly reduced compared with patients treated by stripping of the great saphenous vein. Acute closure was achieved in 93 percent of 141 saphenous veins in the first large series to be reported,[12] and 2-year continued closure exceeds 90 percent, with an acceptable rate of complications[13] (Table 16.1).

Surgical series have shown that undesirable outcomes after saphenous stripping are evident quite early[14] and that even surgical stripping is followed by recurrent varices in 20 percent of limbs.[15] Some 73 percent of limbs destined to be affected by recurrent varicosities at 5 years already show clinical evidence of recurrence at 1 year.[16] Thus, the early results of VNUS Closure seem comparable in their outcome to stripping of the saphenous vein in the long term.

Goldman[9] has taken a lead in endovenous Closure and in use of the 810 nm diode laser as a source of energy to destroy the saphenous vein. He surrounds the saphenous vein with large amounts of dilute local anesthetic containing 0.1 percent lignocaine with adrenaline before commencing RF ablation or laser treatment. Intraoperative ultrasound monitoring ensures that the greater saphenous vein is separated from the skin by the local anesthetic solution, thus avoiding skin burns.

Performing endovenous obliteration of the saphenous vein without dissection of the saphenofemoral junction violates a cardinal rule in saphenous vein surgery. This holds that each of the tributaries must be individually divided. It is advocated by some that each of the tributaries should be dissected back beyond their primary and even secondary tributaries.[17]

Table 16.1   *Results and comparisons of saphenous stripping and VNUS Closure at 12 and 24 months*

	Stripping (%)	Closure (%)
Reflux-free at 12 months	91	93
Reflux-free at 24 months	87	93
Neovascularization at 24 months	52	0
Deep venous thrombosis (DVT)	1	1.0
Skin burn	0	1.9
Infection	8	0.2
Above-knee paresthesia at 12 months	8	3.1

In actual experience, such dissection apparently causes neovascularization.[16] This fact has been uncovered by duplex ultrasound surveillance after saphenous stripping and after ligation (Table 16.2). In contrast, neovascularization has yet to be reported after VNUS Closure when done without groin dissection. Absence of tributary interruption and saphenous transection does not leave a saphenous stump in the groin; therefore,[19] abdominal wall venous drainage is preserved. In addition, the absence of surgical intervention means that no hematoma forms outside the vessels.

The issue of varicose vein recurrence after saphenous vein obliteration by RF ablation without saphenofemoral junction tributary disconnection is not settled. Careful duplex evaluation of saphenous RF ablation by Pichot et al.[19] has revealed marked shrinking and obliteration of the saphenous vein itself but with preservation of tributaries to the saphenofemoral junction. Sixty limbs treated with saphenofemoral junction ligation and division of tributaries have been compared with 120 limbs treated without high ligation.[20] Of the 49 high ligation limbs, 2 percent developed recurrent reflux by 6 months and, in 97 non-high ligation limbs followed for that length of time, 8 percent developed recurrent reflux (not statistically significant). In limbs followed to 12 months, no new instances of reflux developed. Actual recurrence curves did not differ between patients who had or had not undergone saphenofemoral ligation, and the experience predicted a greater than 90 percent freedom from recurrent reflux and varicosities at 1 year for both groups. Decisions on this issue are not final, but it is acknowledged that, should a tributary develop reflux and prove to be a source of recurrent varicosities, the problem can be managed without further surgery by using sclerotherapy. Many surgeons would prefer ambulatory phlebectomy at this point, but in either event, the problem is not a major deterrent to use of endovascular saphenous vein obliteration by RF energy without saphenofemoral ligation.

A significant limitation of VNUS Closure is that it is only used to treat the trunk of the great saphenous vein in the thigh, as described above. The reason for this is that the small saphenous vein lies close to the sural nerve and there is some concern that this nerve may be damaged by heating the adjacent vein. Similarly, in the calf, the saphenous nerve lies close to the saphenous vein and the amount of subcutaneous fat is usually very limited. In these circumstances, both the skin and nerve might be damaged by treating the vein. A common complication following treatment by RF ablation is paresthesia or anesthesia in the treated region. This is usually transient but indicates that cutaneous nerves adjacent to veins are at risk from the heating used to destroy the veins. Varices arising in saphenous tributaries are usually managed by hook phlebectomy or sclerotherapy since these are not amenable to treatment by RF ablation. The necessity to pass a catheter along the saphenous vein in order to treat the vein means that, in general, this method is not suitable for the management of recurrent varicose veins. A possible exception to this are cases where the saphenous vein remains incompetent following previous ligation without stripping. These restrictions on the use of VNUS Closure significantly diminish the number of patients in whom the technique may be used. A randomized controlled study has been conducted to evaluate the advantages of VNUS Closure over surgical stripping of the great saphenous vein.[21] It was found that this technique resulted in more rapid return to normal activities compared with surgery and that the postoperative pain and bruising were less. The differences between the surgery and VNUS Closure groups disappeared after 4 weeks following treatment.

ENDOVENOUS LASER

Radiofrequency energy and light energy are similar because both are part of the electromagnetic spectrum. Delivery of laser light energy to the interior of the greater saphenous vein has been accomplished using a 400–750 Φm sterile bare-tipped quartz fiber.[22,23] Energy from an 810 nm diode laser is utilized to produce non-thrombotic occlusion of the vein (Fig. 16.3). In preliminary reports, obliteration of the saphenous vein has been accomplished in all cases. Only long-term follow-up studies will prove that this, too, is effective treatment.

The technique used is very similar to that employed when treating a saphenous vein by RF ablation. Again, the great saphenous vein is cannulated under ultrasound guidance at about the level of the knee. The laser fiber is passed proximally to the saphenofemoral junction under ultrasound control. The vein is surrounded by a large volume of dilute local anesthetic solution, since any treatment that involves heating the vein to the point of destruction causes pain. The anesthetic solution also ensures that the skin is not heated excessively by the laser energy by introducing a buffer of fluid

Table 16.2 *Neovascularization after comprehensive saphenofemoral junction (SFJ) ligation*

Lead author	No. of limbs	Mean follow-up (years)	Saphenectomy	Recurrent SFJ reflux (clinically relevant)[a]		
				Multiple channels at site of former SFJ	Dominant single channel at site of former SFJ	Circumjunctional connection
Fischer[18]	125	34	Yes	22 [2 (0.9%)]	31 [25 (81%)]	22 [0 (0%)]
Jones[16]	113	2.5	Yes, 53; no, 60	44 [11 (25%)]	12 [12 (100%)]	3 [0 (0%)]
Total	238	2.5 to 34	Yes, 178; no, 60	66 [13 (60%)]	43 [37 (86%)]	25 [0 (0%)]

[a] Clinically relevant defined as sufficiently symptomatic or cosmetically disturbing to cause consideration of re-operation.

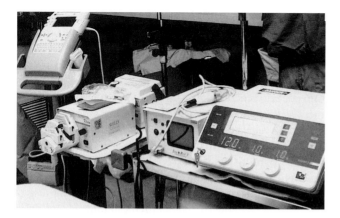

Figure 16.3 *Devices used to ablate the saphenous vein are shown here. From left to right: Sonosite ultrasound monitor, Klein pump for high-volume anesthesia; SiteRite ultrasound for transcutaneous catheter placement; and the Diomed laser light generator.*

Table 16.3 *Comparison of VNUS Closure and laser light treatment of the saphenous vein[a]*

	VNUS Closure	**Laser Diomed 810**
Patients	281	114
Limbs	348	122
DVT	1/348 (0.3%)	1/122 (0.8%)
Superficial phlebitis	0	4/122 (3.2%)
Paresthesias	1/348 at 9 months	1/122 at 6 months
Ecchymosis	1/348 (0.3%)	19/122 (15.6%)
Cost	$850	$120
Return to normal	0–7 days (1.08 days mean)	0–14 days (1.2 days mean)
Patient preference	10	1

[a] Data provided by Nick Morrison, MD. DVT, deep vein thrombosis.

between the vein and the skin. Laser energy is applied and the fiber is slowly withdrawn from the vein, ensuring that all parts of the vein to be treated receive sufficient energy to destroy them. The laser is not used to treat superficial varices and these are managed by hook phlebectomy or by sclerotherapy. Postoperatively, the patient wears a compression stocking for 10–14 days. Moderate bruising is usually seen along the track of the treated vein, but the discomfort experienced by the patient is less than would follow stripping of the saphenous vein.

Short-term comparison of endovenous obliteration of the saphenous vein by closure techniques of RF energy and laser light energy has been accomplished by Nick Morrison. At the time of writing his experience has not been reported but has been graciously provided to us for this volume. A summary of his findings (Table 16.3) favors closure by RF energy if cost is not a consideration.

Laser treatment may result in damage to nerves running adjacent to the vein in a similar way to RF ablation. This had led to the use of this technique to treat the great saphenous vein with only limited use in the small saphenous vein. Superficial varices generally run too close to the skin for this method to be used in view of the risk of skin burns. Therefore, residual varices

are usually managed conventionally by phlebectomy or sclerotherapy. This technique has not been compared directly with surgery in a clinical trial, but the clinical series which have been reported suggest that patients experience greater ease of mobility and less pain than following stripping of the saphenous vein.

MECHANICAL PHLEBECTOMY

Surgery for superficial venous incompetence consists of two major steps. The first, obliteration of the saphenous vein or removal of the saphenous vein from the circulation, has been discussed above. The second step is removal of the varicose veins themselves. While many physicians who treat varices favor sclerotherapy for this step, others prefer to remove the saphenous tributary varicose clusters by hook phlebectomy, stab avulsion, or other surgical techniques. Transilluminated powered phlebectomy has been recently developed to offer a minimally invasive alternative to hook avulsion of varicose veins.[13] The system was developed by Smith & Nephew Endoscopy Division, Inc. and has been called the TriVex system because of its incorporation of three technologies. These are: dissection of varices; direct visualization of the varicose veins by transillumination; and excision by a rotating blade and suction aspiration (Fig. 16.4).[24]

The instrumentation consists of an endoscopic transilluminator and a powered dissector. The endoscopic transilluminator is a two-channel device. One channel is used to distribute large volumes of very dilute local anesthetic solution to achieve tissue tumescence. This local anesthetic is placed alongside and deep to the varicosities. The second channel of this instrument provides light from a 45-degree illuminator to transilluminate the varicose vein clusters in their location subcutaneously. Anesthesia is obtained by infusing as much as 1000 mL of 0.9 percent normal saline to which has been added 50 mL of 1 percent lignocaine and 2 mL of 1:1000 adrenaline. A pressurized infusion set is connected directly to the endoscopic channel.

The second instrument is a Smith & Nephew EP-1 endoscopic powered tissue dissector. This device contains a rotating tubular blade encased in a protective sheath. A lateral cutting window is addressed by the dissector, and varicose veins adjacent to that window are morcellated and withdrawn using wall suction. The tissue dissector is introduced on a plane just deep to the veins and slowly withdrawn along the course of the varicosities. The skin is then stretched between the operator's left hand and the dissector. The window of the tissue dissector is directed along the varicosities and these are subsequently broken up under direct vision. The morcellated tissue fragments are aspirated into the system by a suction device that is connected to the handle of the instrument. The transillumination allows one to confirm that the veins are entirely removed. In practice, the blade rotations can be clockwise, counterclockwise or used in an alternating fashion with speeds ranging from 800 to 2000 revolutions/min.

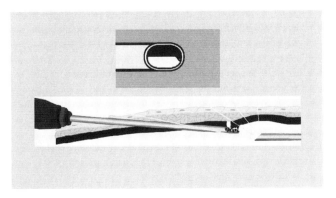

Figure 16.4 *The TriVex device, as illustrated here, consists of two parts. The transilluminator (top and right) allows delivery of high volumes of local anesthesia and visualization of the subcutaneous varices. The powered dissector (left) contains a distal window harboring a rotating blade which morcellates adjacent tissue (varices) and aspirates this under wall suction.*

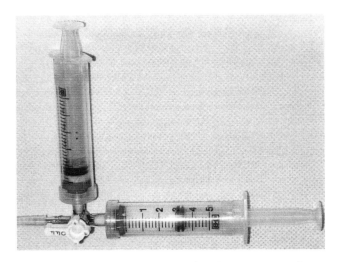

Figure 16.5 *Two syringes connected by a three-way stopcock allow rapid generation of a stable microfoam for endovenous obliteration of varices or the saphenous veins.*

Following vein extraction, further tumescent anesthesia solution is infiltrated liberally along the pathway of the excised varicosities. This is to discourage ecchymosis from hematoma formation and aid in postoperative analgesia.[24]

Spitz, who developed the device, has shown that this technique is significantly quicker, requires fewer incisions, and results in fewer complications when compared with traditional hook phlebectomy.[24] In practice, bruising and ecchymosis are seen in nearly all patients but this resolves within 6–12 weeks. Others have reported paresthesia as well as ecchymosis. A recent study has investigated the efficacy of powered phlebectomy compared with surgery in a randomized controlled trial. This has shown no statistically significant advantage for the speed of the technique compared with surgery.[25] The cosmetic outcome was identical in the two groups at 1 year. The extent of bruising and postoperative pain was similar in the two groups. The main advantage was that fewer incisions were needed in the powered phlebectomy group. Whether this is sufficient advantage to justify the additional cost of the equipment and disposables is debatable.

While this new procedure appears to be a useful adjunct to varicose vein surgery, as with any new procedure, long-term results and cost–benefit analyses will be required.

FOAM SCLEROTHERAPY

Foam sclerotherapy has developed into an important treatment modality over the past 10 years (Fig. 16.5). The technique and its outcomes are presented in detail in Chapters 18 and 19. It is sufficient to say that this method promises to dominate the management of incompetent superficial veins in the future. It offers technical simplicity compared with RF ablation and endovenous laser, as well as greatly reduced costs of treatment.

CONCLUSION

The aim of these new modalities of treatment is to facilitate obliteration of saphenous trunks, whilst minimizing the consequences for the patient. At the same time, there should be no prejudice of the long-term outcome. Both RF ablation and endovenous laser treatment achieve this to a substantial extent. Both are limited as to the veins in which they may be used, and the advantage to the patient appears to be limited to the perioperative period when postoperative sequelae are reduced compared with surgery. Powered phlebectomy offers some limited advantages for the surgeon, but there is little to offer the patient. This technique is probably more invasive than conventional phlebectomy and therefore has potential disadvantages. Time will establish whether these methods remain popular. Further clinical trials will be required to establish the role of these methods and their relationship to foam sclerotherapy.

REFERENCES

1. Sawyer PN, Page JW. Bioelectric phenomena as an etiologic factor in intravascular thrombosis. *Am J Physiol* 1953; **175**: 103–7.
2. Thompson WM, Pizzo S, Jackson DC, Johnsrude IS. The effect of drug-induced thrombocytopenia on direct-current transcatheter electrocoagulation. *Works Prog* 1977; **124**: 831–3.
3. Phillips JF, Robinson AE, Johnsrude IS, Jackson DC. Experimental closure of arteriovenous fistula by transcatheter electrocoagulation. *Radiology* 1975; **115**: 319–21.
4. Brunelle F, Kunstlinger F, Quillard J. Endovascular electrocoagulation with a bipolar electrode and alternating current: a follow-up study in dogs. *Radiology* 1998; **148**: 413–5.
5. Sigel B, Dunn MR. The mechanism of blood vessel closure by high-frequency electrocoagulation. *SG & O* 1965; 823–31.
6. Politowski M, Szpak E, Marszalek Z. Varices of the lower extremities treated by electrocoagulation. *Surgery* 1964; 355–60.

7. Politowski M, Zelazny T. Complications and difficulties in electrocoagulation of varices of the lower extremities. *Surgery* 1966; **59**: 932–4.

8. Weiss RA, Goldman MP. Controlled RF-mediated endovenous shrinkage and occlusion. In: Goldman MP, Weiss RA, Bergan JJ, eds. *Varicose Veins and Telangiectasias: Diagnosis and Management*, 2nd edn. St Louis: Quality Medical Publishing, Inc., 1999.

9. Goldman MP. Closure of the greater saphenous vein with endoluminal radiofrequency thermal heating of the vein wall in combination with ambulatory phlebectomy: preliminary 6-month followup. *Dermatol Surg* 2000; **26**: 105.

10. Chandler JG, Pichot O, Sessa C *et al.* Treatment of primary venous insufficiency by endovenous saphenous vein obliteration. *Vasc Surg* 2000; **34**: 201–14.

11. Whiteley MS, Pichot O, Sessa C *et al.* Endovenous obliteration: an effective, minimally invasive surrogate for saphenous vein stripping. *J Endovasc Surg* 2000; **7**: 11–17.

12. Manfrini S, Gasbarro V, Danielsson G *et al.* Endovenous management of saphenous vein reflux. *J Vasc Surg* 2000; **32**: 330–42.

13. Arumugasamy M, McGreal G, O'Connor A *et al.* The technique of transilluminated powered phlebectomy: a novel, minimally invasive system for varicose vein surgery. *Eur J Vasc Endovasc Surg* 2002; **23**: 180–2.

14. Sarin S, Scurr JH, Coleridge Smith PD. Assessment of stripping the long saphenous vein in the treatment of primary varicose veins. *Br J Surg* 1992; **79**: 889–93.

15. Dwerryhouse S, Davies B, Harradine K, Earnshaw JJ. Stripping the long saphenous vein reduces the rate of reoperation for recurrent varicose veins: five-year results of a randomized trial. *J Vasc Surg* 1999; **29**: 589–92.

16. Jones L, Braithwaite BD, Selwyn D *et al.* Neovascularization is the principal cause of varicose vein recurrence: results of a randomized trial of stripping the long saphenous vein. *Eur J Vasc Endovasc Surg* 1996; **12**: 442–5.

17. Bergan JJ. Saphenous vein stripping by inversion: current technique. *Surg Rounds* 2000; 118–24.

18. Fischer R, Linde N, Duff C *et al.* Late recurrent saphenofemoral junction reflux after ligation and stripping of the greater saphenous vein. *J Vasc Surg* 2001; **34**(2): 236–40.

19. Pichot O, Sessa C, Chandler JG *et al.* Role of duplex imaging in endovenous obliteration for primary venous insufficiency. *J Endovasc Ther* 2000; **7**: 451–9.

20. Chandler JG, Pichot O, Sessa C *et al.* Defining the role of extended saphenofemoral junction ligation: a prospective comparative study. *J Vasc Surg* 2000; **32**: 941–53.

21. Lurie F, Creton D, Eklof B *et al.* Prospective randomized study of endovenous radiofrequency obliteration (closure procedure) versus ligation and stripping in a selected patient population (EVOLVeS Study). *J Vasc Surg* 2003; **38**: 207–14.

22. Boné C. Tratamiento endoluminal de las varices con laser de Diodo. Estudio preliminar. *Rev Patol Vasc* 1999; **v**: 35–46.

23. Navarro L, Min RJ, Boné C. Endovenous laser: a new minimally invasive method of treatment for varicose veins: preliminary observations using an 810 nm diode laser. *Dermatol Surg* 2001; **27**: 117–22.

24. Spitz GA, Braxton JM, Bergan JJ. Outpatient varicose vein surgery with transilluminated powered phlebectomy. *Vasc Surg* 2000; **34**: 547–55.

25. Aremu MA, Mahendran B, Butcher W *et al.* Prospective randomized controlled trial: conventional versus powered phlebectomy. *J Vasc Surg* 2004; **39**: 88–94.

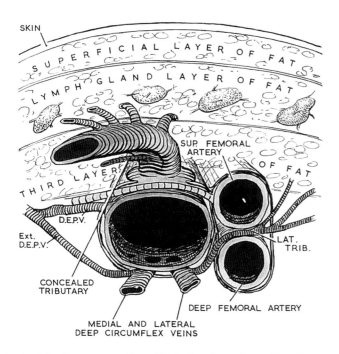

Plate 3.1 *Transverse section of the left sapheno-femoral junction. (See Ch. 3, p. 16)*

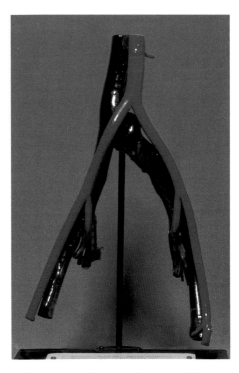

Plate 3.3 *Cadaver corrosion cast of the aorta, inferior vena cava and iliac vessels. Widening and flattening of the termination of the left common iliac vein are clearly seen at the point where it is crossed by the right common iliac artery. (See Ch. 3, p. 21)*

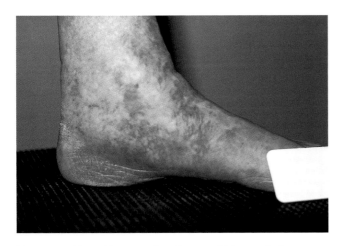

Plate 3.2 *The ankle venous flare (corona phlebectactica), an important physical sign indicating calf perforating vein incompetence. (See Ch. 3, p. 19)*

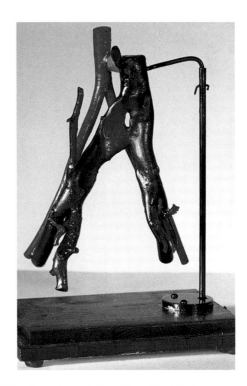

Plate 3.4 *Corrosion cast dissection of the inferior vena cava, aorta and iliac arteries, posterior view, showing a filling defect, representing an intraluminal band, in the left common iliac vein, where it lies posterior to the right common iliac artery. (See Ch. 3, p. 22)*

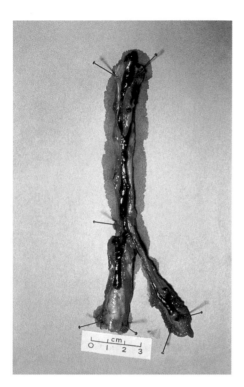

Plate 5.1 *Postmortem dissection of deep veins of calf showing typical deep vein thrombosis. (See Ch. 5, p. 38)*

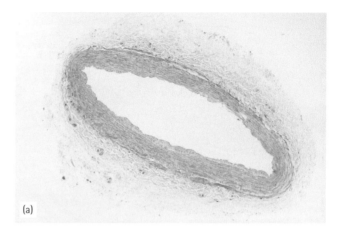

(a)

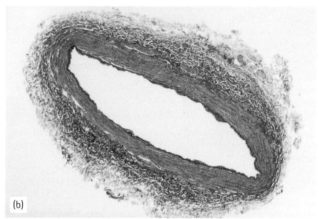

(b)

Plate 6.2 *Normal vein. (a) HEB. (b) Van Giesen elastic stain. (See Ch. 6, p. 51)*

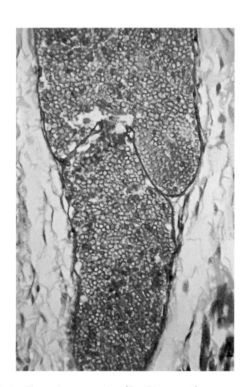

Plate 6.1 *Normal venous valve. (See Ch. 6, p. 50)*

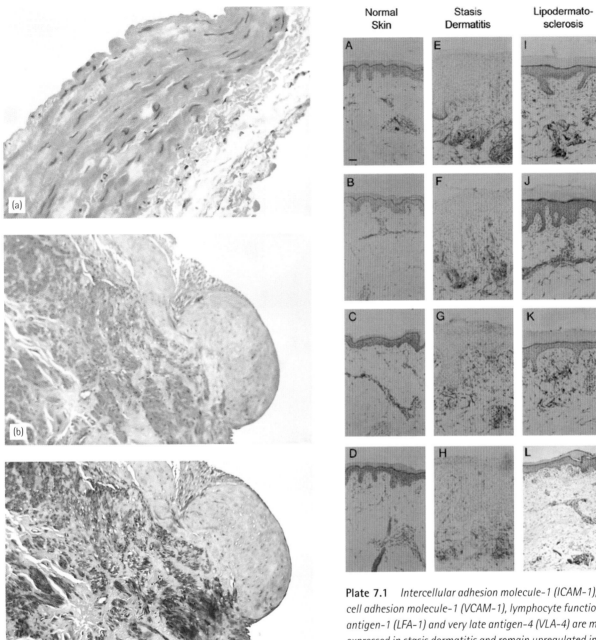

Plate 6.3 *(a) Early localized change. (b, c) Advanced change. (See Ch. 6, p. 51)*

Normal Skin Stasis Dermatitis Lipodermato-sclerosis

ICAM-1

VCAM-1

LFA-1

VLA-4

Plate 7.1 *Intercellular adhesion molecule-1 (ICAM-1), vascular cell adhesion molecule-1 (VCAM-1), lymphocyte function-associated antigen-1 (LFA-1) and very late antigen-4 (VLA-4) are markedly expressed in stasis dermatitis and remain upregulated in lipodermatosclerosis. (×506). Scale bar: (A) 150 mm. (See Ch. 7, p. 58)*

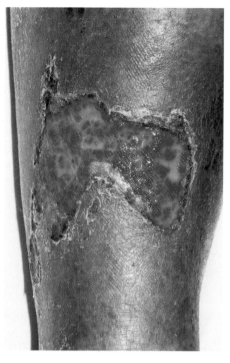

Plate 8.1 *Ulcerated venous hemangioma of leg. (See Ch. 8, p. 67)*

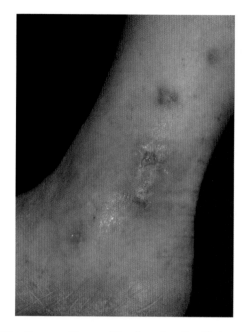

Plate 8.3 *Non-specific vasculitic ulceration. (See Ch. 8, p. 68)*

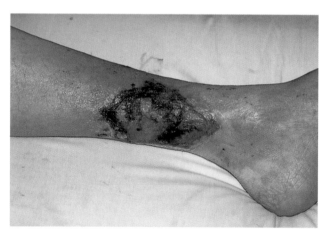

Plate 8.2 *Rheumatoid ulcer; usually indistinguishable from ischemic ulcer. (See Ch. 8, p. 68)*

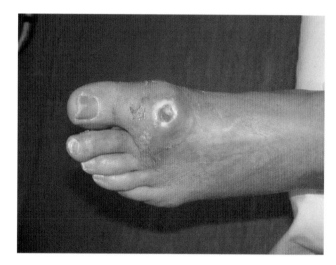

Plate 8.4 *Diabetic foot ulcer. (See Ch. 8, p. 69)*

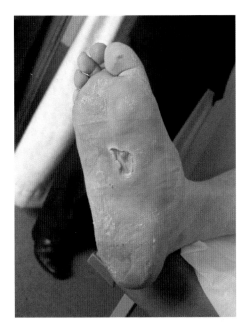

Plate 8.5 *Diabetic foot: pressure ulcer in a Charcot's foot. (See Ch. 8, p. 69)*

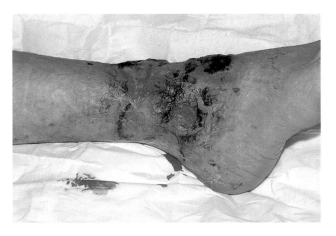

Plate 8.7 *Marjolin's ulcer. This squamous carcinoma developed in an 85-year-old's chronic leg ulcer and required treatment by above-knee amputation and inguinal block dissection. (See Ch. 8, p. 72)*

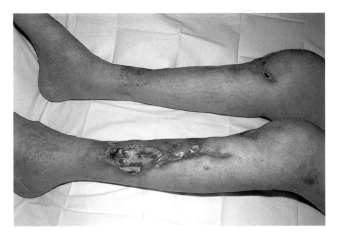

Plate 8.6 *Necrobiosis lipoidica of both shins of an insulin-dependent diabetic woman. (See Ch. 8, p. 69)*

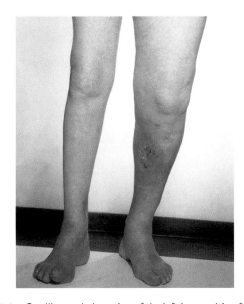

Plate 9.1 *Swelling and ulceration of the left leg resulting from left common iliac vein occlusion. (See Ch. 9, p. 76)*

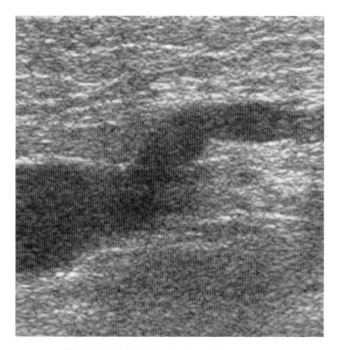

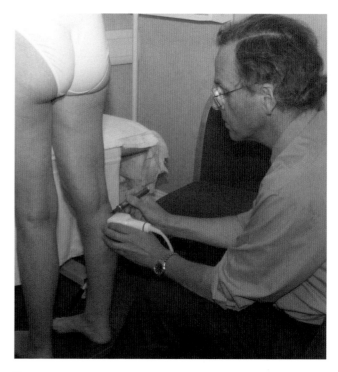

Plate 10A.2 *Preoperative vein localization using duplex ultrasonography. The location of the saphenopopliteal junction (SPJ) and small saphenous vein (SSV) are being marked in the popliteal fossa. (See Ch. 10A, p. 85)*

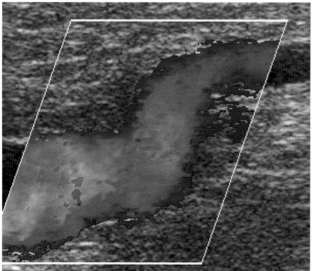

Plate 10A.1 *Duplex ultrasound image of varices arising from a mid-thigh perforating vein. (See Ch. 10A, p. 84)*

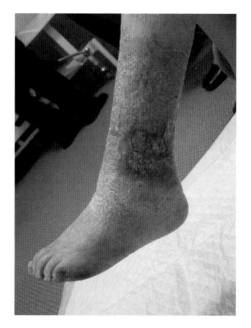

Plate 13.1 *Dermatitis resulting from dressing allergy. (See Ch. 13, p. 123)*

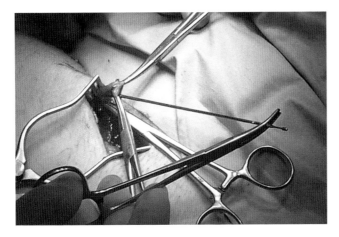

Plate 24.1 *An Oesch pin-stripper is passed down the great saphenous vein following ligation of the saphenofemoral junction. (See Ch. 24, p. 222)*

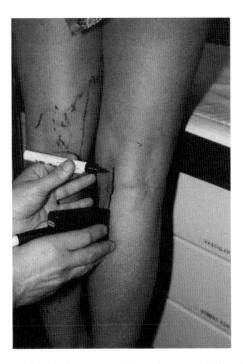

Plate 24.3 *Duplex ultrasonography used preoperatively to locate the saphenopopliteal junction and mark the track of the small saphenous vein. (See Ch. 24, p. 223)*

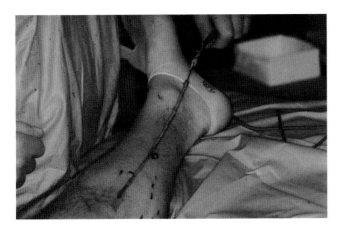

Plate 24.2 *The great saphenous vein is removed by inverting stripping through a 3 mm incision just below the knee. (See Ch. 24, p. 222)*

17

Surgery of perforating veins

MANJU KALRA, PETER GLOVICZKI

INTRODUCTION

Incompetent perforating veins were observed in patients with venous ulceration more than a century ago by John Gay,[1] but surgical interruption of these to prevent ulcer recurrence was first suggested by Linton only in 1938.[2] Linton attributed a key role to 'communicating' veins in the mechanism of venous ulceration, an idea embraced later by Cockett,[3,4] Dodd,[5] and several other investigators.[6–12] The rationale of surgical interruption of perforating veins was to prevent transmission of elevated venous pressure from the deep to the superficial venous system during ambulation, and thereby promote ulcer healing.

In the mid-twentieth century perforator vein ligation using different open techniques was adopted by many surgeons as the panacea to heal venous ulcers. However, a high incidence of wound complications, coupled with conflicting long-term results reported by various investigators, led to virtual abandonment of the open procedures during the 1980s.[13,14] Several modifications to Linton's original operation were proposed; invariably these included the use of shorter skin incisions,[3–6,9,10] or long posterior incision away from damaged skin,[15,16] or multiple medial skin crease incisions,[17] and blind avulsion of the perforators with a shearing instrument.[18] In the mid-1980s, Hauer developed a technique that enabled incompetent perforating vein interruption under direct vision through small incisions made far away from areas of ulcerated or damaged skin.[19] This technique was rapidly adopted and refined by several groups, and in recent years subfascial endoscopic perforator vein surgery (SEPS) has emerged as an effective minimally invasive technique to interrupt perforating veins.[20–30]

SURGICAL ANATOMY OF PERFORATING VEINS

Perforating veins connect the superficial to the deep venous system, either directly to the main axial veins (direct perforators) or indirectly to muscular tributaries or soleal venous sinuses (indirect perforators). The term 'communicating veins' refers to interconnecting veins within the same system. In calf and thigh perforators, venous valves ensure unidirectional flow, from the great and small saphenous systems towards the deep veins. In contrast, perforating veins of the foot are valveless and flow occurs paradoxically from the deep to the superficial venous system.[31–33]

In the mid-calf and distal calf the most important direct medial perforators do not originate from the great saphenous vein (GSV) (Fig. 17.1). This finding was first noted by John Gay in 1866 in a clinical case with venous ulcers, where he demonstrated the posterior arch vein and three perforating veins.[1] The most significant medial calf perforators, termed the Cockett perforators, connect the posterior arch vein (Leonardo's vein) (Fig. 17.1) to the paired posterior tibial veins. Thus, stripping of the greater saphenous vein will not affect flow through these perforators. Three groups of Cockett perforators have been identified. The Cockett I perforator is located posterior to the medial malleolus and may be difficult to reach endoscopically. The Cockett II and III perforators are located 7–9 and 10–12 cm proximal to the lower border of the medial malleolus, respectively (Fig. 17.2).[32] All are found in 'Linton's line', 2–4 cm posterior to the medial edge of the tibia.[33,34] Mozes *et al.*[32] from our group described their anatomy in detail by performing corrosion cast studies in 40 normal limbs from 20 cadavers. They identified an average of 14 medial calf perforating veins (direct and indirect) per limb,

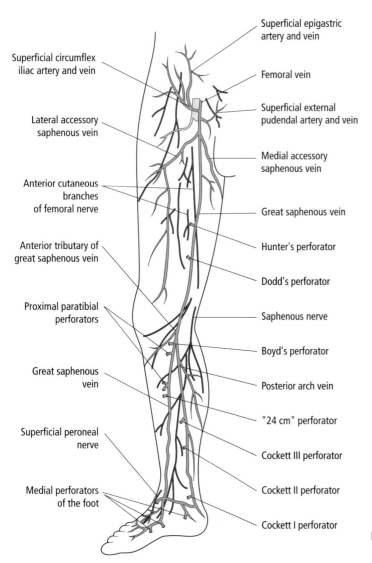

Figure 17.1 *Anatomy of medial superficial and perforating veins of the leg.*

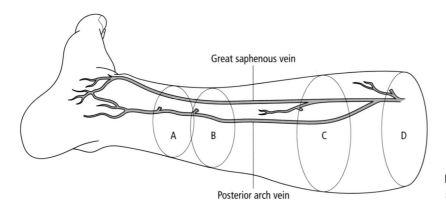

Figure 17.2 *Superficial and perforating veins in the medial side of the leg.*

with a range of seven to 22 veins. However, only three of these were greater than 2 mm in diameter, in concordance with the earlier clinical descriptions of Linton and Cockett, and the fact that only three to five clinically significant incompetent perforators are found in most patients.[21]

The next group of clinically relevant perforating veins are the paratibial perforators, which connect the GSV and its

tributaries to the posterior tibial and popliteal veins. The paratibial perforators are found in three groups, all located 1–2 cm posterior to the medial tibial border. They are located 18–22, 23–27 and 28–32 cm from the inferior border of the medial malleolus, respectively (Fig. 17.1). The 18–22 cm group corresponds to the '24 centimeter' perforator described by Sherman, who used the sole of the foot as his point of reference.[33] There are three additional direct perforating veins that connect the GSV to the popliteal and superficial femoral veins. Boyd's perforator, just distal to the knee, connects the GSV to the popliteal vein.[32] Dodd's and Hunterian perforators are located in the thigh and connect the GSV to the proximal popliteal or the superficial femoral veins (Fig. 17.1). Boyd's perforator may be reached endoscopically, while stripping of the GSV will interrupt the drainage of Dodd's and Hunterian perforators, except in 8 percent of patients with a duplicated saphenous system.

Certain anatomic considerations specific to the endoscopic interruption of medial calf perforators need to be emphasized. In cadaver dissections, Mozes *et al.* noted that only 63 percent of all medial perforators were directly accessible from the superficial posterior compartment.[32] Based on clinical reports, only 32 percent of Cockett II, 84 percent of Cockett III and 43 percent of lower paratibial perforating veins are accessible from the superficial posterior compartment.[35] In order to interrupt all incompetent perforating veins, two additional areas require exploration: the deep posterior compartment and the intermuscular septum in 'Linton's line'. The paratibial and the Cockett veins can be found under the fascia of the deep posterior compartment, while the Cockett II/III veins can also be located within the intermuscular septum (Fig. 17.3). Distally in the subfascial space, the Cockett I perforator usually cannot be visualized or reached because of its retromalleolar position.

In the calf, anterior and lateral perforators are also found and may gain clinical significance in patients with lateral ulceration. The anterior perforators connect tributaries of the great and small saphenous veins directly to the anterior tibial veins. The lateral perforating veins consist of both direct and indirect perforators. In the distal calf, the small saphenous vein is connected by direct perforators to the peroneal veins (Bassi's perforator). The indirect perforators connect tributaries of the small saphenous vein to either the muscular venous sinuses or the gastrocnemius or soleus veins prior to entering the deep axial system.

PATHOPHYSIOLOGY

Although the pathophysiology of chronic venous insufficiency (CVI) at the cellular level remains controversial, most authors agree that venous hypertension in the erect position and during ambulation is the most important factor responsible for the development of skin changes and venous ulcerations. The relationship between venous ulceration and ambulatory venous pressure was first described by Beecher *et al.*[36] in 1936. Subsequent studies have confirmed that ambulatory venous pressure has not only diagnostic but also prognostic significance in CVI.[37–39] Ambulatory venous pressure may be elevated due to primary valvular incompetence (PVI) in superficial, deep and/or perforator veins, or it may be the result of a previous deep venous thrombosis (DVT). Deep venous

incompetence (DVI) is initially compensated by the calf muscle pump, but eventually results in secondary incompetence of valves in perforating veins, and transmission of pressure from the deep to the superficial veins, a fact that was first suggested by Homans[40] and documented by Linton.[2]

Hemodynamic abnormalities in limbs with venous ulceration

Reflux of blood due to primary or post-thrombotic valvular incompetence coupled with calf muscle pump failure, is the most frequent cause of CVI and venous ulceration. While severe isolated incompetence of the superficial system may also lead to sufficiently high ambulatory pressures and the development of ulcers, evidence is increasing that the majority of patients with venous ulcers have multisystem (superficial, deep and/or perforator) incompetence, involving at least two of the three venous systems.[30,41–43] DVI has been reported to occur in a significant number of patients (21–80 percent) in large surgical series of venous ulcer (Table 17.1).[41,44,45] Incompetent calf perforators in conjunction with superficial or deep reflux have been reported in 66 percent of limbs with venous ulceration, and occur more frequently in limbs with complications.[44,46] A Duplex ultrasound study in 91 limbs with venous ulcerations from Boston University revealed isolated superficial vein incompetence (SVI) in only 17 percent and perforator vein incompetence in 63 percent of limbs.[43] Similarly, Lees and Lambert[47] reported perforator incompetence in 60 percent of ulcer patients, and Labrapoulos *et al.* in 56 percent.[42] It is extremely important to obtain an accurate assessment of the underlying pathophysiology in every patient, not only to aid in treatment planning, but also to evaluate and compare results.

Hemodynamic significance of incompetent perforators

While few argue today that incompetent perforators occur in at least two-thirds of patients with venous ulceration, the contribution of incompetent perforators to the hemodynamic derangement in limbs with CVI remains a topic of debate. Cockett and Jones[3] coined the term 'ankle blow-out syndrome' to differentiate perforator incompetence from the usually more benign isolated saphenous incompetence.[48] Indeed, perforator vein incompetence can raise pressures in the supramalleolar network well above 100 mmHg during calf muscle contraction, a phenomenon best described by Negus and Friedgood[10] using the analogy of a 'broken bellows'. Experiments of Bjordal[49] confirmed a net outward flow of 60 mL/min through incompetent perforating veins. Skin changes and venous ulcers almost always develop in the gaiter area of the leg (the area between the distal edge of the soleus muscle and the ankle), where large incompetent medial perforating veins are located, underscoring their importance. Direct estimation of the hemodynamic significance of incompetent perforators is difficult, since isolated perforator vein incompetence in CVI is rare,[42]

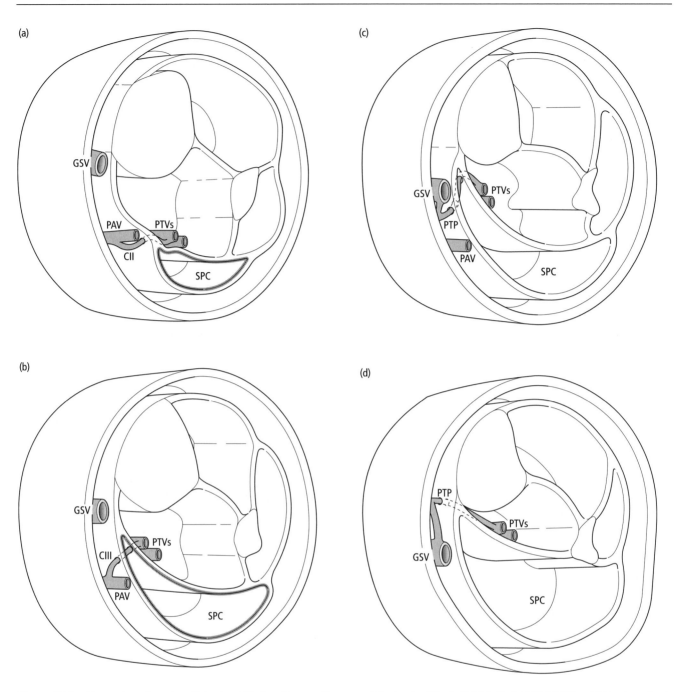

Figure 17.3 *Compartments and medial veins of the leg. Cross-sections are at the levels of Cockett II (a), Cockett III (b), '24 cm' (c) and proximal paratibial perforating veins (d). GSV, greater saphenous vein; PAV, posterior arch vein; PTVs, posterior tibial veins; SPC, superficial posterior compartment; CII, Cockett II; CIII, Cockett III; PTP, paratibial perforator.*

and because incompetent perforators have been observed in as many as 21 percent of normal limbs.[50]

Based on duplex ultrasound studies, several authors have demonstrated a correlation between the number and size of incompetent perforating veins detected by duplex ultrasonography, and the severity of CVI.[51,52] Recently, Delis *et al.*[53] quantified perforator incompetence based on diameter, flow velocities and volume flow, and stressed that incompetent perforators sustain further hemodynamic impairment in the presence of deep reflux.

INDICATIONS FOR PERFORATOR INTERRUPTION

The presence of incompetent perforators in patients with advanced CVI (clinical classes 4–6 of the CEAP classification; see Box 6.1, p. 46) constitutes for us the indication for surgical treatment in a fit patient. While most authors prefer to perform open perforator ligation only after ulcers have healed, a clean, granulating open ulcer is not a contraindication for the

Table 17.1   *Distribution of valvular incompetence in patients with advanced chronic venous disease*

Authors (year)	No. of limbs	Sup. [n (%)]	Perf. [n (%)]	Deep [n (%)]	Sup. + perf. [n (%)]	Sup. + perf. + deep [n (%)]
Schanzer and Pierce[9] (1982)	52	3 (6)	20 (38)	4 (8)	11 (21)	14 (27)
Negus and Friedgood[10] (1983)	77	0 (0)	0 (0)	0 (0)	35 (46)	42 (54)
Sethia and Darke[48] (1984)	60	0 (0)	5 (8)	20 (33)	17 (28)	18 (30)
van Bemmelen et al.[45] (1991)	25	0 (0)	0 (0)	2 (8)	3 (12)	20 (80)
Hanrahan et al.[43] (1991)	91	16 (17)	8 (8)	2 (2)	18 (19)	47 (49)
Darke and Penfold[46] (1992)	213	0 (0)	8 (4)	47 (22)	83 (39)	75 (35)
Lees and Lambert[47] (1993)	25	3 (12)	0 (0)	3 (12)	10 (40)	9 (36)
Shami et al.[74] (1993)	59	0 (0)	0 (0)	19 (32)	31 (53)	9 (15)
van Rij et al.[41] (1994)	120	48 (40)	6 (5)	10 (8)	31 (26)	25 (21)
Myers et al.[44] (1995)	96	15 (16)	2 (2)	7 (8)	25 (26)	47 (49)
Labropoulos et al.[75] (1996)	120	26 (22)	1 (1)	5 (4)	23 (19)	65 (54)
Gloviczki et al.[28] (1999)	146	0 (0)	7 (5)	0 (0)	66 (45)	73 (50)
Total no. of limbs (%)	1084	111 (10)	57 (5)	119 (11)	353 (32)	444 (41)

Sup, superficial incompetence; perf, perforator incompetence; deep, deep vein incompetence.

Table 17.2   *Diagnostic tests to identify the sites of incompetent perforating veins*

Test	Sensitivity (%)	Specificity (%)
Physical examination[34]	60	0
Continuous wave Doppler ultrasonography[34]	62	4
Ascending phlebography[34]	60	50
Duplex scanning[22]	79	100

SEPS procedure. Contraindications include associated chronic arterial occlusive disease, infected ulcer, morbid obesity, non-ambulatory or high-risk patient. Diabetes, renal failure, liver failure or ulcers in patients with rheumatoid arthritis or scleroderma are relative contraindications. Presence of deep venous obstruction at the level of the popliteal vein or higher on preoperative imaging is also a relative contraindication. Patients with extensive skin changes, circumferential large ulcers, recent deep venous thrombosis, severe lymphedema or large legs may not be suitable candidates. SEPS has been performed for recurrent disease after previous perforator interruption; however, it is technically more demanding in this situation. Limbs with lateral ulcerations should be managed by open interruption of lateral or posterior perforators where appropriate.

PREOPERATIVE EVALUATION

Preoperative evaluation includes imaging studies to assess the superficial, deep and perforating veins for incompetence and/or obstruction, and guide the operative intervention. Duplex scanning has 100 percent specificity and the highest sensitivity of all diagnostic tests to predict the sites of incompetent perforating veins (Table 17.2),[22,34] Perforator incompetence

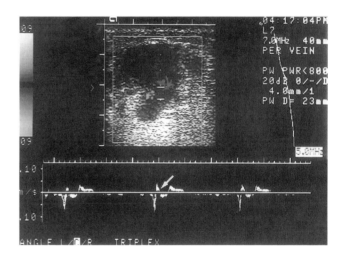

Figure 17.4   *Color Doppler and spectral tracing of an enlarged incompetent perforating vein. Spectral analysis demonstrates bidirectional flow (arrow). (Reproduced with permission from Gloviczki et al.[54])*

is defined by retrograde (outward) flow lasting greater than 0.3 s or longer than antegrade flow during the relaxation phase after release of manual compression.[54] All candidates for SEPS in our practice undergo Duplex ultrasonography of the deep, superficial and perforator systems,[54] and sites of incompetent perforators are marked on the skin the day before surgery (Fig. 17.4). Ascending and descending phlebography is reserved for patients with underlying occlusive disease or recurrent ulceration after perforator division, in whom deep venous reconstruction is being considered. In addition to Duplex scanning, a functional study such as strain gauge or air plethysmography is performed before and after surgery to quantify the degree of incompetence, identify abnormalities in calf muscle pump function, aid in the exclusion of outflow obstruction and assess hemodynamic results of surgical intervention.[12,29]

SURGICAL TECHNIQUES

Open technique of perforator interruption

Linton's radical operation of subfascial ligation,[2] which included long medial, anterolateral and posterolateral calf incisions, was abandoned because of wound complications. In a subsequent report published in 1953, Linton advocated only a long medial incision from the ankle to the knee to interrupt all medial and posterior perforating veins.[55] Several authors proposed modifications to Linton's open procedure to limit wound complications. Cockett advocated ligation of the perforating veins above the deep fascia, a technique distinctly different from the Linton operation.[3] The importance of ligating the perforating veins subfascially was emphasized by Sherman,[33] as the perforating veins branch extensively once they penetrate the deep fascia. Further modifications included the use of shorter medial incisions or a more posteriorly placed stocking seam-type incision.[4,15,16] DePalma[17] observed good results using multiple, parallel bipedicled flaps placed along skin lines to access and ligate the perforating veins above or below the fascia (Fig. 17.5).

The classic papers of Linton[2] and Cockett and Jones[3] reported benefit from open perforator ligation, and this was supported later by data from several other investigators.[6,9,10,56] In the larger series, ulcer recurrence ranged from 12 to 55 percent and averaged 24 percent (Table 17.3),[8,10,11,13] a significant drawback of open perforator ligation. Further controversy over the efficacy of this operation emerged when Burnand et al.[13] reported a 55 percent ulcer recurrence rate in their patients, with 100 percent recurrence in a subset of 23 patients with post-thrombotic (PT) syndrome. Although these data are compelling evidence against perforating vein ablation, ulcer recurrence in the other subset of patients in the same study, those without PT damage of the deep veins, was only 6 percent.

The concept of ablating incompetent perforating veins from a site remote from diseased skin was first introduced by Edwards in 1976.[18] He designed a device called the phlebotome, which is inserted through a medial incision just distal to the knee, deep to the fascia, and advanced to the level of the medial malleolus (Fig. 17.6). Resistance is felt as perforators are engaged and subsequently disrupted with the leading edge. DePalma[17] in the USA published good results with this procedure. Interruption of perforators through stab wounds and hook avulsion is another possibility and accuracy of this blind technique improves with preoperative duplex scanning and perforator mapping. Sclerotherapy of perforating veins and suture ligation of perforators without making skin incisions are among other reported techniques.

Techniques of subfascial endoscopic perforator vein surgery

First introduced by Hauer in 1985, using endoscopic instruments, interruption of incompetent perforators may now be

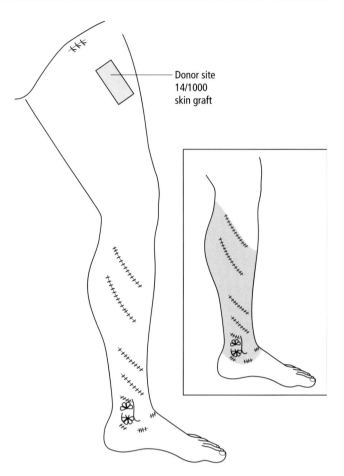

Figure 17.5 *Linton operation modified by DePalma. Note the extent of the area which is dissected as shown in the shaded inset. Also note the submalleolar skin line incisions. (Modified from DePalma.[17])*

performed through small ports placed remotely from the active ulcer or area of skin discoloration.[19–21,57–59] Since its introduction, two main techniques for SEPS have been developed. The first, practiced mostly in Europe, is a refinement of the original work of Hauer[19] by Fischer,[24] with further development by Bergan et al.[20] and by Wittens and Pierik.[22,23] In the early development of the 'single port' technique, available light sources such as mediastinoscopes and bronchoscopes were used. With time a specially designed instrument was devised which uses a single scope with channels for the camera and working instruments, which sometimes makes visualization and dissection in the same plane difficult (Fig. 17.7). Recent developments in instrumentation for this technique now allow for carbon dioxide (CO_2) insufflation into the subfascial plane.

The second technique, using instrumentation from laparoscopic surgery, was introduced in the USA by O'Donnell,[60] and developed simultaneously by Conrad in Australia[26] and our group at the Mayo Clinic.[27] This technique, the 'two port' technique, employs one port for the camera and a separate port for instrumentation, thereby making it easier to work in the limited subfascial space. First the limb is exsanguinated with an elastic bandage such as Esmarch, and a thigh tourniquet

Table 17.3   *Clinical results of open perforator interruption for the treatment of advanced chronic venous disease*

Authors (year)	No. of limbs treated	No. of limbs with ulcer	Wound complications [n (%)]	Ulcer healing [n (%)]	Ulcer recurrence [n (%)][a]	Mean follow-up (years)
Silver et al.[6] (1971)	31	19	4 (14)	–	– (10)	1–15
Thurston and Williams[7] (1973)	102	0	12 (12)	–[b]	11 (13)	3.3
Bowen[8] (1975)	71	8	31 (44)	–	24 (34)	4.5
Burnand et al.[13] (1976)	41	0	–	–[b]	24 (55)	–
Negus and Friedgood[10] (1983)	108	108	24 (22)	91 (84)	16 (15)	3.7
Wilkinson and Maclaren[76] (1986)	108	0	26 (24)	–[b]	3 (7)	6
Cikrit et al.[11] (1988)	32	30	6 (19)	30 (100)	5 (19)	4
Bradbury et al.[12] (1993)	53	0	–	–[b]	14 (26)	5
Pierik et al.[23] (1997)	19	19	10 (53)	17 (90)	0 (0)	1.8
Total no. of limbs (%)	565 (100)	184 (33)	113/468 (24)	138/157 (88)	97/443 (22)	–

[a] Recurrence calculated where data available and percentage accounts for patients lost to follow-up.
[b] Only Class 5 (healed ulcer) patients admitted in study.

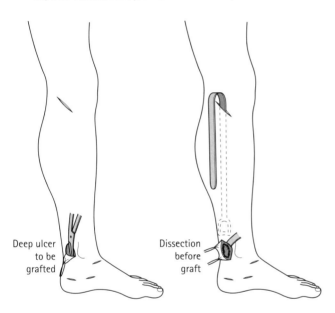

Figure 17.6   *Excision and dissection of a deep ulcer prior to extrafascial shearing operation. The submalleolar incisions allow division of the retro malleolar perforator. (Modified from DePalma.[17])*

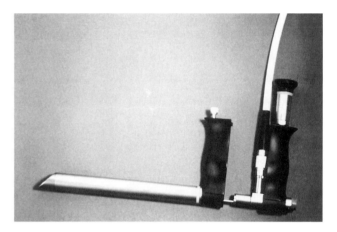

Figure 17.7   *Olympus endoscope for subfascial perforating vein interruption. The scope can be used with or without CO_2 insufflation. It has an 85° field of view and the outer sheath is either 16 or 22 mm in diameter. The working channel is 6×8.5 mm, with a working length of 20 cm. (Reproduced with permission from Bergan et al.[86])*

is inflated to 300 mmHg to provide a bloodless field (Fig. 17.8a). A 10 mm endoscopic port is next placed in the medial aspect of the calf 10 cm distal to the tibial tuberosity, proximal to the diseased skin. Balloon dissection is routinely used to widen the subfascial space and facilitate access after port placement (Fig. 17.8b).[61] The distal 5 mm port is now placed halfway between the first port and the ankle (about 10–12 cm apart), under direct visualization with the camera (Fig. 17.8c). Carbon dioxide is insufflated into the subfascial space and pressure is maintained around 30 mmHg to improve visualization and access to the perforators. Using laparoscopic scissors inserted through the second port, the remaining loose connective tissue between the calf muscles and the superficial fascia is sharply divided.

The subfascial space is widely explored from the medial border of the tibia to the posterior midline, and down to the level of the ankle. All perforators encountered are divided using the harmonic scalpel or, for very large veins, sharply with scissors, after placement of clips (Fig. 17.8d). A paratibial fasciotomy is next made by incising the fascia of the posterior deep compartment close to the tibia, to avoid any injury to the posterior tibial vessels and the tibial nerve (Fig. 17.8e). The Cockett II and Cockett III perforators are located frequently within an intermuscular septum, and this has to be incised before identification and division of the perforators can be accomplished. The medial insertion of the soleus muscle on the tibia may also have to be exposed to visualize proximal paratibial perforators. By rotating the ports cephalad and continuing the dissection up to the level of the knee, the more proximal perforators can also be divided. While the paratibial fasciotomy can aid in distal exposure, reaching the retromalleolar Cockett I perforator endoscopically is usually not possible and, if incompetent, may require a separate small incision over it to gain direct exposure.

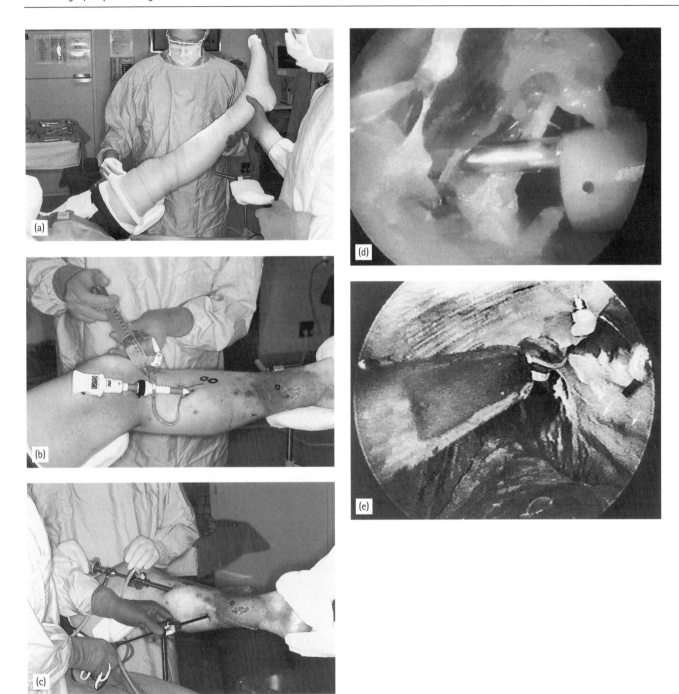

Figure 17.8   *Two port technique of subfascial endoscopic perforator vein surgery (SEPS). (a) A thigh tourniquet inflated to 300 mmHg is used to create a bloodless field. (b) Balloon dissection is used to widen the subfascial space. (c) SEPS is performed using two ports: a 10 mm camera port and a 5 or 10 mm distal port inserted under video control. Carbon dioxide is insufflated through the camera port into the subfascial space to a pressure of 30 mmHg to improve visualization and access to perforators. (d) The subfascial space is widely explored from the medial border of the tibia to the posterior midline and down to the level of the ankle, and all perforators are interrupted using clips or harmonic scalpel. (e) A paratibial fasciotomy is routinely performed to identify perforators in the deep posterior compartment. (Reproduced with permission from Gloviczki et al.[87])*

After completion of the endoscopic portion of the procedure, the instruments and ports are removed, the CO_2 is manually expressed from the limb and the tourniquet is deflated. Twenty millilitres of 0.5 percent bupivicaine solution is instilled into the subfascial space for postoperative pain control. Stab avulsion of varicosities in addition to high ligation and stripping of the greater and/or lesser saphenous vein, if incompetent, is performed. The wounds are closed and the limb is elevated and wrapped with an elastic bandage. Elevation is maintained at 30° postoperatively for 3 h after which ambulation is permitted. Unlike the in-hospital stay after an open Linton procedure, this is an outpatient procedure and

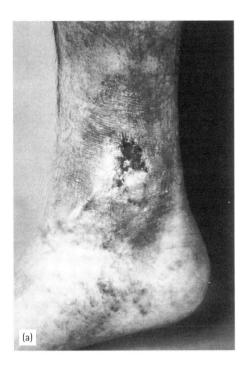
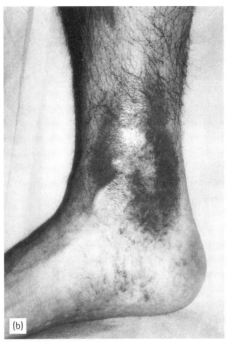

Figure 17.9 *(a) A 36-year-old male with post-thrombotic ulcer on the right ankle, before endoscopic division of six medial perforating veins. (b) The same leg 10 months later shows the healed ulcer. (Reproduced with permission from Gloviczki et al.[87])*

patients are discharged the same day or next morning following overnight observation.

EFFICACY OF SEPS

Clinical results

In the absence of prospective, randomized trials, there is no level I evidence to support the performance of SEPS in patients with advanced CVI and venous ulcers. In fact, the optimal treatment for these patients, whether surgical or medical, is not well defined. Presently, prospective randomized multicentre trials are being designed in North America as well as in Europe. Until results of such studies are available, one can only draw on the experience of investigators in the field, and retrospective as well as prospective data from single institutions.

Encouraging early results with SEPS were reported by several authors, with accelerated ulcer healing after ablation of the incompetent superficial and perforator systems without intervention to the deep veins, even in patients with combined deep, perforator and superficial incompetence (Figs 17.9 and 17.10).[21,57,58,62,63] Results from several centres are available and are summarized in Table 17.4. Unfortunately, analysis of available results is difficult with only the most recent publications using the CEAP classification scheme proposed by the International Consensus Committee on Chronic Venous Disease,[64] and reporting sufficient technical details, especially the performance of a paratibial fasciotomy. Despite these limitations, valuable insight can be gained from the growing literature.

The North American (NASEPS) registry provided uniform evaluation and reporting of results following SEPS in 146 patients with advanced CVI from 17 centres in North America.[21] Concomitant superficial venous surgery was performed in 71 percent of patients. Wound complication rate was 6 percent, and one deep venous thrombosis occurred at 2 months after surgery The mid-term (24 months) results of the NASEPS registry demonstrated an 88 percent cumulative ulcer healing rate at 1 year.[28] The median time to ulcer healing was 54 days. Cumulative rate of ulcer recurrence was significant – 16 percent at 1 year, 28 percent at 2 years – but still compared favourably with results of non-operative management (Table 17.5).

In the largest series from a single institution, Nelzen *et al.*[65] reported prospectively collected data from 149 SEPS procedures in 138 patients. However, only 45 percent of limbs had venous ulceration (C6, 36 limbs; C5, 31 limbs) and deep venous insufficiency was present in only 7 percent of limbs. Concomitant saphenous vein surgery was performed in 89 percent of limbs. During a median follow-up of 32 months, 32 of 36 ulcers healed, more than half (19/36) within 1 month. Three ulcers recurred, one of which subsequently healed during follow-up. At a median follow-up of 7 months following surgery, 91 percent of patients were satisfied with the results of the operation.

A recent study analysed extended results in 103 consecutive SEPS procedures performed at the Mayo Clinic over a 7-year period.[66] Venous ulceration affected 74 percent of limbs (C6, 42 limbs; C5, 34 limbs) and deep venous incompetence was present in 89 percent of limbs. Concomitant superficial reflux ablation was performed in 74 limbs (72 percent). Thirty-eight out of 42 ulcers healed with a median time to ulcer healing of 35 days; all four ulcers that failed to heal were in PT limbs. On life-table analysis, 90 day and 1 year cumulative ulcer healing rates were 80 and 90 percent, respectively. One- and 5-year cumulative ulcer recurrence rates were 4 and 27 percent, respectively.

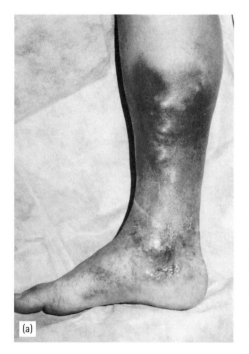

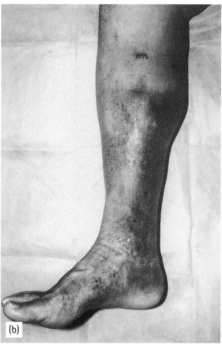

Figure 17.10 *(a) Right leg of a 64-year-old male with a 2-year history of ulcer and severe post-thrombotic syndrome. (b) Postoperative picture at 6 weeks shows healed ulcer and incisions following subfascial endoscopic perforator vein surgery (SEPS), stripping and avulsion of varicose veins. Three years later the patient is asymptomatic, does not use elastic stockings and had no ulcer recurrence. (Reproduced with permission from Gloviczki et al.[87])*

Table 17.4 *Clinical results of SEPS for the treatment of advanced chronic venous disease*

Authors (year)	No. of limbs treated	No. of limbs with ulcer[a]	Concomitant saphenous ablation [n (%)]	Wound complications [n (%)]	Ulcer healing [n (%)]	Ulcer recurrence [n (%)][b]	Mean follow-up (months)
Jugenheimer and Junginger[25] (1992)	103	17	97 (94)	3 (3)	16 (94)	0 (0)	27
Pierek et al.[57] (1995)	40	16	4 (10)	3 (8)	16 (100)	1 (2.5)	46
Bergan et al.[20] (1996)	31	15	31 (100)	3 (10)	15 (100)	(0)	–
Wolters et al.[77] (1996)	27	27	0 (0)	2 (7)	26 (96)	2 (8)	12–24
Padberg et al.[62] (1996)	11	0	11 (100)	–	–[c]	0 (0)	16
Pierek et al.[78] (1997)	20	20	14 (70)	0 (0)	17 (85)	0 (0)	21
Rhodes et al.[29] (1998)	57	22	41 (72)	3 (5)	22 (100)	5 (12)	17
Gloviczki et al.[28] (1999)	146	101	86 (59)	9 (6)	85 (84)	26 (21)	24
Illig et al.[71] (1999)	30	19	–	–	17 (89)	4 (15)	9
Nelzen[65] (2000)	149	36	132 (89)	11 (7)	32 (89)	3 (5)	32
Total no. of limbs (%)	614 (100)	273 (44)	416/567 (73)	34/556 (6)	246/273 (90)	41/392 (10)	–

[a] Only class 6 (active ulcer) patients are included.
[b] Recurrence calculated for Class 5 and 6 limbs only, where data available and percentage accounts for patients lost to follow-up.
[c] Only class 5 (healed ulcer) patients were admitted in this study.

The major advantage of SEPS is the lower wound complication rate compared with traditional open surgical techniques.[21,23] In an uncontrolled trial that compared 37 SEPS procedures with 30 antedated open perforator ligations, SEPS resulted in lower calf wound morbidity, shorter hospital stay and comparable short-term ulcer healing.[67] A single prospective randomized study by Pierik et al.[23] in 39 patients reported wound complications in 53 percent of patients undergoing open perforator ligation versus 0 percent in the SEPS group, with no ulcer recurrence in either group over a mean follow-up of 21 months. In a subsequent communication 4 years later, the authors reported that long-term ulcer recurrence in the open perforator ligation group (22 percent) was not significantly different from that in the SEPS group (12 percent).[68]

All the above data support the use of SEPS rather than open ligation, yet do not address the role of SEPS in the management of advanced CVI and venous ulceration.

Defining the role of SEPS in ulcer healing

Since concomitant ablation of superficial reflux is often performed at the same time as SEPS, clinical benefit attributed directly to perforator interruption has been difficult to assess. It must be pointed out that the majority (greater than two-thirds) of patients reported in the above studies underwent

Table 17.5 *Ulcer recurrence or new ulceration following medical treatment*

Authors (year)	No. of limbs treated	No. of limbs with ulcer	Ulcer recurrence [n (%)][a]	Mean follow-up (months)
Anning[56] (1956)	100	100	59 (59)	64
Monk and Sarkany[79] (1982)	83	83	58 (69)	12
Kitahama *et al.*[80] (1982)	65	59	8 (14)	12
Negus[81] (1985)	109	109	22 (30)	43
Mayberry *et al.*[82] (1991)	113	113	24 (33)	30
Erickson[83] (1995)	99	99	52 (58)	10
DePalma and Kowallek[84] (1996)	11	11	11 (100)	24
Samson and Showalter[85] (1996)	53	53	23 (43)	28
Total	549 (100)	518/549 (94)	241/488 (52)	27

[a]Percentage accounts for patients lost to follow-up.

concomitant saphenous vein stripping and branch varicosity avulsion (Table 17.4), making it impossible to ascertain how much clinical improvement can be attributed to the addition of SEPS. The NASEPS registry demonstrated improved ulcer healing in limbs that underwent SEPS with saphenous vein stripping, compared with limbs that underwent SEPS alone; 3- and 12-month cumulative ulcer healing rates of 76 and 100 percent vs. 45 and 83 percent ($P < 0.01$), respectively.[28] Ulcer recurrence was not significantly different among the two groups. We attempted to study this in our recent analysis of 103 limbs.[66] Ulcer healing was significantly delayed in limbs undergoing SEPS alone, compared with limbs that underwent SEPS with superficial reflux ablation; 90-day cumulative ulcer healing rate was 49 vs. 90 percent ($P = 0.02$). Cumulative ulcer recurrence at 5 years was also higher in limbs that underwent SEPS alone (53 percent), compared with those undergoing SEPS with superficial reflux ablation (19 percent) ($P = 0.01$; Fig. 17.11). However, the number of limbs in the SEPS-alone group was considerably smaller, with a relative predominance of PT limbs. All 29 limbs undergoing SEPS alone had previously undergone saphenous vein ligation and stripping, and had recurrent or persistent ulcers, automatically placing them in a higher-risk category and creating a selection bias. The question regarding the absolute benefit of SEPS will not be answered until such time that patients can be prospectively randomized to undergo saphenous vein stripping alone, or saphenous vein stripping with SEPS. The Dutch prospective randomized study has been completed and results will be available soon.

Results in post-thrombotic syndrome

Another group of patients generating significant controversy constitutes those with post-thrombotic syndrome. In all the above communications, limbs with PT syndrome fared poorly compared with limbs with primary valvular incompetence (PVI). Cumulative ulcer recurrence in the first Mayo Clinic series was 60 vs. 0 percent at 3 years in PT and PVI limbs, respectively, and 46 vs. 20 percent at 2 years in the NASEPS registry ($P < 0.05$).[28,69] The results of the recent Mayo Clinic series which comprised a larger group of patients with longer follow-up support this earlier observation.[66] All ulcers in

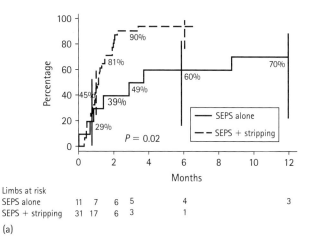

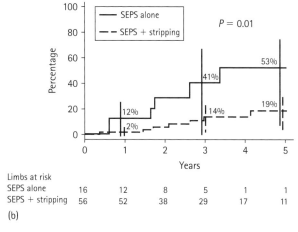

Figure 17.11 *(a) Cumulative ulcer healing based on the extent of venous surgery – 11 limbs following subfascial endoscopic perforator vein surgery (SEPS) alone and 31 limbs following SEPS with saphenous vein stripping. (b) Cumulative ulcer recurrence based on extent of venous surgery – 16 limbs following SEPS alone and 56 limbs following SEPS with saphenous vein stripping.*

limbs with PVI healed; all four ulcers that did not heal were in PT limbs. Cumulative 5-year ulcer recurrence in PT limbs was 56 vs. 15 percent in limbs with PVI ($P = 0.001$; Fig. 17.12). However, despite the high ulcer recurrence rate, patients with

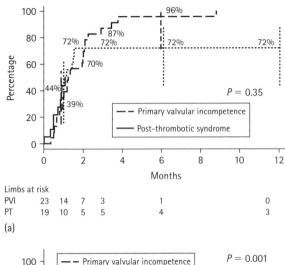

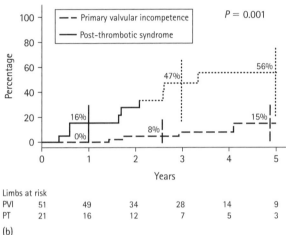

Figure 17.12 *(a) Cumulative ulcer healing based on the etiology of chronic venous insufficiency – 23 limbs with primary valvular incompetence (PVI) and 19 limbs with post-thrombotic syndrome (PT). The dotted line represents SEM > 10%. (b) Cumulative ulcer recurrence based on the etiology of chronic venous insufficiency – 51 limbs with primary valvular incompetence and 21 limbs with post-thrombotic syndrome. The dotted line represents SEM > 10%.*

PT syndrome had marked symptomatic improvement, with significant improvement in the clinical scores following SEPS and superficial reflux ablation (9.5 to 3; Fig. 17.13). In addition, recurrent ulcers were small, superficial, single more often than multiple, and healed easily with conservative management.

Hemodynamic results

Several investigators have studied the effect of superficial reflux ablation and perforator ligation on venous hemodynamics and have attempted to evaluate the hemodynamic significance of perforator ligation. In 1972, Bjordal *et al.* showed normalization of direct venous pressures on occlusion of the GSV alone in patients with PVI, but not following occlusion of large perforating veins alone.[49] Venous pressures in patients with PT syndrome failed to normalize following all these maneuvers. Åkesson *et al.*[70] reported a significant decrease in ambulatory

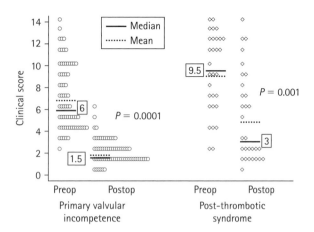

Figure 17.13 *Preoperative and postoperative clinical scores based on the etiology of chronic venous insufficiency – 73 limbs with primary valvular incompetence and 30 limbs with post-thrombotic syndrome.*

foot venous pressure following saphenous vein ligation and stripping in patients with recurrent ulcers, but there was no further hemodynamic improvement following perforator ligation performed 3 months later.

While most studies, including the NASEPS registry, lacked sufficient hemodynamic data to support the clinical results, functional improvement after perforator interruption has been reported. Bradbury *et al.*[12] used foot volumetry and duplex scanning to assess hemodynamic improvement after saphenous and perforator ligation in 43 patients with recurrent ulcers. Expulsion fraction and half-refilling time (T_{50}) improved significantly after surgery in the 34 patients with no ulcer recurrence at 66 months. Recent air plethysmographic studies by Padberg *et al.*[62] have documented persistent hemodynamic improvement up to 2 years following perforator ligation with concomitant correction of superficial reflux. Illig *et al.*[71] reported a slight improvement in venous refill time following 30 SEPS procedures with superficial reflux ablation in 28 patients.

Rhodes *et al.*[29] studied hemodynamic consequences of incompetent perforator vein interruption, using strain gauge plethysmography to assess calf muscle pump function, venous incompetence and outflow obstruction before and within 6 months following SEPS. Both calf muscle pump function and the degree of venous incompetence improved significantly following SEPS, with or without superficial reflux ablation. The improvement in venous incompetence (measured by refill rate) correlated strongly with clinical improvement. A similar significant improvement in calf muscle pump function and the degree of venous incompetence was seen in the subgroup of patients with DVI ($n = 24$). As with clinical improvement, the hemodynamic benefit as a direct consequence of perforator ligation was not evident. In the subset of patients that underwent SEPS alone ($n = 7$), without concomitant superficial reflux ablation, no significant improvement in hemodynamic status could be demonstrated. This was most likely due to both the small number of patients in this group, and the relative predominance of PT limbs.

Patients with PVI demonstrate significantly better hemodynamic improvement, compared with PT limbs.[28,29] Proebstle et al.,[72] using light reflection rheography before and 8 weeks following SEPS, had very similar results to the Mayo Clinic series, showing significant improvement in limbs with PVI. Similar to findings of Burnand et al.,[14] and Stacey et al.,[73] neither we nor the University of Ulm group were able to show significant hemodynamic improvement in PT patients. It is important to note, however, that the number of patients studied in this subgroup has been low (less than 15 in all reported studies).[72,73] The overall benefits in these patients are clearly not of the same magnitude as in those with PVI.

CONCLUSION

The optimal treatment of patients with advanced CVI and especially venous ulcers is not established. Our knowledge about the efficacy and applicability of SEPS is far from complete, and the need for prospective randomized studies comparing saphenous vein stripping with saphenous vein stripping with SEPS has been expressed by many investigators in the field. Less invasive occlusion of perforating veins with sclerotherapy using duplex guidance may change the technique of perforator vein interruption. Based on presently available data, patients who benefit from SEPS are those with ulcers due to primary valvular incompetence of the superficial and perforating veins, with or without deep venous incompetence. These patients are good candidates, and derive maximum benefit in terms of accelerated ulcer healing and an estimated 80–90 percent chance of freedom from ulcer recurrence in the long-term. Despite subjective symptomatic and objective clinical score improvement, the role of SEPS continues to be controversial in patients with post-thrombotic syndrome, as only 50 percent of patients can be predicted to be free from ulcer recurrence in the long term. Patients with ulcer recurrence following SEPS, and recurrent or persistent perforators documented on duplex ultrasound, warrant a repeat perforator interruption. Those without perforator incompetence should be considered for deep venous reconstruction.

REFERENCES

1. Gay J. *Lettsomian Lectures 1867. Varicose Disease of the Lower Extremities*. London: Churchill, 1868.
2. Linton RR. The operative treatment of varicose veins and ulcers, based upon a classification of these lesions. *Ann Surg* 1938; **107**: 582–93.
3. Cockett FB, Jones BD. The ankle blow-out syndrome: a new approach to the varicose ulcer problem. *Lancet* 1953; **i**: 17–23.
4. Cockett FB. The pathology and treatment of venous ulcers of the leg. *Br J Surg* 1956; **44**: 260–78.
5. Dodd H. The diagnosis and ligation of incompetent perforating veins. *Ann R Coll Surg Engl* 1964; **34**: 186–96.
6. Silver D, Gleysteen JJ, Rhodes GR et al. Surgical treatment of the refractory postphlebitic ulcer. *Arch Surg* 1971; **103**: 554–60.
7. Thurston OG, Williams HT. Chronic venous insufficiency of the lower extremity. Pathogenesis and surgical treatment. *Arch Surg* 1973; **106**: 537–9.
8. Bowen FH. Subfascial ligation of the perforating leg veins to treat post-thrombophlebitic syndrome. *Am Surg* 1975; 148–51.
9. Schanzer H, Peirce EC. A rational approach to surgery of the chronic venous statis syndrome. *Ann Surg* 1982; **195**: 25–9.
10. Negus D, Friedgood A. The effective management of venous ulceration. *Br J Surg* 1983; **70**: 623–7.
11. Cikrit DF, Nichols WK, Silver D. Surgical management of refractory venous stasis ulceration. *J Vasc Surg* 1988; **7**: 473–8.
12. Bradbury AW, Stonebridge PA, Callam MJ et al. Foot volume try and duplex ultrasonography after saphenous and subfascial perforating vein ligation for recurrent venous ulceration. *Br J Surg* 1993; **80**: 845–8.
13. Burnand K, Thomas ML, O'Donnell T, Browse NL. Relation between postphlebitic changes in the deep veins and results of surgical treatment of venous ulcers. *Lancet* 1976; **i**: 936–8.
14. Burnand KG, O'Donnell TF Jr, Thomas ML, Browse NL. The relative importance of incompetent communicating veins in the production of varicose veins and venous ulcers. *Surgery* 1977; **82**: 9–14.
15. Rob C. G. *Surgery of the Vascular System*. University Minn Vascular Symposium, 1972; 272.
16. Lim RC J, Blaisdell FW, Zubrin J et al. Subfascial ligation of perforating veins in recurrent stasis ulceration. *Am J Surg* 1970; **119**: 246–9.
17. DePalma RG. Surgical therapy for venous stasis surgery. *Surgery* 1975; **76**: 910–17.
18. Edwards JM. Shearing operation for incompetent perforating veins. *Br J Surg* 1976; **63**: 885–6.
19. Hauer G. [Endoscopic subfascial discussion of perforating veins – preliminary report.] *Vasa* 1985; **14**: 59–61.
20. Bergan JJ, Murray J, Greason K. Subfascial endoscopic perforator vein surgery: a preliminary report. *Ann Vasc Surg* 1996; **10**: 211–9.
21. Gloviczki P, Bergan JJ, Menawat SS et al. Safety, feasibility, and early efficacy of subfascial endoscopic perforator surgery: a preliminary report from the North American registry. *J Vasc Surg* 1997; **25**: 94–105.
22. Pierik EG, Toonder IM, van Urk H, Wittens CH. Validation of duplex ultrasonography in detecting competent and incompetent perforating veins in patients with venous ulceration of the lower leg. *J Vasc Surg* 1997; **26**: 49–52.
23. Pierik EG, van Urk H, Hop WC, Wittens CH. Endoscopic versus open subfascial division of incompetent perforating veins in the treatment of venous leg ulceration: a randomized trial. *J Vasc Surg* 1997; **26**: 1049–54.
24. Fischer R. Surgical treatment of varicose veins; endoscopic treatment of incompetent Cockett veins. *Phlébologie* 1989; 1040–1.
25. Jugenheimer M, Junginger T. Endoscopic subfascial sectioning of incompetent perforating veins in treatment of primary varicosis. *World J Surg* 1992; **16**: 971–5.
26. Conrad P. Endoscopic exploration of the subfascial space of the lower leg with perforator interruption using laparoscopic equipment: a preliminary report. *Phlebology* 1994; **9**: 154–7.
27. Gloviczki P, Cambria RA, Rhee RY et al. Surgical technique and preliminary results of endoscopic subfascial division of perforating veins. *J Vasc Surg* 1996; **23**: 517–23.

28. Gloviczki P, Bergan JJ, Rhodes JM et al. Mid-term results of endoscopic perforator vein interruption for chronic venous insufficiency: lessons learned from the North American subfascial endoscopic perforator surgery registry. The North American Study Group. J Vasc Surg 1999; **29**: 489–502.

29. Rhodes JM, Gloviczki P, Canton LG et al. Endoscopic perforator vein division with ablation of superficial reflux improves venous hemodynamics. J Vasc Surg 1998; **28**: 839–47.

30. Rhodes JM, Gloviczki P, Canton LG et al. Factors affecting clinical outcome following endoscopic perforator vein ablation. J Vasc Surg 1998; **176**: 162–7.

31. Lofgren EP, Myers TT, Lofgren KA, Kuster G. The venous valves of the foot and ankle. Surg Gynecol Obstet 1968; **127**: 289–90.

32. Mozes G, Gloviczki P, Menawat SS et al. Surgical anatomy for endoscopic subfascial division of perforating veins. J Vasc Surg 1996; **24**: 800–8.

33. Sherman RS. Varicose veins: further findings based on anatomic and surgical dissections. Ann Surg 1949; **130**: 218–32.

34. O'Donnell TFJ, Burnand KG, Clemenson G et al. Doppler examination vs clinical and phlebographic detection of the location of incompetent perforating veins: a prospective study. Arch Surg 1977; **112**: 31–5.

35. O'Donnell TF Jr. Surgery for incompetent perforating veins at the turn of the millennium. In: Yao JST, Pearce WH, eds. Current Techniques in Vascular Surgery. New York: McGraw-Hill, 2001; 487–515.

36. Beecher HK, Field ME, Krogh A. The effect of walking on the venous pressure at the ankle. Skand Arch Physiol 1936; **73**: 133–40.

37. DeCamp PT, Ward JA, Ochner A. Ambulatory venous pressure studies in post-phlebitic and other disease states. Surgery 1951; **29**: 365–77.

38. Warren R, White D. Venous pressures in the saphenous system in normal, varicose and post-phlebitic extremities. Surgery 1948; **26**: 435–41.

39. Nicolaides AN, Hussein MK, Szendro G et al. The relation of venous ulceration with ambulatory venous pressure measurements. J Vasc Surg 1993; **17**: 414–9.

40. Homans J. The operative treatment of varicose veins and ulcers, based upon a classification of these lesions. Surg Gynecol Obstet 1916; **22**: 143–58.

41. van Rij AM, Solomon C, Christie R. Anatomic and physiologic characteristics of venous ulceration. J Vasc Surg 1994; **20**: 759–64.

42. Labropoulos N, Leon M, Geroulakos G et al. Venous hemodynamic abnormalities in patients with leg ulceration. Am J Surg 1995; **169**: 572–4.

43. Hanrahan LM, Araki CT, Rodriguez AA et al. Distribution of valvular incompetence in patients with venous stasis ulceration. J Vasc Surg 1991; **13**: 805–12.

44. Myers KA, Ziegenbein RW, Zeng GH, Matthews PG. Duplex ultrasonography scanning for chronic venous disease: patterns of venous reflux. J Vasc Surg 1995; **21**: 605–12.

45. van Bemmelen PS, Bedford G, Beach K, Strandness DE Jr. Status of the valves in the superficial and deep venous system in chronic venous disease. Surgery 1991; **109**: 730–4.

46. Darke SG, Penfold C. Venous ulceration and saphenous ligation. Eur J Vasc Surg 1992; **6**: 4–9.

47. Lees TA, Lambert D. Patterns of venous reflux in limbs with skin changes associated with chronic venous insufficiency. Br J Surg 1993; **80**: 725–8.

48. Sethia KK, Darke SG. Long saphenous incompetence as a cause of venous ulceration. Br J Surg 1984; **71**: 754–5.

49. Bjordal RI. Circulation patterns in incompetent perforating veins of the calf in venous dysfunction. In: May R, Partsch J, Staubesand J, eds. Perforating Veins. Baltimore: Urban & Schwarzenberg, 1981; 77–8.

50. Sarin S, Scurr JH, Smith PD. Medial calf perforators in venous disease: the significance of outward flow. J Vasc Surg 1992; **16**: 40–6.

51. Sandri JL, Barros FS, Pontes S et al. Diameter-reflux relationship in perforating veins of patients with varicose veins. J Vasc Surg 1999; **30**: 867–74.

52. Stuart WP, Adam DJ, Allan PL et al. The relationship between the number, competence, and diameter of medial calf perforating veins and the clinical status in healthy subjects and patients with lower-limb venous disease. J Vasc Surg 2000; **32**: 138–43.

53. Delis KT, Husmann M, Kalodiki E et al. In situ hemodynamics of perforating veins in chronic venous insufficiency. J Vasc Surg 2001; **33**: 773–82.

54. Gloviczki P, Lewis BD, Lindsey JR, McKusick MA. Preoperative evaluation of chronic venous insufficiency with Duplex scanning and venography. In: Gloviczki P, Bergan JJ, eds. Atlas of Endoscopic Perforator Vein Surgery. London: Springer-Verlag, 1998; 81–91.

55. Linton RR. The post-thrombotic ulceration of the lower extremity: its etiology and surgical treatment. Ann Surg 1953; **138**: 415–32.

56. Anning ST. Leg ulcers the results of treatment. Angiology 1956; **7**: 505–16.

57. Pierik EG JM, Wittens CHA, van Urk H. Subfascial endoscopic ligation in the treatment of incompetent perforator veins. Eur J Vasc Endovasc Surg 1995; **5**: 38–41.

58. Sparks SR, Ballard JL, Bergan JJ, Killeen JD. Early benefits of subfascial endoscopic perforator surgery (SEPS) in healing venous ulcers. Ann Vasc Surg 1997; **11**: 367–73.

59. Wittens CH, Pierik RG, van Urk H. The surgical treatment of incompetent perforating veins [Review; 63 refs]. Eur J Vasc Endovasc Surg 1995; **9**: 19–23.

60. O'Donnell TF. Surgical treatment of incompetent communicating veins. Atlas of Venous Surgery. Philadelphia: WB Saunders, 2000; 111–24.

61. Allen RC, Tawes RL, Wetter A, Fogarty TJ. Endoscopic perforator vein surgery: creation of a subfascial space. In: Gloviczki P, Bergan JJ, eds. Atlas of Endoscopic Perforator Vein Surgery. London: Springer-Verlag, 1998; 153–62.

62. Padberg FT J, Pappas PJ, Araki CT et al. Hemodynamic and clinical improvement after superficial vein ablation in primary combined venous insufficiency with ulceration. J Vasc Surg 1996; **24**: 711–8.

63. Murray JD, Bergan JJ, Riffenburgh RH. Development of open-scope subfascial perforating vein surgery: lessons learned from the first 67 patients. Ann Vasc Surg 1999; **199**: 372–7.

64. Porter JM, Moneta GL. Reporting standards in venous disease: an update. International Consensus Committee on Chronic Venous Disease. J Vasc Surg 1995; **21**: 635–45.

65. Nelzen O. Prospective study of safety, patient satisfaction and leg ulcer healing following saphenous and subfascial endoscopic perforator surgery. Br J Surg 2000; **87**: 86–91.

66. Kalra M, Gloviczki P, Noel AA et al. Subfascial endoscopic perforator vein surgery in patients with post-thrombotic venous insufficiency – is it justified? Vasc Endovasc Surg 2002; **36**: 41–50.

67. Stuart WP, Adam DJ, Bradbury AW, Ruckley CV. Subfascial endoscopic perforator surgery is associated with significantly less morbidity and shorter hospital stay than open operation (Linton's procedure). Br J Surg 1997; **84**: 1364–5.

68. Sybrandy JE, van Gent WB, Pierik EG, Wittens CH. Endoscopic versus open subfascial division of incompetent perforating veins in the treatment of venous leg ulceration: long-term follow-up. *J Vasc Surg* 2001; **33**: 1028–32.

69. Rhodes JM, Gloviczki P, Canton LG *et al.* Factors affecting clinical outcome following endoscopic perforator vein ablation. *Am J Surg* 1998; **176**: 162–7.

70. Akesson H, Brudin L, Cwikiel W *et al.* Does the correction of insufficient superficial and perforating veins improve venous function in patients with deep venous insufficiency? *Phlebology* 1990; **5**: 113–23.

71. Illig KA, Shortell CK, Ouriel K *et al.* Photoplethysmography and calf muscle pump function after subfascial endoscopic perforator ligation. *J Vasc Surg* 1999; **30**: 1067–76.

72. Proebstle TM, Weisel G, Paepcke U *et al.* Light reflection rheography and clinical course of patients with advanced venous disease before and after endoscopic subfascial division of perforating veins. *Dermatol Surg* 1998; **24**: 771–6.

73. Stacey MC, Burnand KG, Layer GT, Pattison M. Calf pump function in patients with healed venous ulcers is not improved by surgery to the communicating veins or by elastic stockings. *Br J Surg* 1988; **75**: 436–9.

74. Shami SK, Sarin S, Cheatle TR *et al.* Venous ulcers and the superficial venous system. *J Vasc Surg* 1993; **17**: 487–90.

75. Labropoulos N, Delis K, Nicolaides AN *et al.* The role of the distribution and anatomic extent of reflux in the development of signs and symptoms in chronic venous insufficiency. *J Vasc Surg* 1996; **23**: 504–10.

76. Wilkinson GE Jr, Maclaren IF. Long term review of procedures for venous perforator insufficiency. *Surg Gynecol Obstet* 1986; **163**: 117–20.

77. Wolters U, Schmit-Rixen T, Erasmi H, Lynch J. Endoscopic dissection of incompetent perforating veins in the treatment of chronic venous leg ulcers. *Vasc Surg* 1996; **30**: 481–7.

78. Pierik EG, van Urk H, Wittens CH. Efficacy of subfascial endoscopy in eradicating perforating veins of the lower leg and its relation with venous ulcer healing. *J Vasc Surg* 1997; **26**: 255–9.

79. Monk BE, Sarkany I. Outcome of treatment of venous stasis ulcers. *Clin Exp Dermatol* 1982; **7**: 397–400.

80. Kitahama A, Elliott LF, Kerstein MD, Menendez CV. Leg ulcer. Conservative management or surgical treatment? *J Am Med Assoc* 1982; **247**: 197–9.

81. Negus D. Prevention and treatment of venous ulceration. *Ann R Coll Surg Engl* 1985; **67**: 144–8.

82. Mayberry JC, Moneta GL, Taylor LMJ, Porter JM. Fifteen-year results of ambulatory compression therapy for chronic venous ulcers. *Surgery* 1991; **109**: 575–81.

83. Erickson CA. Healing of venous ulcers in an ambulatory care program: the role of chronic venous insufficiency and patient compliance. *J Vasc Surg* 1995; **22**: 629–36.

84. DePalma RG, Kowallek DL. Venous ulceration: a cross-over study from nonoperative to operative treatment. *J Vasc Surg* 1996; **24**: 788–92.

85. Samson RH, Showalter DP. Stockings and the prevention of recurrent venous ulcers. *Dermatol Surg* 1996; **22**: 373–6.

86. Bergan JJ, Ballard JL, Sparks S. In: Gloviczki P, Bergan JJ, eds. *Atlas of Endoscopic Perforator Vein Surgery*. London: Springer-Verlag, 1998; 141–9.

87. Gloviczki P, Canton LG, Cambria RA, Rhee RY. Subfascial endoscopic perforator vein surgery with gas insufflation. In: Gloviczki P, Bergan JJ, eds. *Atlas of Endoscopic Perforator Vein Surgery*. London: Springer-Verlag, 1998; 125–38.

18

Sclerotherapy in the treatment of varicose veins

PHILIP D. COLERIDGE SMITH

INTRODUCTION

Sclerotherapy is a long established method of treating varicose veins. It is currently used to obliterate veins ranging from less than 1 mm in diameter to over 10 mm. The first use of injection therapy was performed in 1840 with a solution of absolute alcohol.[1] Since then a number of compounds have been used as sclerosants for the treatment of varicose veins and telangiectases. Sodium tetradecyl sulfate (STS) is in widespread use at present. This is an anionic surface-active substance which was introduced more than half a century ago.[2,3] A range of techniques of sclerotherapy have been published by different authors and have been in use with various modifications for many years.[4–6] In general, these comprise injection of sclerosant into the vein followed by the application of compression bandaging. A recent Cochrane review was unable to conclude that any particular technique of injection or compression led to an advantage in outcome.[7]

MECHANISM OF ACTION OF SCLEROTHERAPY

Sclerotherapy refers to the introduction of a foreign substance into the lumen of a vessel, causing thrombosis and subsequent fibrosis. This procedure performed on telangiectases is referred to as microsclerotherapy.[8] The mechanism of action for sclerosing solutions is that of producing endothelial damage (endosclerosis) that evolves in endofibrosis. The extent of damage to the blood vessel wall determines the effectiveness of the solution. Total endothelial destruction results in the exposure of subendothelial collagen fibres, causing platelet aggregation, adherence, and release of platelet-related factors. This series of events initiates the intrinsic pathway of blood coagulation by activating factor XII. Ideally, sclerosing solutions should not otherwise cause activation or release of thromboplastic activity because this would initiate the extrinsic pathway of blood coagulation.[9]

Excessive thrombosis is detrimental to the production of endofibrosis because it may lead to recanalization of the vessel and excessive intravascular and perivascular inflammation and its resulting sequelae. This can be prevented, or at least minimized, with post-sclerotherapy compression. However, thrombosis usually occurs to some degree as a result of sclerotherapy.

TECHNIQUE OF SCLEROTHERAPY

The use of compression sclerotherapy in the treatment of varicose veins depends not only on the solution which is used but also on the technique used to treat the varicose veins. The method of managing the patient is very important in the final outcome.

According to Fegan,[10] as soon as the exact points at which the injections should be placed have been decided, the patient sits upright on a couch with the leg horizontal. The pressure in the veins in this position is sufficient to make venepuncture possible but low enough to obviate the danger of bleed-back along the needle tract. The most distal incompetent perforating vein should be injected first, followed by the next most distal and so on until all the selected sites have been injected. This progression allows for the veins to empty completely before each injection.

Of even greater importance than the concentration of sclerosing solution in the syringe is the concentration within the vein.[11] Stemmer *et al.* expanded on this principle by demonstrating in polyvinyl tubes that the local conditions of 'time and space' regarding contact of the sclerosing solution with the vessel wall were important determinants of therapeutic outcome.[12] They demonstrated that the zone of contact diminishes as the calibre of the vessel increases. In tubes with a diameter less than or equal to 4 mm, the liquid flowed in a laminar fashion. In tubes with a diameter greater than or equal to 8 mm, turbulent flow was produced. In tubes 6 mm in diameter, a mixed flow occurred, with a transition between a laminar and turbulent appearance. In contrast, the calibre and position of the needle, the speed of injection, and the viscosity of the solution did not seem to influence the time of contact of the sclerosing solution with the tube.

Guex[13] calculated that the concentration of sclerosing solution is based on the diameter of the vein. He used a formula where the mean concentration of solution is equal to the volume of injected sclerosing solution multiplied by the concentration of sclerosing solution and the number of injections divided by the radius of the injected vein. Thus, if 0.5 mL is injected into a varicose vein 2 mm in diameter, the sclerosing solution will fill a 16 cm length of vein. In reality, the concentration of sclerosing solution at the injection site is maximal and decreases with distance from each point when small volumes of solution are injected. The concentration of sclerosing solution along the entire course of the vein can be equalized either by injecting a larger volume into a single site or by injection of small volumes in multiple sites. A study by Cornu-Thenard[14] confirmed Guex's formula and recommended 0.5 mL injections be placed every 6–10 cm along the varicose vein.

Another important principle in performing sclerotherapy is that the amount of sclerosing solution injected into a single site should not be more than 1.0 mL (usually 0.5 mL). Venographic studies of direct injections into varicosities of the leg have demonstrated that if more than 1.5 mL of solution is injected at single site, it is likely to spill over into the deep veins.[15,16] In addition, the patient should not move the leg for a few minutes so that the sclerosing solution can remain in contact with the varicose vein, because any movement of the leg will rapidly move the sclerosing solution into the deep venous system.

In addition to injection techniques, post-treatment techniques are important. After injections of varicose or telangiectatic veins, the treated veins are immediately compressed to minimize significant thrombosis. The patient is instructed to walk immediately after the injection session to help prevent deep vein thrombosis and reduce venous reflux into the treated veins. Calf muscle movement produces a rapid blood flow in the deep venous system, which dilutes sclerosing solution that may have migrated into the area.

Post-sclerosis compression is perhaps the most important advance in sclerotherapy treatment of varicose veins since the introduction of relatively safe synthetic sclerosing agents in the 1940s. Primarily, compression eliminates thrombophlebitic reaction and substitutes a 'sclerophlebitis' with the production of firm fibrous cord.[17]

One of the first descriptions of a method of sclerotherapy that resembles the techniques used today was published in a monograph by Dr R. Thornhill in 1929.[18] The essence of the treatment was initial clinical examination of the patient to establish the sources of varicose vein filling. The apparatus used to make the injections included a syringe which had been modified to include a small glass window between the syringe and the needle. This was used to aspirate blood from the vein to be injected in order to confirm that the tip of the needle was in the lumen of the vein. Thornhill used a solution of quinine and urethane to treat veins. He found this effective without resulting in undue complications when injected intravenously. He described an 'empty vein' technique which he achieved by first inserting the needle in the vein with the help of a tourniquet and then deflating the tourniquet to empty the vein. Blood was emptied from the vein on either side of the injection site with a rubber roller before the injection began. Following injection of veins, he would ensure that the patient lay supine for 5–10 min but did not systematically apply compression bandaging or stockings.

McPheeters and Anderson[4] also described an 'empty vein' technique in 1939 which was used to minimize the tendency to thrombophlebitis caused by sclerotherapy. By 1956, compression bandaging over rubber pads was used to maintain veins which had been treated in a compressed state, minimizing the extent of thrombus within the lumen of these vessels.[19] In 1963 Fegan[20] published his technique of sclerotherapy based on rigorous clinical examination of patients to establish the location of the feeding veins, followed by injection using an empty vein technique. Compression was applied to the treated limbs by wrapping the leg in a bandage over rubber pads followed by the application of an elastic stocking. He considered that maintenance of compression for at least 6 weeks was required to achieve a good outcome. His strategies were based on clinical experience as well as histological investigation of varicose veins treated by sclerotherapy.

ULTRASOUND GUIDANCE OF INJECTIONS

Continuous-wave (CW) Doppler ultrasound has been in use for the study of blood flow in veins in health and disease for many years.[21] In France, where enthusiasm for the use of sclerotherapy has remained strong, this led Schadeck and Vin[22] to improve the efficacy of their treatment by using a Doppler ultrasound probe to assist with placing injections of STS in the great saphenous vein. In the late 1980s, ultrasound imaging combined with blood flow measurement (duplex ultrasonography) was introduced for the diagnosis of venous disease of the lower limb,[23] although this was on a limited scale. Subsequently, ultrasound imaging was used to guide the placing of injections into incompetent saphenous trunks.[24–29] This method of treatment was found to achieve obliteration of the saphenous trunks in a substantial proportion of patients, resulting in long-term relief from varices. Duplex ultrasound examination demonstrated recanalization of veins in up to one-quarter of patients at 1 year.[30] Nevertheless, ultrasound-guided injection for varicose veins remains a widely performed treatment, especially in southern European countries as well as in Australia and New Zealand.

FOAM SCLEROTHERAPY

In 1944, Orbach described the 'air block' technique. In this, a small volume of air is included in the syringe with the sclerosant. This is injected ahead of the sclerosant in order to prevent blood diluting the sclerosant and reducing its efficacy. In 1950, Orbach[31] published a further paper describing the use of a foam which he created by vigorously shaking a syringe containing air and sclerosant to produce a froth. He modestly records that this method was also suggested by Foote.[32] He investigated the efficacy of this in comparison with liquid alone using an animal model in the tail veins of mice. His experiments demonstrated that STS foam was 3.5 to four times more effective than the solution when comparing the weight of sclerosant injected. In the same article, he described the outcome of 115 injections given to patients using the foam technique. Four to six injections per session were given without discomfort to the patient and with good efficacy. The author used this method widely and mentions in 1956 that he had carried out over 2000 treatments.[19] Other practitioners in this field took up the technique at the time, including Sigg[33] who mentions 15 000 injections given in his own practice. A few subsequent papers show that the method of sclerotherapy using foam was employed by a number of physicians in the 1950s and 1960s.[34–36] Fegan[37] refers to the use of STS as a foam in the management of vulval varices of pregnancy in his book on sclerotherapy, originally published in 1967.

The next significant advance came in 1993 when Cabrera *et al.*[38] suggested that foam could be created using carbon dioxide mixed with a detergent sclerosant. Cabrera published a further article in 1997 describing his experience in 261 limbs with long saphenous varices and eight patients with vascular malformations (Fig. 18.1). He had used sclerotherapy with foam, guiding his injections by ultrasound imaging. Some of the varicose veins reached 20 mm in diameter. He considered that foam, which he had created from polidocanol a non-ionic detergent sclerosant, greatly extended the range of vein sizes which could be managed by sclerotherapy using liquid sclerosants. He felt that the increased efficacy of foam was attributable to its displacement of blood from the treated vein, thus increasing the contact time between the sclerosant and the vein. He used a 'microfoam', i.e. a foam made of very small bubbles. His method of preparing this foam was not published.

Frullini and Cavezzi have reported similar data in a series of 453 patients. Early observations showed that 93 percent of veins remained occluded after treatment with foam. The sclerosants used in this series were polidocanol and STS. A number

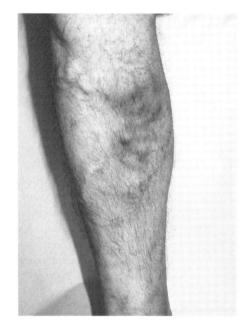

Figure 18.1 *Large saphenous varices arising from incompetence of the great saphenous vein. This type of varicose vein was treated by Cabrera in his clinical series.*

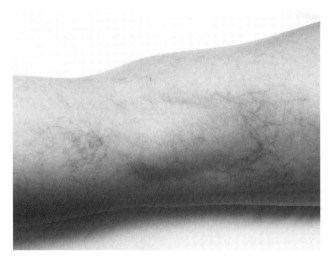

Figure 18.2 *Small varicose veins: telangiectases and reticular veins (<3 mm diameter). This type of vein was treated by Vin using foam sclerotherapy.*

of instances of limited calf vein thrombosis have been observed following foam sclerotherapy. Cavezzi *et al.*[39] subsequently published a detailed analysis of the efficacy of foam sclerotherapy in 194 patients. They report a good outcome after treatment in 93 percent of patients.

Foam sclerotherapy has also been investigated in the management of small varices, including reticular veins and telangiectases (Fig. 18.2). In 1999, Henriet[40] reported his results in 10 000 patients with reticular varices and telangiectases of the lower limb treated between the years 1995 and 1998. He found that the outcome of foam treatment in small varices was excellent and that reduced volumes and concentrations of sclerosant could be employed compared with liquid sclerosants.

Benigni *et al.*[41] reported the findings of a pilot study comparing liquid and foam sclerosants. They measured the outcome using a visual analogue scale to describe the improvement in appearance and found that foam sclerotherapy resulted in a 20 percent improved appearance compared with liquid sclerosant.[41] Both of these groups used foam made from polidocanol.

A series of authors has described methods of preparing 'home-made' foam which may be used for ultrasound-guided sclerotherapy. Monfreux[42] described a method necessitating a glass syringe that produced small quantities of polidocanol foam which he used in a series of patients with truncal varicose veins. Sadoun and Benigni[43] described a method of preparing foam using a plastic syringe avoiding the need for reusable glass syringes. Subsequently, Tessari[44] described a method of preparing foam using two disposable syringes and a three-way tap (Fig. 18.3).[44] This method can be used to produce large quantities of foam suitable for treating saphenous trunks and large varices. Frullini[45] has added his own method of producing foam to this increasing list based on that of Fluckinger.[46]

In summary, foam sclerotherapy using polidocanol and STS has become widely used in recent years. Its popularity is based on an improved efficacy compared with liquid sclerosants, enabling far lower doses of sclerosant to be used. It is a technique which is popular in southern European countries as well as in Australia and New Zealand.[47] The majority of practitioners prepare their own foam using the Tessari[44] method.

Reason for increased efficacy of foam

Detergent sclerosants such as polidocanol and STS become protein-bound and inactivated when mixed with blood. Therefore the importance of avoiding this in the treatment method is important. Fegan emphasized the need for an 'empty vein' technique in which he elevated the limb and maintained the segment empty by manual compression.[10] If a sclerosant is injected into a vein containing blood, it will become mixed with the blood and efficacy of the treatment will be reduced (Fig. 18.4). When a foam sclerosant is injected, it tends to remain separate from the blood and fills the vein completely, displacing blood from the vein (Fig. 18.5). Since the volume

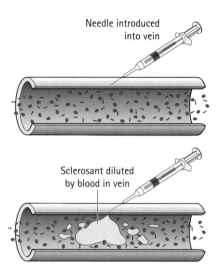

Figure 18.4   *Liquid sclerosants mix with blood in the vein which is being treated, resulting in inactivation of the sclerosant.*

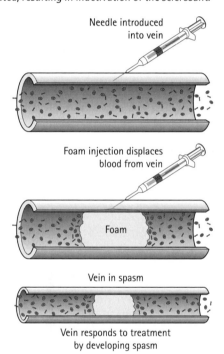

Figure 18.5   *Foam sclerosants displace blood from the vein under treatment and completely fill it, making treatment more effective.*

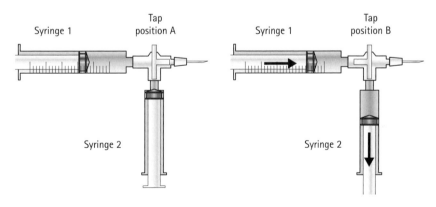

Figure 18.3   *Tessari's method for creating sclerosant foam.[44] A mixture of air and sclerosant is passed between the two syringes about 20 times to create a foam comprising very small bubbles.*

of the foam is much greater than the original volume of the sclerosant from which it was prepared, it is relatively easy to completely fill a vein which is to be treated, ensuring that all endothelium is exposed to the sclerosant and destroyed. This is facilitated by elevating the limb being treated in order to empty the superficial veins, a technique long established in sclerotherapy.

Efficacy and safety of treatment

No randomized clinical trial comparing this technique with surgery has so far been published. However, a large multicentre trial is currently in progress in Europe comparing surgery with a commercial pharmaceutical foam (Varisolve, Provensis, UK). The clinical series of Cabrera and Frullini indicate that 80–90 percent of saphenous trunks remain occluded after 3 years when treated by foam sclerotherapy. This is in keeping with the author's experience of this technique[48] (Fig. 18.6).

Adverse reactions to this treatment include the development of pigmentation in relation to treated veins, superficial thrombophlebitis and thrombosis in deep calf veins. All of these complications are common to conventional sclerotherapy and can be addressed by standard means. Some concern remains about the intravenous injection of a foam based on air. No serious complication of foam sclerotherapy has been reported and the volumes of air used during treatment are small. In a few patients, the development of a scotoma has been detected following treatment. It has been hypothesized that this may be attributable to air embolism to the visual cortex via a patent foramen ovale. However, conventional sclerotherapy may occasionally also produce this problem. In any case, complete resolution of the visual field defect has occurred within an hour or two in all cases so far encountered.

RESULTS OF TREATMENT IN PATIENTS WITH VARICOSE VEINS

Reid and Rothnie[49] studied the effect of compression sclerotherapy on varicose veins of 974 patients. They grouped the various types of varicose veins according to their clinico-anatomical appearance. The sclerosants used were 3 percent STS and 5 percent ethanolamine sulfate. A good response to treatment was seen in 85 percent or more of the patients treated in most groups. The good response to treatment was slightly lower (76 percent) in pregnant women, probably as a result of the tendency of sclerosed veins to re-open as the pregnancy progressed. Very often, in the pregnant women, a regression of the varicose veins was seen after pregnancy and these investigators adopted a policy to treat only those patients with marked symptoms.

There were no significant reactions immediately following the injection. Ulceration, probably as a result of leakage or injection of the material outside the vein, occurred in a number of patients receiving STS. Ulceration was not seen in those patients receiving ethanolamine sulfate. On the assumption that the two compounds were injected with comparable skill, this would suggest that STS causes greater irritation than ethanolamine sulfate.

Doran and White,[50] compared the efficacy of Fegan's method[51] and surgery for the treatment of varicose veins. They randomly selected 331 patients with varicose veins uncomplicated by ulceration. Of this total, 182 patients were treated primarily by Fegan's method and 149 were operated upon. In the Fegan group, 98 had bilateral varicose veins, and in 84 the varicosities were restricted to one leg. In the group that underwent surgery, 73 had bilateral varicose veins and in 76 they were unilateral. Presented as individual limbs, the Fegan group

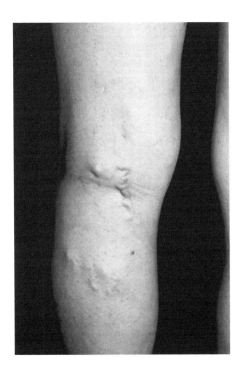
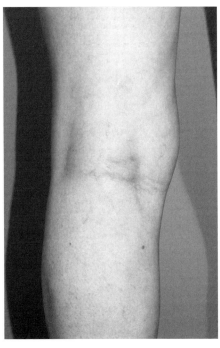

Figure 18.6 *Outcome of foam sclerotherapy: before (left) and 1 year following treatment (right).*

contained 280 and the operative group 222. The results showed that the initial response of varicose veins to compression sclerotherapy using 3 percent STS was likely to be superior to that after surgery. In patients with incompetence at the saphenofemoral junction and who underwent surgery, 49.6 percent of the limbs on which long saphenous stripping was done required injections at the end of the first year compared with 23.7 percent of those who received sclerotherapy as their primary treatment. When comparing all limbs treated, fewer limbs treated by sclerotherapy required additional treatment at the end of the first year, than those operated upon, irrespective of site. The investigators concluded that the initial response of varicose veins to Fegan's sclerotherapy method is better than surgery. They did not investigate the long-term results, due to the difficulty of maintaining the efficiency of follow-up.

In another study comparing sclerotherapy with surgery in the treatment of varicose veins, Chant et al.[52] treated a total of 215 randomly selected patients. The group was subdivided into 115 receiving sclerotherapy using Fegan's method and 100 undergoing surgery. The patients were seen 6 months and 1, 2 and 3 years after treatment started. The number of patients with bilateral varicose veins was not mentioned in the paper. However, in the analysis of results, the investigators reduced any bias that might occur by randomly selecting one of the treated legs. The outcome of the study was that there was no significant difference between the treatments during the whole of the study period; no further treatment was required for 78–89 percent of the patients receiving sclerotherapy and 86–93 percent of those patients receiving surgery.

In four random trials on 418 patients, Hobbs[53] used a modification of Fegan's method to compare injection sclerotherapy (211 patients), using 3 percent STS, with surgery (207 patients) as an effective treatment of varicose veins. The patients were assigned to one of four groups according to the venous systems involved:

- group I – great saphenous system only
- group II – small saphenous system only
- group III – great saphenous system plus incompetent perforating veins
- group IV – lower leg perforating vessels only.

Each leg was further classified as mild, moderate or severe. The patients were reviewed for up to 27 months (average 12) following treatment. The results after 12 months showed that for groups I and II, injection sclerotherapy was comparable to surgery (approximately 50–60 percent cured using either technique). For those patients in groups III and IV, injection sclerotherapy (56–59 percent cured) appeared to be significantly superior to surgery (12 and 13 percent cured). Of the 211 patients receiving injection sclerotherapy, there were 14 cases of complications. These included skin staining or necrosis (six cases), overdose effects (five cases), allergic reaction (one case), acute flare-up of rheumatism (one case), attacks of recurrent boils (one case). With the 207 patients receiving surgical treatment, there were 40 cases of complications following surgery. These included cutaneous nerve

injury (21 cases), delayed wound healing (15 cases), deep vein thrombosis (two cases), minor pulmonary embolism (one case) and anesthetic collapse (one case). The investigators concluded that, for the treatment of diffuse dilated superficial veins, injection sclerotherapy was most effective and results from surgery were poor. Dilated superficial veins plus incompetent perforating vein surgery would need to be supported by injection sclerotherapy in order to achieve a complete cure. Incompetence of the great saphenous system can be effectively treated by either method.

By 1974, Hobbs[54] had reviewed the results of surgical treatment and sclerotherapy of varicose veins over a 6-year follow up, including those patients reported in the above-mentioned study. The group size had increased to 250 in each of the surgery and sclerotherapy groups. In total, 404 legs had been treated by injection and 275 legs by surgery. The results revealed that whilst injection sclerotherapy was superior to surgery up to 2 years post-treatment, the failure rate increased over the next 4 years to achieve a level greater than that seen following surgery. It should be stated here that the cure rate was not particularly high for either treatment at 6 years (7 percent sclerotherapy and 20 percent surgery).

Patients with below-knee saphenous varicose veins, without clinical evidence of saphenofemoral incompetence, were treated either by surgery ($n = 195$) or injection compression sclerotherapy ($n = 74$). STS 3 percent solution was used as the sclerosant. Examinations of the legs 2–3 years after treatment showed that surgery was significantly more successful ($P < 0.01$) than sclerotherapy.[55] In all patients, the success rate for surgery was 71 percent compared with 47 percent for sclerotherapy.

Varicose veins and their treatment can be a problem during pregnancy. Abramowitz[56] described the successful use sclerotherapy (STS, 3 percent solution) in the treatment of varicose veins during pregnancy. No injections were given during the first trimester of pregnancy and patients seen during the last 6 weeks of pregnancy were excluded. Sclerotherapy was compared with the use of elastic hosiery in a total of 101 patients, 45 receiving sclerotherapy and 56 being given elastic hosiery. The results showed that sclerotherapy was far superior, 32 (71 percent) achieving a good result, compared with five (9 percent) using elastic hosiery. No serious complications arose following the use of STS.

MANAGEMENT OF SMALL VARICES AND TELANGIECTASES

Sodium tetradecyl sulfate became widely used in the 1950s after its introduction in 1946 by Reiner.[2] In 1978, Tretbar[57] first reported the injection of a 1 percent solution into spider angiomata. He noted excellent results in virtually all 144 patients treated. He also noted an unspecified number of episodes of epidermal necrosis without significant sequelae and a 30 percent incidence of post-sclerosis pigmentation resolved within a few months. In 1982 Shields and Jansen[58] were the first to describe microsclerosis of telangiectases with STS in the dermatological literature. They injected STS 1 percent into 105 patients and reported only one episode of necrosis in more than 600 treatments in vessels less than 5 mm in diameter. There were no systemic reactions, and the majority of post-sclerosis skin pigmentation resolved in 3–4 months. However, as more experience with its use in the treatment of leg telangiectases occurred, even further dilutions (0.1–0.3 percent) were recommended, both to achieve clinical efficacy and to limit adverse sequelae.

Thibault[59] has recently reported on his 2-year experience with STS used to treat varicose veins and telangiectases. He evaluated 2665 patients in a 2-year prospective study and found excellent results with minimal adverse sequelae. Using minimally effective sclerosing concentrations, he found a 0.15 percent incidence of significant or severe pigmentation that was identical to the rate found with another sclerosing solution, polidocanol. Four patients (0.15 percent) developed uncomplicated anaphylactoid reactions, with two patients (0.07 percent) developing urticaria.

CONCLUSIONS ON EFFICACY

The treatment of varicose veins has generally been undertaken by surgery, compression therapy or injection. Surgery is effective, yet it carries the risk that is associated with the use of general anesthesia. It is especially hazardous for obese patients. Compression therapy using elastic stockings or bandages manages the problems of skin changes and aching from varices but is not a permanent solution. The introduction of injection therapy using sclerosants provided an opportunity to treat varicose veins with very little risk to the patient.

In recent years, ultrasound imaging has been used to guide the placing of injections. This requires competence at ultrasonography of the venous system as well as knowledge of the standard techniques of sclerotherapy.

The use of foam sclerosants has been employed in the injection of telangiectases, reticular varices, saphenous varices and saphenous trunks. Ultrasound guidance is often used to place injections into saphenous trunks.

The majority of complications following sclerotherapy are relatively minor and are self-limiting. Thrombophlebitis and pigmentation over the injected vein usually resolve spontaneously without intervention. Occasionally, clot has to be evacuated from an injected vein. Paresthesia may arise if a peripheral sensory nerve is affected. As with many of the potential hazards of this technique, the correct use of the sclerosant is important and those wishing to practice sclerotherapy should receive training from an experienced operator.

Injection outside a vein is to be avoided, since this may result in a small ulcer at the injection site. Intra-arterial injection of sclerosants will result in severe ischemia of the region of limb supplied by the artery which has been injected. If this is a major axial limb vessel, then gangrene of the foot may occur.[60] This is a rare complication and can be avoided by a careful technique.

Allergic reactions to sclerosants are relatively few, but a number of cases of anaphylaxis have been reported. Those practicing sclerotherapy should have suitable drugs available to them in their treatment room in order to manage any severe allergic reaction.

Deep vein thrombosis may occur following sclerotherapy for varicose veins. This probably reflects use of a technique which allows a significant quantity of sclerosant to enter the deep veins of the leg. The technique of treatment is important, with the volume of injection limited to that which is considered safe, i.e. in the range of 0.5–1.0 mL at any one injection site. The use of firm compression bandaging following treatment and post-sclerotherapy walking exercise may also reduce the risk of deep vein thrombosis. Some patients are especially prone to venous thrombosis. In patients with a history of previous DVT or in whom duplex ultrasound examination has shown evidence of previous venous thrombosis, consideration should be given to the use of an alternative method of managing varicose veins. This remains an infrequent complication of sclerotherapy but one with potentially fatal consequences should pulmonary embolism result. Only a few case reports appear to have been published in the literature on this subject with no case series.[61,62] Recent publications concerning the outcome of foam sclerotherapy have reported a small number of cases of thrombosis limited to calf veins and no proximal venous thrombosis affecting the popliteal vein or femoral vein.[38,39] Calf vein thrombosis occurred in less than 1 percent of patients. Henriet[40] reported no case of deep vein thrombosis or pulmonary embolism in his series of 10 000 patients. Patients undergoing sclerotherapy should be advised to seek urgent medical advice should they develop any symptom suggestive of deep vein thrombosis following treatment by sclerotherapy.

The major complications of sclerotherapy are infrequently encountered and most minor undesirable events can be minimized by the use of an appropriate technique, which can only be achieved by proper training.

The efficacy of sclerotherapy is difficult to assess since few long-term studies have been done to address this issue. Hobbs[54] compared the efficacy of sclerotherapy to surgery in patients with truncal incompetence of the great saphenous vein. Although good results were found initially, with no difference between sclerotherapy and surgery after 10 years' follow-up, he found a much higher rate of recurrence in patients who had undergone sclerotherapy than in those undergoing surgical treatment. From the surgical literature, it has been found that failure to control venous reflux in the great saphenous vein by stripping leads to a higher recurrence rate than when the saphenous vein has been stripped.[63] In one series it was found that even direct sclerotherapy to the great saphenous vein failed to occlude this vein permanently in 80 percent of cases.[64] In another series there was 24 percent recurrence of varices and 27 percent recurrence of great saphenous vein reflux 2 years following ultrasound-guided injection of the long saphenous vein.[65] The reason for the less satisfactory long-term outcome following sclerotherapy is that, although the local varices are successfully treated, the great saphenous vein may recanalize in a substantial proportion of patients. This leads to an earlier return of varices than would have been the case had surgery been used. One solution here is to manage patients with truncal saphenous incompetence using surgical techniques instead, whilst reserving sclerotherapy for those patients in whom the great saphenous vein is competent or has been removed at surgery. The recent re-introduction of foam sclerotherapy has greatly increased the efficacy of sclerotherapy of saphenous trunks, with recanalization rates of 15 percent reported after 1–3 years.[38,39,66] In the long term this may result in clinical recurrence of varicose veins at a similar rate to that of surgery. The rate of recurrence of varicose veins following surgery is difficult to estimate since very wide variation in recurrence has been reported in different studies following surgery. The definition of requirement for further surgery resulted in an overall recurrence rate of 15 percent in the study mentioned above and was much greater in the patients in whom the long saphenous vein had not been stripped.[63]

Surgery involves significant postoperative morbidity with bruising, hematomas, postoperative pain, sensory nerve injury, lymphatic injury and surgical scars as well as the risks of general anesthesia. The risk of DVT following surgical treatment in varicose veins is in the range 0.1–1 percent.[67] The risks of complications following surgery for recurrent varicose veins increase further, and therefore it is highly desirable to avoid surgery for this problem. Sclerotherapy remains of similar difficulty for recurrent or primary varices and it is therefore not so imperative to avoid recurrence when treating patients by sclerotherapy. Further injections can easily be given to treat any recurrence without the need for general anesthesia or risking postoperative complications.

CONCLUSIONS

Sclerotherapy is a widely used and effective method of treating varicose veins, including telangiectases, reticular veins and saphenous varices. The use of foam sclerotherapy offers significant advantages when managing larger varices. This allows lower doses of the active compound to be injected, with improved results especially in larger veins. It appears that tens of thousands of patients have already been managed in this way, with adverse reactions from the treatment being no different from those of conventional liquid sclerotherapy and with less perioperative morbidity than following surgery.

REFERENCES

1. Schneider W. Contribution to the history of the sclerosing treatment of varices and to its anatomo-pathologic study. *Phlébologie* 1965; **18**: 117–30.

2. Reiner L. The activity of anionic surface active compounds in producing vascular obliteration. *Proc Soc Exp Biol Med* 1946; **62**: 49–54.

3. Hirschman SR. Sclerotherapy of varicose veins with Sotrodecol. *N Y State J Med* 1947, June 15.

4. McPheeters HO, Anderson JK. *Injection Treatment of Varicose Veins and Haemorrhoids*. Philadelphia: FA Davies, 1939.

5. Tournay R. La technique des injections sclérosants intravariqueuses. *Concours Med* 1928; **26**: June.

6. Riddle P. *Injection Treatment of Varicose Veins*. Philadelphia: WB Saunders, 1940; 136.

7. Tisi PV, Beverley CA. Injection sclerotherapy for varicose veins (Cochrane Review). In: *The Cochrane Library, Issue 2*: Oxford: Update Software, 2003.

8. Green D. Compression sclerotherapy techniques. *Dermatol Clin* 1989; **7**: 137–46.

9. Goldman MP. *Sclerotherapy Treatment of Varicose and Telangiectatic Leg Veins*, 2nd edn. St Louis: Mosby Yearbook, 1995.

10. Fegan WG. Compression sclerotherapy. *Ann R Coll Surg* 1967; **41**: 364–9.

11. Merlen JF, Curri SB, Saout J, Coget J. Histologic changes in a sclerosed vein, *Phlébologie* 1978; **31**: 17–34.

12. Stemmer R, Kopp C, Voglet P. Étude physique de l'injection sclérosante. *Phlébologie* 1969; **22**: 149–72.

13. Guex J-J. Indications for the sclerosing agent polidocanol. *J Dermatol Surg Oncol* 1993; **19**: 959–61.

14. Cornu-Thenard A. Sclerotherapy of varicose veins: value of measurement of vessel diameter before the first injection. Paper presented at the second annual International Congress of the North American Society of Phlebology, New Orleans, February 25, 1989.

15. Vin F. Principles, technique, and results of treatment of the greater saphenous vein by sclero-therapy. Paper presented at the second annual International Congress of the North American Society of Phlebology, New Orleans, February 25, 1989.

16. Kinmonth JB, Robertson DJ. Injection treatment of varicose veins. radiological and histological investigations of methods. *Br J Surg* 1949; **36**: 294.

17. Reid RG, Rothnie NG. Treatment of varicose veins by compression sclerotherapy. *Br J Surg* 1968; **55**: 889–95.

18. Thronhill R. Varicose veins and their treatment by 'empty vein' injection. London: Baillière, Tindall & Cox, 1929; 64.

19. Orbach EJ. Varicose veins. In: Samuels SS, ed. *Diagnosis and Treatment of Vascular Disorders*. Baltimore: Williams & Wilkins, 1956; 475–540.

20. Fegan WG. Continuous compression technique of injecting varicose veins. *Lancet* 1963; **ii**: 109–12.

21. Sumner DS, Baker DW, Strandness DE Jr. The ultrasonic velocity detector in a clinical study of venous disease. *Arch Surg* 1968; **97**: 75–80.

22. Schadeck M, Vin F. Resultats du traitement de 192 spaphenes internes par sclerose de la junction sapheo-femorale controles au Doppler. In: Negus D, Jantet G, eds. *Phlebology '85*. London: John Libbey, 1986; 132–6.

23. Schadeck M. Doppler et échotomographie dans la sclérose des veines saphènes. *Phlébologie* 1986; **39**: 697–716.

24. Brizzio E, Avramovic A, De Simone J. Appreciation de l'effet sclerosant avec l'emploi de l'échographie veineuse et le Doppler. *IX World Congress of Phlebology Abstr., Kyoto September 1986, FP 19-5*. 1986; 25.

25. Schadeck M. Etude par Doppler et Echotomographie de l'évolution des veines saphènes sous traitement sclérosant. Communication au 19 ème Congrès de Pathologie Vasculaire. Paris, 14 March 1985.

26. Knight RM, Vin F, Zygmunt JA. *Ultrasonic Guidance of Injections into the Superficial System.* In: Davy A, Stemmer R, eds. *Phlébologie 89.* Montrouge: John Libbey Eurotext Ltd, 1989; 339–41.

27. Schadeck M, Allaert F. Sclerotherapy of the long saphenous vein: methodology and results controlled by echo-Doppler on 300 patients. In: Davy A, Stemmer R, eds. *Phlebologie '89.* Montrouge: John Libbey Eurotext, 1989; 836–8.

28. Schadeck M, Allaert F. Echotomographie de la sclérose. *Phlébologie* 1991; **44**: 111–30.

29. Vin F. Echo-sclérothérapie de la veine saphène externe. *Phlébologie* 1991; **44**: 79–84.

30. Kanter A, Thibault P. Dermatol saphenofemoral incompetence treated by ultrasound-guided sclerotherapy. *Surgery* 1996; **22**: 648–52.

31. Orbach EJ. The thrombogenic activity of foam of a synthetic anionic detergent (sodium tetradecyl sulfate NNR). *Angiology* 1950; **1**: 237–43.

32. Foote RR. *Varicose Veins.* London: Butterworth, 1949; 1–225.

33. Sigg K. The treatment of varicosities and accompanying complications. *Angiology* 1952; **3**: 355.

34. Ree A. Ethanolamine foam in the treatment of varicose veins. A new treatment. *Acta Dermatovenerolog* 1953; **33**.

35. Flückiger P. Nicht-operative retrograde Varizenverödung mit Varsylschaum. *Schweizer Med Wochenschr* 1956; **48**.

36. Brücke H, Mayer H. Zur Ätiologie und Behandlung der Varizen der unteren Extremität 1957.

37. Fegan G. *Varicose Veins: Compression Sclerotherapy.* London: Heinemann Medical, 1967; 1–114.

38. Cabrera Garido JR, Cabrera Garcia Olmedo JR, Garcia Olmedo Dominguez. Nuevo meodo de esclerosis en las varices tronculares. *Pathologia Vasculares* 1993; **1**: 55–72.

39. Cavezzi A, Frullini A, Ricci S, Tessari L. Treatment of varicose veins by foam sclerotherapy: two clinical series. *Phlebology* 2002; **17**: 13–8.

40. Henriet JP. Expérience durant trois années de la mousse de polidocanol dans le traitement des varices réticulaires et des varicosités. *Phlebologie* 1999; **52**: 277–82.

41. Benigni JP, Sadoun S, Thirion V et al. Télangiectasies et varices réticulaires traitement par la mousse d'aetoxisclérol à 0.25% présentation d'une étude pilote. *Phlebologie* 1999; **52**: 283–90.

42. Monfreux A. Traitement sclérosant des troncs saphènies et leurs collatérales de gros calibre par le méthode mus. *Phlébologie* 1997; **50**: 351–3.

43. Sadoun S, Benigni JP. The treatment of varicosities and telangiectases with TDS and Lauromacrogol foam. *XIII World Congress of Phlebology Abstract Book* 1998; 327.

44. Tessari L. Nouvelle technique d'obtention de la scléro-mousse. *Phlébologie* 2000; **53**: 129.

45. Frullini A. New technique in producing sclerosing foam in a disposable syringe. *Derm Surg* 2000; **26**: 705–6.

46. Flückinger P. Nicht-operative retrograde Varizenverödung mit Varsylschaum. *Schweiz Med Wochenschr* 1956; **48**.

47. Varcoe P. Ultrasound guided sclerotherapy. *Aust NZ J Phlebol* 2000; **4**: 117.

48. Coleridge Smith P, Wright D, Tristram S. Foam sclerotherapy of saphenous trunk varices. *Phlebology* 2002; **17**: 75.

49. Reid RG, Rothnie NG. Treatment of varicose veins by compression therapy. *Br J Surg* 1968; **55**: 889–95.

50. Doran FS A. White M. A clinical trial designed to discover if the primary treatment of varicose veins should be by Fegan's method or by operation. *Br J Surg* 1975; **62**: 72–6.

51. Fegan WG. Continuous uninterrupted compression technique of injecting varicose veins. *Proc R Soc Med* 1960; **53**: 837–40.

52. Chant AD, Jones HO, Weddell JM. Varicose veins: a comparison of surgery and injection/compression sclerotherapy. *Lancet* 1972; **ii**: 1188–91.

53. Hobbs JT. The treatment of varicose veins. A random trial of injection compression therapy versus surgery. *Br J Surg* 1968; **55**: 777–80.

54. Hobbs JT. Surgery and sclerotherapy in the treatment of varicose veins. *Arch Surg* 1974; **109**: 793–6.

55. Freedman DL. The value of sclerocompression in treatment of below-knee varicose veins. *Opuscula Med* 1980; **25**: 92–6.

56. Abramowitz I. The treatment of varicose veins in pregnancy by empty vein compression sclerotherapy. *SA Med J* 1973; **47**: 607–10.

57. Tretbar LL. Spider angiomata: treatment with sclerosant injections. *J Kansas Med Soc* 1978; **79**: 198.

58. Shields JL, Jansen GT. Therapy for superficial telangiectasias of the lower extremities. *J Dermatol Surg Oncol* 1982; **8**: 857.

59. Thibault PK. Sclerotherapy of varicose veins and telangiectasias: a 2-year experience with sodium tetradecyl sulfate. *Aust NZ J Phlebol* 1999; **3**: 25–30.

60. Fegan WG, Pegum JM. Accidental intra-arterial injection during sclerotherapy of varicose veins. *Br J Surg* 1974; **61**: 124–6.

61. Yamaki T, Nozaki M, Sasaki K. Acute massive pulmonary embolism following high ligation combined with compression sclerotherapy for varicose veins report of a case. *Dermatol Surg* 1999; **25**: 321–5.

62. McMaster P, Everett WG. Fatal pulmonary embolism following compression sclerotherapy for varicose veins. *Postgrad Med J* 1973; **49**: 517–8.

63. Dwerryhouse S, Davies B, Harradine K, Earnshaw JJ. Stripping the long saphenous vein reduces the rate of reoperation for recurrent varicose veins: five-year results of a randomized trial. *J Vasc Surg* 1999; **29**: 589–92.

64. Bishop CC, Fronek HS, Fronek A et al. Real-time color duplex scanning after sclerotherapy of the greater saphenous vein. *J Vasc Surg* 1991; **14**: 505–8.

65. Kanter A, Thibault P. Saphenofemoral incompetence treated by ultrasound-guided sclerotherapy. *Dermatol Surg* 1996; **22**: 648–52.

66. Tessari L, Cavezzi A, Frullini A. Preliminary experience with a new sclerosing foam in the treatment of varicose veins. *Dermatol Surg* 2001; **27**: 58–60.

67. Bohler K, Baldt M, Schuller-Petrovic S et al. Varicose vein stripping – a prospective study of the thrombotic risk and the diagnostic significance of preoperative color coded duplex sonography. *Thromb Haemost* 1995; **73**: 597–600.

19

Echosclerotherapy for the management of saphenous reflux

KENNETH MYERS, AMY CLOUGH, JAYNE CHAMBERS, MICHELE RODEH

INTRODUCTION

Many patients with complications from venous disease including leg ulcers have underlying predominant superficial reflux rather than deep venous disease.[1–3] Accordingly, treatment for leg ulceration may include control of superficial saphenous reflux. Traditionally, this has been by surgical ligation and stripping, with varying attitudes towards treating calf perforators. In recent years, an alternative treatment has been ultrasound-guided echosclerotherapy. This chapter explores possible indications, techniques and medium-term outcome for this technique illustrated by a personal experience of 308 patients followed by ultrasound surveillance.

Patients with ulceration are frequently older and less favourable candidates for an operation under general anesthesia. Many have already had surgery and are unlikely to be enthusiastic about another operation. The condition of the skin in the leg frequently makes any below-knee surgery prone to wound breakdown. If there is active ulceration, then surgery at any level carries an increased risk of infection. For these reasons, non-operative alternatives are highly attractive, provided that they are effective. This is particularly so if control of the refluxing vein can be performed early even when the ulcer is still present, rather than waiting for it to heal prior to an operation.

Sclerotherapy has been practiced for at least 100 years.[4–6] In a landmark study, Hobbs[5] showed that conventional sclerotherapy was inferior to surgery for truncal saphenous reflux, including reflux at the saphenofemoral junction. Clearly, pruning the branches is inadequate and long-term control relies on destroying the saphenous trunk. Ultrasound-guided echosclerotherapy was introduced to permanently obliterate the saphenous veins.[7]

The technique uses ultrasound to guide the needle to the vein and to follow passage of sclerosant. Many now consider that it is the preferred option for treating varicose veins. Early reports suggest that success rates compare favourably with those for surgery.[3,8–13] The outcome appears to have been improved by techniques to prepare the sclerosant as a foam, first introduced by Cabrera et al. in Spain.[10,11]

SELECTION OF SUITABLE PATIENTS

Older patients are well suited to this type of treatment rather than surgery, particularly if they have cardiovascular or other systemic disease. Accordingly, it is highly suited to patients with venous ulceration.

Contraindications to echosclerotherapy include pregnancy, past deep vein thrombosis or thrombophilia. Associated lower limb arterial disease is not necessarily a contraindication, although severe arterial disease is always treated first. We have little concern about losing the vein from subsequent echosclerotherapy since varicose veins have been shown to have poor patency rates when used as arterial bypass grafts.[14]

PREOPERATIVE CLINICAL ASSESSMENT

The first consultation involves taking a full medical history and performing clinical examination of the venous system to establish the severity and general nature of the problem. A history is taken for heart disease or other circulatory disorders, risk factors for arterial disease, and bleeding or clotting disorders. A history of severe allergic disorders or asthma may influence the choice of sclerosant. The oral contraceptive pill or hormone replacement therapy should be stopped for a time before treatment if this is thought to put the patient at greatly increased risk of venous thrombosis. We do not consider that warfarin or aspirin therapy needs to be stopped. The clinical examination attempts to determine which saphenous system or perforator veins are responsible for the varices and to localize the complications of lipodermatosclerosis or past or present ulceration.

Clinical assessment alone is insufficient to plan treatment and all patients require a precise diagnosis obtained from a venous duplex ultrasound scan. We no longer use the hand-held continuous-wave Doppler unit to evaluate the pathology. Reticence to rely on clinical judgment and the hand-held Doppler has been supported by studies from Mercer *et al.*[15] and Wills *et al.*[16] who found that combined clinical and continuous-wave Doppler assessment misses 25–30 percent of communications between deep and superficial veins when compared with duplex ultrasound.

The second consultation involves detailed discussion of the findings from the scan and the proposed treatment. If echosclerotherapy is advised then the limbs are measured to be fitted with a pair of class 2 compression stockings. The patient is advised not to apply moisturizer to the legs on the day of treatment, and to wear slacks or loose trousers and sandals or loose shoes to allow for the thickness of the bandages.

As well as discussion, each patient is given a pamphlet that details the anatomy, physiology, pathology, results and potential complications in lay terms. For medicolegal reasons, patients are required to sign a consent form for treatment that states that they have read the pamphlet. Whether this is sufficient in law has yet to be tested by the authors.

PREOPERATIVE VENOUS DUPLEX ULTRASOUND EXAMINATION

The scan is of use only if performed by a skilled vascular sonographer who thoroughly understands the requirements after considerable experience of working with the sclerotherapist. We use an ATL HDI3000 or HDI5000 duplex ultrasound scanner (Philips Medical Systems, Andover, MA, USA). Scanning is performed with the patient standing or on a tilt table supported with weight taken on the opposite limb. We routinely examine for reflux or obstruction at both saphenous junctions and in superficial veins, deep axial veins from the ankle to the groin, and thigh and calf perforators. All sources

of reflux from deep to superficial veins are recorded. Reflux is defined as reverse flow for more than 1 s after release of a calf squeeze or during the Valsalva maneuver, although most incompetent valves allowed reflux for 3 s or more. Diameters are measured at incompetent saphenous junctions and at representative sites along refluxing saphenous veins. Whether or not the saphenopopliteal junction is present is recorded and the level of the junction relative to the knee crease is noted if it is present. Outward flow through calf or thigh perforators with a calf squeeze or isometric calf contraction is noted, diameters of refluxing perforators are measured at the level of the deep fascia, and their levels are noted relative to the malleoli for the calf and the knee crease for the thigh.

PREPARATION AND ACTION OF FOAMED SCLEROSANTS

Sclerosants act to denude vein endothelium promoting thrombosis, and subsequent compression reduces the volume of thrombus to allow subsequent fibrosis to obliterate the lumen. Initially, sclerosants for echosclerotherapy were injected as a liquid but this has various constraints. Only a limited fluid volume can be administered to stay within the toxic dose limit and this volume is frequently inadequate to fill the veins. Fluid sclerosant stays in contact with the endothelium for a very short time before flowing away. The fluid sclerosant mixes with blood, leading to the possibility of considerable thrombus in the veins.

These problems are greatly reduced by techniques to convert the sclerosant into foam. Foam largely displaces blood from the lumen and immediately causes the vein to spasm so that less thrombosis develops. Foam does not flow as a liquid sclerosant would so that it stays in contact with the vein wall for a prolonged period, shown by ultrasound for up to 30 min after injection. This allows the sclerosant to be diluted since it will be acting for much longer so that a smaller total volume of sclerosant is used. Diluted sclerosant is far less likely to cause local tissue damage. Finally, foam is easy to see on ultrasound since it is highly echogenic, allowing precise placement of an appropriate volume.

Sclerosants readily make foam, as they are detergents. Cabrera *et al.*[10,11] have developed a technique to stabilize the foam but this has not yet become available commercially. We use a modification of an Italian technique to prepare foam.[13,17] We now combine diluted sodium tetradecyl sulfate (STS) with air. Foam is produced with two 5 mL syringes connected by a three-way tap, one containing 2 mL of diluted sclerosant and the other containing 3 mL of air, and these are vigorously syringed from one to the other some five to 10 times. A filter is inserted on the air syringe to remove particulate matter. The fluid aliquot is usually made by diluting 4 mL of 3 percent STS with 4 mL of normal saline to produce a 1.5 percent solution to provide a total available volume of 20 mL of foam. If there is a history of past allergies or asthma then 3 percent ethoxysclerol (aetherosclerol) is used because of a probable decreased risk of an anaphylactic reaction. The volumes that we use are higher than used by many other sclerotherapists but comparable with that used by Cabrera *et al.,*[11] and we have not observed any significant pulmonary, visual or cerebral effects in this series.

Foam consists of microbubbles that are 0.1–0.5 mm in diameter. Foam characteristics are not dependent on the sclerosant chosen. A considerable part of foam will become liquid again within a few minutes so that injection should be made promptly after it is foamed. Foaming is prolonged by bringing the sclerosant to blood temperature or at least to room temperature, as well as by the vigor and number of passages between syringes.

TECHNIQUES FOR INJECTIONS

The procedure is performed by the sclerotherapist with a sonographer and nurse present as well. However, many skilled sclerotherapists make the procedure more simple and cost-effective by operating the ultrasound probe as well as making up foam without assistance.

There has been past debate as to whether to commence serial injections from proximal to distal or vice versa. The present techniques make this irrelevant since the principle now is to simply fill up the full length of the affected saphenous vein and its tributaries.

This can be achieved by injecting the saphenous vein directly or injecting superficial tributaries. Whichever technique is selected, a tilt table is used with a reverse Trendelenburg position to approximately 30°. This makes it more simple to puncture the vein and it also keeps foam distally within superficial veins until injection is completed. When sclerotherapy is complete, foam causes such intense spasm that the vein does not fill with blood in the treated segments, even when placed in a dependent position. The sonographer flattens the table and compresses the saphenous junction when it is confirmed that the superficial veins have been filled. Otherwise, foam can be seen to dribble through the junction for a short time, but it is only necessary to occlude its outflow for 2–3 min before foam becomes adherent and sequestrated. Care is taken to avoid extravasation because it will cause appreciable pain that lasts for approximately 1 hour. However, diluted foam does not appear to cause tissue damage, and extravasation ulceration has not been observed in the present series. On completing the injections, we apply a three-layer compression bandage as we are convinced that this gives better compression than a stocking, at least for the crucial first 24 hours. This is often part of ongoing treatment for complications of active eczema or ulceration.

It is usual policy to inject only one leg at a time. Injecting both legs could mean that too much foam is given at one time, there is more inconvenience from having both legs bandaged rather than one, and inevitable discomfort from injections is magnified if it involves both legs. If both legs require treatment, then the options are to alternate echosclerotherapy from leg to leg at weekly intervals or to complete treatment for one limb before commencing treatment for the other.

We use one or more of several techniques, as described below.

Saphenous puncture under ultrasound guidance

This is usually reserved for limbs with saphenous reflux without prominent superficial varices. We inject as far distal to the saphenous junction as possible where the diameter is still sufficient for the vein to be easily punctured. Foam predominantly passes proximally from the puncture site.

Our preference is to hold the probe to show the vein in the longitudinal view to guide the needle, for this shows a length of foam in the vein as it is injected. The sonographer must hold the probe exactly perpendicular to the skin and the sclerotherapist must place the needle exactly in the midline of the probe axis to guide the needle (Fig. 19.1). An alternative approach that we occasionally use is to hold the probe to show the vein in transverse section and approach with the needle from one or other side. The advantage is that the probe can be shifted up or down to bring the needle into view if it has not been placed correctly, but it does not show any length of the vein.

A 1.5-inch long 25-gauge needle is used to allow a sufficient length to be viewed on the screen. The 25-gauge needle is easily seen with B-mode using modern ultrasound machines (Fig. 19.2). In general, the deeper the vein, the more distance there is to view and guide the needle, but it can be difficult to reach the vein in an obese thigh. A 5 mL syringe containing foamed sclerosant is connected to the needle and blood is aspirated to confirm the needle is in the lumen. Foam is injected slowly and the screen is watched carefully to confirm it is flowing along the

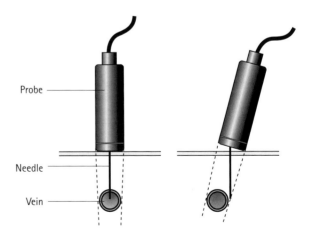

Figure 19.1 *The probe is held vertical and the needle placed in the midline of the probe to give a clear view (left). Otherwise, there is parallax and the needle passes across the beam, making it difficult to see its tip (right).*

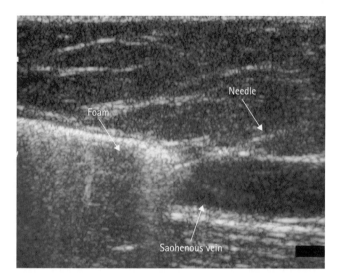

Figure 19.2 *The B-mode appearance in the longitudinal view showing a great saphenous vein, the needle with the tip in the lumen, and foam being injected to pass proximally.*

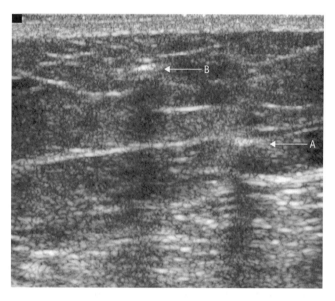

Figure 19.3 *The B-mode appearance in a transverse view of foam in the great saphenous vein deep to its characteristic layer of fascia (A) and tributaries superficial to the fascia (B).*

vein, and injection is immediately stopped if extravasation is seen. The injection causes turbulence which probably further helps to displace blood rather than mixing with it (Fig. 19.2).

Once 5 mL has been injected, the sonographer scans to see whether foam has reached the saphenous junction. If not, it is gently massaged up along the vein until it appears at the saphenous junction. If it does not fill the vein, a further injection is made just above the upper limit, although this can be more difficult due to venous spasm. It is unusual to require more than 10 mL of foam. The sonographer then gently occludes the junction with the probe to prevent foam from entering the deep veins. If foam is observed in deep veins, the patient is told to exercise the calf muscles and the sclerotherapist massages the limb to promote deep flow. With this regime, we have not yet encountered any occlusive deep venous thrombosis above the level of the tibial veins. With the junction occluded, it is then easy to massage foam back down the saphenous vein and its tributaries unless they contain competent valves.

Injection through tributaries without ultrasound guidance of the needle

We favour this technique if the limb has large tributaries as it is simpler and just as effective. A strategic vein is chosen that appears to have the best chance of leading to the saphenous vein and other tributaries. The sonographer does not need to show the tributary at the time of injection but is required to follow foam to confirm it is passing in the desired direction. If not, the sonographer can direct flow of sclerosant by compressing other veins. When the saphenous vein is filled, the point of connection of the tributary to the saphenous vein is compressed to direct flow into other varicosities. Large thigh and calf perforators are compressed by the probe or by a finger, whether they are incompetent or not. The sonographer then

follows the saphenous and superficial veins along the limb in transverse section to confirm they contain foam (Fig. 19.3). It may be necessary to inject up to 20 mL of foam in limbs with large varicose veins.

There is a perception that tributaries belong to either the great or small saphenous circulations, but experience with injecting foam shows that it frequently passes from one system to the other, often in an unpredictable manner. The direction that foam takes is frequently different from the path of reflux shown by the preoperative duplex scan. Injecting great saphenous tributaries to control great saphenous reflux frequently fills the small saphenous vein as well, even though it was not showing reflux. It is common to fill most veins through one injection site and rarely necessary to inject more than three or four sites. If filling is incomplete, it is best to reschedule the patient to complete the process a week later.

A 23-gauge butterfly needle is preferred to puncture the tributary. Once there is reflux in the needle, a 5 mL syringe containing foam is attached. For a right-handed operator, the left hand steadies the needle using the thumb and index finger to hold the hub and syringe, the middle finger to steady the wings on the skin, and the ring and little fingers placed gently on the vein beyond the needle to feel that there is no extravasation. If this is detected, injection is immediately stopped, the needle is removed and a new butterfly needle is used to puncture at a different site.

Injection into tributaries with ultrasound guidance

It may be necessary to inject a superficial tributary that is not clearly visible. The most common reason is to obliterate superficial tributaries draining from one or more incompetent perforators in limbs with complications. Our policy is to attempt to prevent foamed sclerosant entering a perforator because of concern that it might cause adjacent deep vein thrombosis. A site is chosen to inject the tributary as far distal to the perforator as possible. A shorter 3/4-inch, 25-gauge needle may be preferred. The probe is used to guide the needle and this is the most difficult procedure performed since there is very little room at the corner of the ultrasound field to see the needle and determine the angle to place it in the lumen. However, once aspiration is confirmed, 5 mL of foam is injected very slowly and with minimal pressure. The probe is then shifted to the perforator site, injection is stopped as soon as foam is seen at its superficial end, and digital compression is applied for 2–3 min. The procedure may need to be repeated for a tributary proximal to the perforator.

Catheter–directed echosclerotherapy

For limbs with large-diameter saphenous veins >5–6 mm, we favour control by endovenous laser therapy (EVLT) or radiofrequency ablation (VNUS closure). These ensure that the entire length from the saphenous junction to the puncture site is destroyed. We advise against the above techniques for echosclerotherapy for large veins because of concern that they are likely to fail and because of the volume of foam required. However, financial and other considerations may lead the patient to reject EVLT or VNUS closure, and in these cases we offer catheter-directed echosclerotherapy.

A point is chosen towards the distal end of the refluxing saphenous vein. Holding the probe in the longitudinal view, 1 mL of 1 percent plain xylocaine is injected along the center of its axis and a 1 mm longitudinal puncture is made and slightly dilated. A 19-gauge angiogaphy needle punctures the vein and an empty attached 5 mL syringe confirms aspiration of blood. The syringe is removed and a standard 0.035-inch-diameter safety-J guide wire is inserted and followed by ultrasound to the saphenous junction (Fig. 19.4). The needle is removed and a 5F Van Andel or Hinck catheter is passed over the wire to the junction. The wire is removed, the saphenous junction is compressed by the sonographer, and 10 mL of 1.5 percent foamed sclerosant is slowly infused as the catheter is withdrawn.

Variations of this catheter technique have been well described by Grondin and Soriano[8] and by Min and Navarro[9].

Other techniques

Many sclerotherapists are not yet ready to accept the technique using foam, probably out of concern that it might be causing an increased incidence of macroscopic or microscopic thromboembolism. The conventional technique requires multiple injections of more concentrated sclerosant but this is not a major drawback. Alternative approaches have been described, such as sclerotherapy through an angioscope.[18] Others have combined flush saphenous ligation with sclerotherapy[19] and

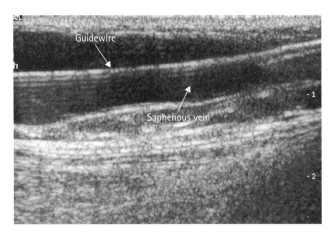

Figure 19.4   *The B-mode appearance in a longitudinal view of the great saphenous vein with a guidewire in place prior to catheter echosclerotherapy.*

we have no reason to dispute this approach, although we consider that it is unnecessary, while we would strongly advise a few days' delay between the two procedures because of concern about injecting sclerosants with the patient anaesthetized.

SELECTION OF THE VEINS TO BE TREATED

Any vein of any size can be treated by echosclerotherapy. There is a suggestion that results worsen for increasing vein diameters[20] and we favour alternative endovenous techniques for veins with diameter >5–6 mm, although this has not discouraged other proponents of the technique.[10,11]

Whichever system is involved, tributaries are marked out with an indelible pen so that they can be checked by the sonographer to confirm that all have been filled with foam. If it is chosen to inject the saphenous vein, the puncture site is marked distinctively. Calf and thigh perforators are similarly marked distinctively.

The great saphenous vein

This is the vein most often treated. Our experience with duplex scanning is that most have reflux from saphenofemoral incompetence, but that one-third of females and 20 percent of males have reflux from pelvic or abdominal veins with a competent saphenofemoral junction.[2,3] However, we treat both variations with the same technique. Using direct saphenous puncture, injection is commenced from the lowest level that shows reflux from the preoperative scan.

A frequent variant well suited to echosclerotherapy is reflux in thigh tributaries from saphenofemoral incompetence without great saphenous reflux, and these are treated by tributary injection without injecting the saphenous vein. For patients with both thigh tributaries from the saphenofemoral junction and great saphenous reflux, it is usually necessary to use both saphenous and tributary injections. For saphenous reflux with varices from more distal tributaries, injection is directly into the tributary in the hope that this will fill up the great saphenous vein as well.

The small saphenous vein

The small saphenous vein is ideally suited to echosclerotherapy. Indeed, it may well be more effective than surgery, as many surgeons simply ligate the vein, flush and excise a short segment without stripping, owing to concern about damage to adjacent nerves, and this leads to a high rate of recurrence.[22]

Our experience with duplex scanning is that one-third of saphenopopliteal junctions lie higher up than the conventional 3–4 cm above the knee skin crease. One-quarter of limbs do not have a saphenopopliteal junction with the small saphenous continuing up as the vein of Giacomini to end in the great saphenous, deep veins or pelvic veins.[2,3] These variations are noted from the preoperative scan, and the level of the junction is marked if present. The small saphenous is almost always treated by saphenous injection, although superficial tributaries occasionally need to be injected.

Calf perforators

There are varying views about using echosclerotherapy to control refluxing calf perforators. Some sclerotherapists deliberately place the needle into the perforator to obtain precise sclerosis, but we are concerned that this could carry a higher risk of regional deep vein thrombosis. Accordingly, we aim to control superficial varices draining from the perforator compressing the perforator itself to prevent foam entering the deep system.

POSTOPERATIVE MANAGEMENT AND EARLY REVIEW

Patients are rested for 10–15 min after the bandages are applied to allow foamed sclerosant to continue to act on the wall. They are then told to walk gently for 10–15 min before returning to make the follow-up appointment. It is recommended that they be driven home with the leg elevated. They are asked to walk regularly over the next few days but to avoid excessive exercise, even though there is no evidence that these influence the outcome. If walking is difficult due to age or the local condition in the leg, the patient is instructed regarding foot and calf exercises to improve calf muscle pumping.

By 48 hours, patients can remove the bandages and apply the class 2 compression stockings for 2–3 weeks depending on the size of the varices. Stockings are worn through the day, removed at night and replaced in the morning after a shower.

The first review is at 3–5 days when a duplex scan checks that the full length of the saphenous vein and tributaries have been obliterated. If the proximal vein is not occluded, it is reinjected with 5 mL of 1.5 percent foam even if it is not refluxing. Similarly, if occlusion extends the full length but is

only partial then injection is repeated, although it can be difficult to find the lumen and it is important to inject very slowly to prevent distension and pain. Further varicosities are injected with 0.6 percent foam. Repeat injection was required a second time in 20 percent of our patients and a third time in 5 percent. The limb is examined for superficial lumps that are pricked with a 21-gauge needle to release 'trapped blood'.

Patients are told verbally and in the pamphlet that the following features are expected and do not need to be reported prior to the first visit:

- mild pain with tender lumps usually improved by walking and mild analgesics
- discoloration over surface veins that will fade within 4–8 weeks
- mild phlebitis that occurs in about 20 percent and is treated by compression.

LATE SURVEILLANCE

Whatever treatment is used, recurrence rates for veins in the treated region or new veins are very high.[21] Because of this, we now consider that patients require ongoing surveillance. We review all patients at 6 weeks, 6 months, 1 year and then annually. At each visit, patient satisfaction is noted, the legs are examined for minor or major recurrences, and a duplex scan of the treated limb is performed. There is a dilemma as to what to do if the duplex scan shows recurrence without evidence to the patient or doctor that varicose veins have reappeared. The usual policy is to advise the patient that more varicosities are likely to develop, that no further treatment is required for the present, but that the patient should return before the next scheduled visit if varicosities appear, or be prepared for more injections at the next annual visit. Patients are almost universally grateful that an aggressive attitude towards ongoing treatment is recommended, as most are aware of the problems of large neglected recurrent veins from the experience of family or friends who are reluctant to return for repeat surgery.

RESULTS OF TREATMENT

A personal series of 308 patients treated by echosclerotherapy over the past 4 years is described. Both limbs were injected in 104 patients (34 percent) so that 412 limbs were treated. Both saphenous veins were treated in the same limb in 55 limbs (13 percent) so that 467 veins can be analysed for follow-up. It was elected to repeat treatment for 73 veins so that a total of 540 procedures were performed. Details relating to patient and treatment characteristics are shown in Table 19.1.

Medium–term success rates

Success is considered to be absence of reflux in the treated vein from the duplex scan. In most limbs considered to be failures by this definition, the severity and extent of reflux

Table 19.1 *Characteristics for patients treated by echosclerotherapy*

Characteristic	Number	Percent
Sex		
Male	64	21
Female	244	79
Limbs		
Right	198	48
Left	214	52
CEAP (clinical)[a]		
C2–3	366	89
C4–6	46	11
Vein treated		
Great saphenous	296	63
Small saphenous	102	22
Major tributaries	69	15
Technique for injection		
Saphenous	312	58
Tributary	218	40
Catheter	10	2

[a] CEAP, see Box 6.1, page 46.

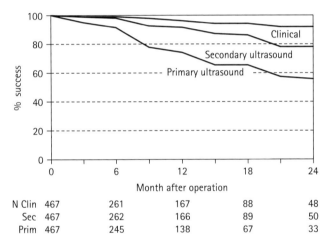

Figure 19.5 *Life-table analysis for success rates after echosclerotherapy.*

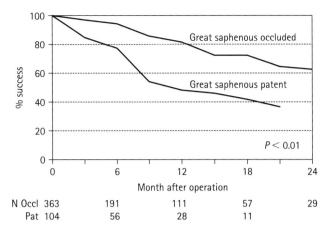

Figure 19.6 *Life-table analysis for primary success rates after echosclerotherapy according to whether the first postoperative scan at 1 week showed that the proximal vein was patent or occluded.*

were considerably less than before treatment, but any degree of recurrent reflux into the treated vein is defined as failure. Non-saphenous recurrence in patients treated for saphenous reflux is not considered to be a failure for the technique although the details will be analysed.

Results are presented using life-table analysis (Fig. 19.5). Although many patients were referred from considerable distances away, there are only 52 patients (17 percent) who have been lost to follow-up at varying times over the 4-year period. The primary ultrasound success rate is a modest 56 percent at 2 years. Recurrence appears to be at a steady rate through this time with no reason to believe that it will slow in the future. However, after allowing for patients who were treated by further repeat echosclerotherapy, the secondary ultrasound success rate improves to 78 percent at 2 years. Most but

not all who were treated again had signs of early recurrent varicose veins. Patients are warned that the technique may well have to be repeated at intervals and this is well accepted. The resultant clinical success rate without evidence of anything more than reticular veins or telangiectases is greater than 90 percent at 2 years.

Multivariate and univariate analysis of covariates

Cox regression multivariate analysis was performed for clinical features as well as technical aspects and none were shown to influence medium-term results. There were insufficient veins >8 mm diameter to evaluate the effect of vein size properly. Not included in the multivariate analysis was the state of the vein at the first visit after treatment. However, univariate life-table analysis showed a significantly worse result if the proximal segment of the saphenous vein was patent rather than occluded to the saphenous junction (Fig. 19.6). It is for this reason that we are now aggressive towards reinjecting the top end if required until it is occluded.

Sites of recurrence

Conventional surgical wisdom is that it is essential to ligate all tributaries in the vicinity of either saphenous junction. Conversely, followers of the CHIVA technique consider that it is important to preserve low pelvic or abdominal veins that drain to the saphenofemoral junction, arguing that this is physiological whereas their ligation forces drainage to veins in the thigh to increase the risk of recurrence.[22] With echosclerotherapy, just as for EVLT or VNUS closure, pelvic and abdominal tributaries are not sclerosed or occluded and this is a drawback or advantage according to which school the surgeon belongs.

This is analysed according to sites of recurrence for the failures. For saphenous recurrence after treating great saphenous

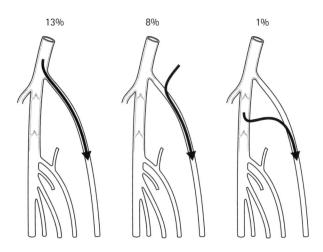

Figure 19.7 *Sites of saphenous recurrence after treatment for great saphenous reflux.*

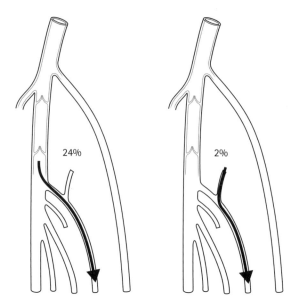

Figure 19.9 *Sites of saphenous recurrence after treatment for small saphenous reflux.*

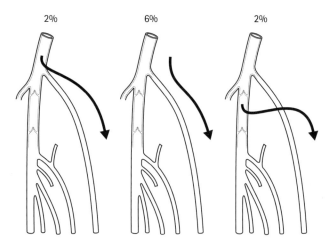

Figure 19.8 *Sites of non-saphenous recurrence after treatment for great saphenous reflux.*

reflux, almost two-thirds were due to recanalization in the great saphenous vein, while approximately one-third were due to recurrences from pelvic or abdominal veins (Fig. 19.7). On the other hand, more than half of non-saphenous recurrences to thigh tributaries arise from pelvic or abdominal veins (Fig. 19.8). A study of tributaries at the saphenofemoral junction after VNUS closure shows similar results.[23] We have previously shown that recurrence after great saphenous surgery most frequently comes from pelvic or abdominal veins, to either the long saphenous or major tributaries.[24] Most recurrences after small saphenous echosclerotherapy were from recanalization of the vein (Fig. 19.9).

COMPLICATIONS

Patients are advised both verbally and in the pamphlet that the following complications can occur:

Allergic reaction is rare with diluted foam. It can present immediately as an anaphylactic reaction or as a delayed allergic skin reaction. In the present series, we encountered one mild case of anaphylaxis that rapidly responded to treatment with intravenous hydrocortisone. Both cortisone and adrenaline are held available for treatment.

Severe thrombophlebitis is difficult to define but has occurred in less than 10 percent since the introduction of the foam technique in the present study. The severe spasm that occurs after injecting foam is considered to reduce thrombosis and thrombophlebitis.

Pigmentation along the treated veins can take up to 12 months to fade, with permanent staining of cosmetic significance in less than 5 percent in this series. Persistent pigmentation has been effectively managed by laser treatment in some.

Skin ulceration is rare with diluted foam and has not been observed in this series. Most injection ulcers encountered in the past with conventional sclerotherapy were small and healed over a few weeks, leaving a small pale scar.

Deep vein thrombosis. For the 540 procedures performed in this series, the 1-week follow-up scan revealed a short length of thrombus in the posterior tibial vein in five limbs (0.9 percent) and in the gastrocnemius veins in six limbs treated for small saphenous reflux (1.1 percent). In each case, treatment was with therapeutic doses of low-molecular-weight heparin once daily with compression as an outpatient. None progressed with weekly duplex scan review and each recanalized within 2–3 weeks so that treatment was then ceased. No major deep vein thrombosis at a more proximal level has occurred. The frequency of deep vein thrombosis after stripping varicose veins is not known.

Intra-arterial injection. This is a rare complication that has not occurred with treatment by any experienced sclerotherapist in Australia to the best of our knowledge. Opponents of echosclerotherapy have frequently quoted inadvertent injection into a major artery as a reason to avoid the technique. In practice, any competent sclerotherapist working with a competent sonographer and using high-quality B-mode ultrasound systems has about as much chance of making this mistake as the surgeon has of inadvertently stripping the superficial femoral artery. For the beginner (who should always perform the first 20 cases or more under supervision), some reassurance may be gained by using color from the duplex scanner to confirm venous rather than arterial flow in the selected vessel. However, the experienced team rarely turn on the color and rely on good-quality B-mode. Inadvertent arterial injection could be more likely using continuous-wave Doppler blindly for guidance, a practice to be deplored. Injecting an artery adjacent to an incompetent perforator might be more likely if the intention is to inject the perforator itself, but we avoid this technique.

OTHER REPORTS

Kanter and Thibault[12] used ultrasound surveillance to show excellent medium-term results after non-foamed echosclerotherapy with no serious complications. They considered that most recurrences occurred early in the first year, usually from recanalization into the great saphenous vein. In a multivariate analysis, Kanter[20] found that vein diameter was the only influence that adversely affected outcome, although he did not consider that this was a contraindication to the technique. In a large series of 500 patients using the catheter technique, Grondin and Soriano[8] found good long-term success and recorded post-injection pain in 20 percent, superficial thrombophlebitis in 6 percent, and no cases of deep vein thrombosis, pulmonary embolism, extravasation ulceration or intra-arterial injection.

Italian workers have reported an 88 percent initial success rate for foamed echosclerotherapy in 170 patients with moderate- to large-diameter veins.[13,17] Cabrera et al.[10,11] reported results for treating 300 great saphenous veins by foamed echosclerotherapy, all with vein diameters >9 mm at the saphenofemoral junctions, and all assessed at 3 years with duplex ultrasound. Absolute success shown by duplex scanning was 81 percent at 3 years and there were no serious complications.

There have been few studies of recurrence rates after surgery defined by ultrasound. We reported virtually identical results for echosclerotherapy, surgery and VNUS closure assessed by ultrasound, although the selection criteria for the three groups were different.[3]

CONCLUSIONS

Hobb's[5] unique randomized study which showed that conventional sclerotherapy was unsatisfactory for limbs with saphenous reflux may or may not be relevant to newer techniques with foamed echosclerotherapy. The case to show that echosclerotherapy gives significantly better results than conventional sclerotherapy has yet to be proven. Similarly, it has yet to be proven that foamed echosclerotherapy gives better results than using liquid sclerosant.

The many reported clinical studies after surgery will show a far lower recurrence rate than for objective studies with duplex ultrasound. Presumably, ultrasound recurrence will eventually be followed by clinical recurrence, but the interval between the two has yet to be established. It may well be that the recurrence rate after echosclerotherapy is higher than after surgery, but it can be argued that this simply means a more frequent need for repeat echosclerotherapy, at an early stage if the patient complies with surveillance.

Accordingly, our results, which are similar to other reports, encourage us to consider that echosclerotherapy with foam, repeated at times if necessary, is highly effective and particularly applicable to the control of superficial venous disease in patients with leg ulcers.

REFERENCES

1. Myers KA, Ziegenbein RW, Zeng GH, Matthews PG. Duplex ultrasonography scanning for chronic venous disease: patterns of venous reflux. *J Vasc Surg* 1995; **21**: 605–12.
2. Myers KA. Duplex ultrasound exploration for diagnosis and evaluation of chronic venous diseases. *Arteres Veins* 1997; **16**: 190–204.
3. Myers KA, Wood S, Lee V, Koh P. Variations of connections to the saphenous systemsin limbs with primary varicose veins: a study of 1481 limbs by duplex ultrasound scanning. *J Phlebol* 2002; **2**: 11–7.
4. Thornhill R. Varicose veins and their treatment by 'empty veins' injection. London: Baillière, Tindall and Cox, 1929.
5. Hobbs JT. Surgery and sclerotherapy in the treatment of varicose veins. A random trial. *Arch Surg* 1974; **109**: 793–6.
6. Fegan WG. Continuous compression technique of injecting varicose veins. *Lancet* 1963; **ii**: 109–12.
7. Knight RM. Treatment of superficial venous disease with accurate sclerotherapy. *Proceedings of the Canadian Society of Phlebology.* Whistler, British Columbia, Canada. 1991.
8. Grondin L, Soriano J. Echosclerotherapy, a Canadian study. In: Raymond-Martimbeau P, Prescott R, Zummo M, eds. *Phlébologie '92,* Paris: John Libbey Eurotext, 1992.
9. Min RJ, Navarro L. Transcatheter duplex ultrasound-guided sclerotherapy for treatment of greater saphenous vein reflux: preliminary report. *Dermatol Surg* 2000; **26**: 410–4.
10. Cabrera J, Cabrera J Jr, Garcia-Olmedo MA. Sclerosants in microfoam. A new approach in angiology. *Int Angiol* 2001; **20**: 322–9.
11. Cabrera J, Cabrera J Jr, Garcia-Olmedo MA. Treatment of varicose long saphenous veins with sclerosant in microfoam form: long-term outcomes. *Phlebology* 2000; **15**: 19–23.
12. Kanter A, Thibault P. Saphenofemoral incompetence treated by ultrasound-guided sclerotherapy. *Dermatol Surg* 1996; **22**: 648–52.
13. Frullini A, Cavezzi A. Sclerosing foam in the treatment of varicose veins and telangiectases: history and analysis of safety and complications. *Dermatol Surg* 2002; **28**: 11–5.

14. Davies AH. Vein factors that affect the outcome of femorodistal bypass. *Ann R Coll Surg Engl* 1995; **77**: 63–6.

15. Mercer KG, Scott DJ, Berridge DC. Preoperative duplex imaging is required before all operations for primary varicose veins. *Br J Surg* 1998; **85**: 1495–7.

16. Wills V, Moylan D, Chambers J. The use of routine duplex scanning in the assessment of varicose veins. *Aust NZ J Surg* 1998; **68**: 41–4.

17. Tessari L, Cavezzi A, Frullini A. Preliminary experience with a new sclerosing foam in the treatment of varicose veins. *Dermatol Surg* 2001; **27**: 58–60.

18. Van Cleef JF, Desvaux P, Griton P, Cloarec M. Sclerose de la saphene externe sous controle endoscopique. *Phlebologie* 1991; **44**: 131.

19. Vin F, Chlier F, Allaert FA. Sclerotherapy section of incompetent short saphenous veins: indications, techniques, results. *Ann Chir* 1997; **51**: 773–9.

20. Kanter A. Clinical determinants of ultrasound-guided sclerotherapy outcome. Part I. The effects of age, gender, and vein size. *Dermatol Surg* 1998; **24**: 131–5.

21. Perrin MR, Guex JJ, Ruckley CV *et al.* Recurrent varices after surgery (REVAS), a consensus document. REVAS group. *Cardiovasc Surg* 2000; **8**: 233–45.

22. Zamboni P, Marcellino MG, Cappelli M *et al.* Saphenous vein sparing surgery: principles, techniques and results. *J Cardiovasc Surg* 1998; **39**: 151–62.

23. Chandler JG, Pichot O, Sessa C *et al.* Defining the role of extended saphenofemoral junction ligation: a prospective comparative study. *J Vasc Surg* 2000; **32**: 941–53.

24. Myers KA, Zeng GH, Ziegenbein RW, Matthews PG. Duplex ultrasound scanning for chronic venous disease: recurrent varicose veins in the thigh after surgery to the long saphenous vein. *Phlebology* 1996; **11**: 125–31.

20

The place of deep vein reconstruction: indications, techniques, results

ROBERT L. KISTNER, FEDOR LURIE, BO EKLOF

INTRODUCTION

Deep venous reconstruction, a development of the past 50 years, is a consequence of the evolving appreciation of the pathological processes that affect the veins in the lower limbs. Early contributions of Homans,[1] Linton,[2] Cockett[3] and others were instrumental in focusing attention on the pathological sequelae of thrombophlebitis. Through the imaginative use of venography in the 1940s, Gunnar Bauer[4] in Sweden was able to discern the pathological findings in both primary and secondary deep vein reflux and to separate reflux from obstructive states in the deep veins. He was the first to describe primary deep valve incompetence, which he termed 'idiopathic' incompetence. Physiological studies of venous pressure and of venous volume were widely reported using various techniques, but the most significant development has been the non-invasive use of imaging by ultrasound which has resulted in the sophisticated duplex scan technology available today. The ability to perform a non-invasive study of the entire deep venous system in the lower extremity safely, economically, and painlessly has made it possible to observe the veins *in situ* without disturbing normal flow. The effects produced by venous hemodynamics can now be observed at will in the veins of the erect human in health and disease. This is necessary because there is no satisfactory animal model that can be used to substitute for the human to study venous physiology and pathology.

In 1954,[5,6] an era of development began for new techniques in the treatment of chronic venous insufficiency of the lower extremity and this has continued up to the present time. The first bypass procedure for post-thrombotic obstruction in the iliac vein was reported 1960 with Palma and Esperon's[7]

report. This was followed by experimentation with saphenopopliteal bypass of the femoral vein described by Dale,[8] Husni[9] and Gruss.[10] In the 1970s, new developments focused on deep vein reconstruction for venous reflux. The importance of primary reflux disease was added to the already well appreciated problems of obstruction and reflux secondary to post-thrombotic disease. Deep vein valve reconstruction was first performed for primary reflux in 1968 and the first clinical series was reported in 1975.[11] This was followed by development of the transposition operation[12] and by transplantation of arm vein segments containing competent valves[13] to treat reflux in post-thrombotic disease. Subsequent reports have included variations on these techniques and reports of clinical case series to present the results of treatment of deep vein reflux and obstruction.

CLINICAL BASIS FOR CONSIDERATION OF DEEP VENOUS RECONSTRUCTION

The decision to consider deep vein reconstruction begins with the effect of the venous problem on the life status of the patient. While ulceration and advanced skin changes (CEAP classes C4–6; see Box 6.1, p. 46) are the most dramatic problems that seriously impact the ability to work or maintain a normal lifestyle, there are those whose swelling or pain is so severe that they cannot lead the lifestyle or perform the work they would otherwise choose. The need for reconstruction may be equally as compelling in any of these indications, and the results as good in one as the other. The prime indication for deep venous reconstruction is the presence of lifestyle-limiting sequelae due to chronic venous disease when conventional treatment of superficial and perforator veins has failed.

Treatment always begins with the principles of external compression, elevation, and rest that are universally accepted in chronic venous disease management. These can be invoked without definitive tests and may provide control of the symptoms in all forms of reflux and many cases of obstruction.

When these principles do not control the problem, surgical treatment may be considered. The initial surgical approaches are conventional saphenous vein stripping and perforator interruption, as indicated by objective diagnostic imaging techniques. When surgery is to be done, diagnosis has to be accurate to guide the type and site of the procedure. If patients fail to respond to the combination of conventional surgical and best medical care and are still affected by pain, swelling, or skin changes to a degree that impairs the quality of life, the choice is whether to insist that they change their lifestyle and adapt to the disease, or consider repair of reflux and disobliteration or bypass of the obstructed deep veins. In the latter approach, the attempt is to fit the disease to the individual's lifestyle rather than permitting the disease to dictate lifestyle limitations, and this requires advanced surgical techniques to achieve the desired result.

Since prospective controlled trials comparing different treatments ranging from external compression through definitive surgical repair of affected venous valves or venous segments have not yet been performed, level I evidence is lacking for the validity of deep venous reconstruction. There are several series that present results with the various techniques of deep vein reconstruction.[14–17] These provide a baseline that establishes the ability to perform deep venous surgery, the risks associated with deep repairs, and the expectations of early and long-term results in specific clinical cases.

While comparative trials of surgical versus non-surgical treatment in advanced stages of chronic venous disease (CVD) are yet to be reported in detail, DePalma and Kowallek[18] described an experiment with crossover treatment of 10 complicated venous ulcer cases which showed the relative value of accurate surgical intervention in the deep veins in these cases when compared with conventional non-surgical management by compression. Their report is reinforced in many of the published series of deep vein reconstruction where the reconstructions were limited to recurrent cases of advanced CVD. These showed significant percentages of long-term good results in 'end-stage' venous disease after correcting specific deep vein abnormalities, and have relevance to the case material in DePalma and Kowallek's series. The question is no longer whether successful deep vein reconstruction is feasible but rather when deep vein reconstruction will yield better short- and long-term outcomes than more conventional methods. This important question will require prospective studies of comparable cases.

Classification of chronic venous disease

Now that there are specific methods to correct problems with reflux and different ones to bypass obstruction, and because

valves that are afflicted with primary incompetence can be repaired while those that are destroyed by phlebitis must be corrected by a valve substitution procedure, it is necessary to know specific details about the venous problem in each case before a surgical plan can be chosen. These details include the cause of the clinical problem and its severity; whether it is a result of congenital, primary, or secondary (post-thrombotic) disease; whether it involves the superficial, perforator, or deep veins, or any combination of these; and to know segment-by-segment whether the vein is patent and, if so, whether it is competent. These elements have been collected under the CEAP classification,[19,20] which outlines six **c**linical states, three **e**tiologic conditions (congenital, primary, and secondary), three **a**natomic divisions (superficial, perforator, and deep), and three **p**athophysiologic states (obstruction, reflux, both) that can occur in 18 separate segments of the abdominal and lower extremity veins (Box 6.1, p. 46). The use of this complete system is basic to the understanding of chronic venous states in sufficient detail to permit the choice of appropriate deep reconstruction techniques.

Diagnostic work–up for venous reconstructive surgery

The work-up for deep reconstruction is more complex than for other treatment methods because of the need to determine the sites of reflux and obstruction of the affected limb segment by segment. This amount of information is needed by the surgeon to develop a total picture of the venous abnormalities in the extremity, from which a surgical approach to the individual problems can be designed. The therapeutic aim of the surgeon is to improve the venous return in a measure appropriate to the patient's needs, recognizing that it is seldom possible to restore the venous system to a completely normal state. The demands to be placed on the extremity are different for a 30-year-old labourer and for a man of 60 years, and the choice of surgical procedure may vary accordingly.

The work-up falls logically into three phases as described below.

Phase I: clinical assessment

A complete history and physical examination pertinent to the lower extremity venous system is necessary, including information about prior thromboses in both the patient and the family. The physical examination should include a continuous-wave (CW) Doppler assessment by the physician. In this phase, the clinical importance of the venous problem will be determined and will be the basis upon which decisions are made about the potential need for deep venous reconstruction after the diagnostic work-up is completed.

Phase II: vascular laboratory phase

All patients who are candidates for venous surgery require a duplex scan of the extremity veins in order to establish the accuracy of the CW findings and to check for anatomical variations, sites of obstruction, and severity of reflux. The duplex scan should evaluate for both patency and competence in all venous segments of the extremity. Newer developments in ultrasound image technology have established this as the most important test in chronic venous disease.

Plethysmography and venous pressure studies can be useful for differentiating dominant reflux from dominant obstruction and for quantifying venous reflux. The limitations of these studies are that they lack specificity. Venous pressure is a global test that identifies the venous system to be abnormal but does not differentiate the site or the cause of the problem. Plethysmography is helpful in differentiating reflux from obstruction, and provides a degree of quantification of both, but is not a guide for surgical treatment. The weakest aspect of the venous work-up is that there is no accurate test to assess different degrees of obstruction to the venous return.

Phase III: radiographic (invasive) phase

The place of ascending and descending venography has decreased as the sophistication of duplex scanning has improved, but these are still critical tests for the individual who is being evaluated for reconstructive surgery. The ascending venogram provides the optimal map of the deep veins. It is useful for separating primary from secondary disease, for identifying collateral pathways, and for determining anatomic variations. The descending venogram shows the valve stations in the deep and superficial veins and tests their competence, and continues to be a key source of information in the planning of a reconstructive operation on the deep veins.

The surgical plan

There are multiple surgical procedures available for deep vein reconstruction because a variety of pathological processes occur in several sites in the extremity, each requiring different corrective procedures. The choice of the actual surgical procedure requires a thorough consideration of the pathology present, its location amongst the venous segments, and the requirements that will be placed upon the repaired extremity as a result of the patient's occupation, age range, and other clinical factors. Since a permanent cure of the venous pathology is rarely possible in deep venous disease, the aim of treatment is to provide sufficient functional capacity for the individual's lifestyle for as long as it may be needed.

Pathologically, reflux occurs in both primary and secondary disease while obstruction is limited to secondary disease. There are different operations for obstruction and for reflux, and there are different opportunities for reconstruction of reflux in primary disease and in secondary post-thrombotic disease. The work-up must provide the details of location of the disease and the differentiation of primary from secondary cause. While treatment of pure obstructive problems is the subject of another chapter, any treatment of secondary reflux requires consideration of at least partial obstruction since the essence of secondary disease is a mixture of initial obstruction and subsequent reflux due to the recanalization process.

The algorithm in Fig. 20.1 provides a guide to the surgical choices appropriate for different chronic venous states. The

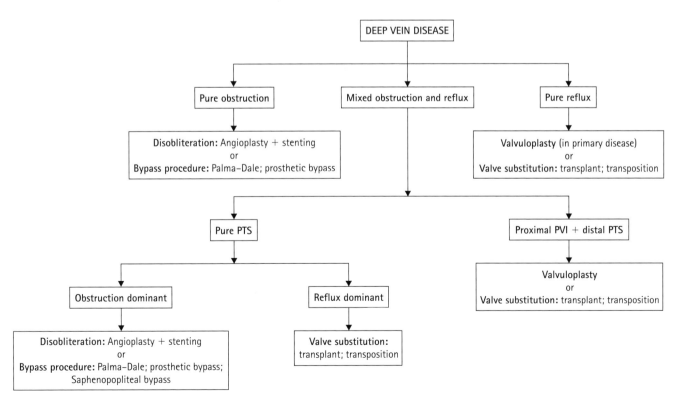

Figure 20.1 *Algorithm for choice of deep venous reconstruction. PTS, post-thrombotic syndrome; PVI, primary valve incompetence.*

basic factors are whether treatment is for reflux or obstruction and whether the process is due to primary or secondary disease. The important category of mixed reflux and obstruction is present in most cases of post-thrombotic disease, or may occur when the femoral vein valves are incompetent from primary disease while the tibial-popliteal veins are incompetent from recanalized post-thrombotic changes. The operations that can be used may be multiple and the choice will depend upon the experience of the surgeon as well as the reported results in the literature. For these reasons, the venous surgeon needs to develop a facility with different techniques to manage the broad scope of venous reconstructive cases.

SURGERY FOR VENOUS REFLUX

Reflux in the deep veins occurs as primary reflux, secondary reflux, or a combination of the two. Primary reflux is the most frequent cause of venous insufficiency,[21,22] and may affect the superficial, perforator, and deep veins. It is most prevalent in the superficial veins and seems to originate there. With the passage of time, it tends to involve the perforator and deep veins. Pathologically, it is a degenerative process in the vein wall with histological findings of increased collagen, fragmented elastic, and decreased muscularis, associated with valvular

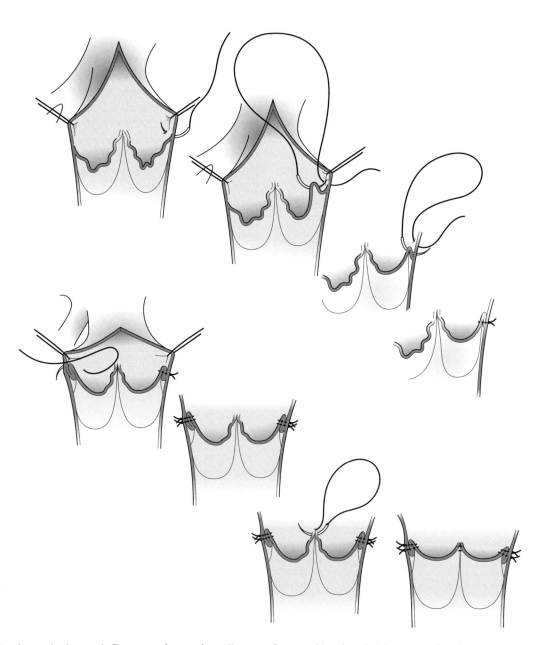

Figure 20.2   *Internal valve repair. First suture (top row): needle passes from outside vein to inside at apex of medial commissure; engages edge of cusp; passes through valve cusp and through vein wall at apex of commissure; first suture tied on outside of vein. Sutures at lateral commissure and at posterior wall (lower row).*

reflux.[23] While it may be found at any age, primary reflux tends to become a progressive clinical problem in older age groups after many years of existence as minimally symptomatic varicose veins.

Primary reflux

Primary disease in the deep veins becomes particularly important when axial reflux occurs from the common femoral vein through the popliteal vein into the calf veins. The valves in primary disease are morphologically normal structures in which the leading edges of the cusps are elongated, or become poorly apposed for any reason. When the valve cusp edges no longer appose because of their length or their position, reflux occurs under physiologic flow conditions.

INTERNAL REPAIR OF PRIMARY REFLUX

The surgical procedure that has been most effective for primary deep reflux is direct intraluminal repair accomplished by interrupted sutures that shorten the leading edge of the valve cusp (Fig. 20.2). This repair is precise and addresses the source of the incompetence directly. The several approaches to the valve and variations of the venotomy described in the literature all achieve successful internal repair[24–26] and all have produced similar results in the reported series (Table 20.1).

The basic tenet of deep valve repair for reflux is to introduce at least one competent valve between the heart and the foot in each axial venous pathway. Some surgeons have preferred more than one valve in a segment while others have not. The chosen valve should be below the common femoral level to prevent circus flow amongst the branches below the repair, e.g. PFV (profunda femoris vein) to femoral vein flow distal to a repaired common femoral valve. The deep axial segments in the lower extremity veins include femoral-popliteal-crural, profunda femoral-popliteal-crural, and non-standard connections between the superficial veins and deep veins such as GSV (great saphenous vein) popliteal-crural. It has been recognized (refer to Eriksson[27]) that repair of the femoral-popliteal pathway without repair of an incompetent profunda-popliteal-crural pathway will yield poor results. For this reason repair at the popliteal level is useful when both the femoral and the profunda veins are incompetent, as in many cases of secondary reflux and some cases of primary reflux.

Table 20.1 illustrates seven series[16,17,27–30] of deep primary valve repairs reported in the 1990s, comprising 394 total repairs. These were performed by the three dominant methods of repair and each series yielded comparable results. The follow-up in each series was long. The good to excellent results (good = asymptomatic with use of elastic stockings; excellent = asymptomatic without elastic stockings) were found in 62–75 percent of cases over the very long term (>8 years) in each series. The factor that correlated best with a long-term good result was competence of the repaired valve.[17,30] Seventy-two percent of internal valvuloplasty repairs remained competent by imaging studies at 1–8 years.

Although these series are examples of level 5 evidence (except one series,[28] which had a control group and is level 3 evidence), there is a strong consistency in these independently performed case series where the only facet common to all of the series was the creation of at least one competent valve in each axial pathway of these advanced cases. For the most part, these were end-stage cases of chronic venous insufficiency representing CEAP classes 4, 5, and 6 disease. Most of the cases had been failures of conventional care, including a high percentage of cases with prior surgery of the superficial and perforator veins. The lack of a control group is partially addressed by the prior treatment failure in nearly all of these cases so that these series have some of the elements of cross-over treatment. This body of literature on internal primary valve repair is the strongest evidence for the validity of deep valve repair to date.

EXTERNAL REPAIR OF PRIMARY DEEP REFLUX

External repair[24] refers to a surgery in which the valve is restored to competence by sutures placed on the outside of the vein wall without the need for a venotomy (Fig. 20.3). This repair is very attractive because it is simpler and safer, since it requires less dissection around the vein, avoids opening the vein and thereby renders anticoagulation less necessary, and minimizes the chance for postoperative thrombosis. However, it is a less precise repair and has been followed by a significantly higher recurrence rate of valve reflux and clinical recurrence of symptoms in several series.[14,17,30] External repair is important

Table 20.1 *Results of internal valvuloplasty*

Authors	Year reported	No. limbs	FU (months)	Good results (%)	Competent value
Eriksson[27]	1990	27	6–108	70	70
Masuda and Kistner[17]	1994	32	48–252	73	77
Lurie[28]	1997	49	36–108	–	85
Perrin[29]	1997	75	24–96	–	85
Perrin[14]	2000	83	12–96	80	79
Raju et al.[30]	1996	68	12–144	62	76
Sottiurai[16]	1997	143	9–168	75	75

FU, follow-up.

as an adjunct to internal repair, and it can often be performed in situations where internal repair is technically very difficult, as in a scarred area or in a deep dissection. Its use as the procedure of choice when internal repair could also be performed might be considered questionable.

External repair with cuffs has been reported both as a stand-alone repair (Jessup and Lane[32]) and as an adjunct to other repairs to prevent dilation of the repaired vein at the valve site (Raju). The studies on external wrapping of deep veins have not been controlled sufficiently to know if the external wraps help or hurt the long-term competence of the valve repaired by either internal or external approach.

Angioscopic repair was reported in 1991 by Gloviczki et al.[33] and has been adopted by several centres[33–35] with enthusiastic reports. Long-term follow-up in significant numbers is still in process.[34]

HOW MANY VALVES SHOULD BE REPAIRED, AND AT WHICH SITES?

There is significant disbelief about the validity of repair of a single valve in the long axial segment from the heart to the ankle that normally contains multiple valves. The reply to this concern is that a single competent valve in the thigh or popliteal vein decreases the column of reflux by at least 50 percent and is adequate to provide a state of compensation, even though the system is not repaired to its full normal status. It would be reassuring to repair more than one valve in the axial segment if this can be done safely and expeditiously, but the proof that this will improve the clinical result has not been

forthcoming to date. The definitive finding about multiple repairs has been the importance of repair of at least one valve in each axial pathway, as shown by increased clinical failure when one system is left unrepaired.[36] Sometimes it is convenient to add a second repair to an adjacent valve when two valves are easily exposed by performing an external repair below or above an internal repair.

ALTERNATIVE METHODS OF PRIMARY VALVE REPAIR

The potential use of transposition of a venous segment, transplantation of a vein-valve segment, or use of a substitute valve such as a cryopreserved valve could apply to primary disease as well as secondary disease, but is not frequently indicated because direct valve repair techniques are preferable. These techniques are discussed below under repair of secondary reflux.

Secondary reflux

Secondary reflux refers to reflux in the post-thrombotic vein which is a result of recanalization or scarring in a given vein segment. The pathology is very different from primary reflux because the post-thrombotic vein lumen is usually scarred and distorted, and the valves are morphologically abnormal in contrast to the normal morphology in primary disease. Often, there are segments of occluded veins and others of refluxing veins, and within the refluxing vein there may be partial obstructions due to post-thrombotic scarring. The extent of

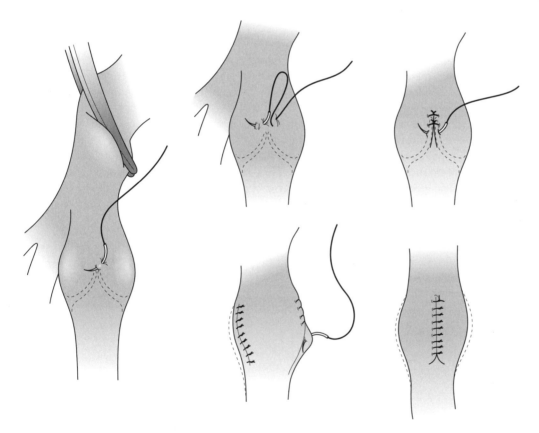

Figure 20.3 *External valve repair. First suture engages one cusp margin, and then another, and is then tied outside the vein. Multiple sutures coapting cusp margins in both commissures.*

damage to the valves is very variable, ranging from nearly normal with a small scar to totally destroyed valve stations that may not even be recognizable. The potential for repair of these valves is very poor.

The range and complexity of findings in the post-thrombotic limb are great. These vessels are more difficult to work with than primary veins because they are thickened and distorted, and because there is a tendency for post-thrombotic veins to develop new thromboses. The post-thrombotic changes involve the deep veins primarily and the superficial veins secondarily. In contrast to primary disease, the saphenous vein is frequently normal when the post-thrombotic deep veins are severely diseased.

Restoration of competence to the venous segment requires a substitution procedure which provides a new valve. The two principal methods are transplantation of a vein that contains a competent valve, or transposition of the diseased post-thrombotic vein to an adjacent segment that contains a competent valve which can serve as the outflow tract of the diseased vein. The other possibility is a cryopreserved venous graft with a competent valve.

TRANSPLANTATION PROCEDURE

This operation was devised[13] to provide a substitute valve for post-thrombotic veins where the native vein is not repairable. In this procedure, a vein segment that contains a competent valve from another extremity, usually the arm, is resected and transplanted into the popliteal or the femoral vein. The usual harvest site is the axillary-brachial vein of the arm where the resected segment does not result in noticeable harm to the extremity, and the size match to the popliteal or the femoral vein is satisfactory (Fig. 20.4).

There are eight series of these operations[16,29,30,37,38,40] (Table 20.2) that total 282 limbs and in whom the follow-up extends from 18 to 72 months. The percentage of good clinical results is variable from author to author over a range of 31–92 percent. In five of the seven series, the good results are below 50 percent in the first 2 years while the other two[37,39] have excellent results at 18–64 months. The reason for these widely divergent results is not clear but it may be related to the site where the transplant is placed because the popliteal vein

was the site of placement in the two better series. There is a tendency for these transplants to dilate over time so an initial successful procedure may fatigue in follow-up.

TRANSPOSITION PROCEDURE

The transposition operation was devised[41] to provide a valved outlet vein for an incompetent post-thrombotic vein. In these cases, an adjacent vein is found that contains a competent valve,

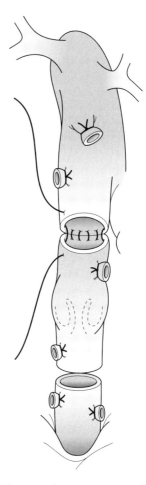

Figure 20.4 *Valve transplantation. The superficial femoral valve segment is excised and replaced by an axillary valve segment.*

Table 20.2 *Results of vein–valve transplantation*

Authors	Year reported	No. of limbs	FU (months)	Clinical success (%)	Ulcer recurrence
Nash[38]	1988	23	18	31	?
Eriksson[37]	1990	35	60	90+	18
Raju *et al.*[30]	1996	44	24	36	54
O'Donnell	1997	15	64	92	21
Perrin[29]	1997	30	60	48	67
Sottiurai[16]	1997	33	74	39	?
Taheri[40]	1997	102	60	45	?
Perrin[14]	2000	32	12–124	62	39

FU, follow-up.

such as a competent profunda vein next to an incompetent femoral vein. The incompetent segment is disconnected from its proximal channel and anastomosed to the side or the end of the competent segment. This permits the valve of the competent segment to serve the incompetent segment as well (Fig. 20.5).

There are four series of these repairs[16,17,29,42] (Table 20.3) totalling 70 cases and with follow-up of 18–120 months. Recurrence is found in 45–75 percent of cases in these reports. These modest results have been a surprise since the procedure is quite simple and only requires one anastomosis.

The transposition operation is useful in certain conditions when an adjacent competent vein is available.

Mixed reflux and obstruction

An important group of cases exists with combinations of reflux and obstruction. This occurs when a patient with primary reflux in the femoral vein develops a distal vein thrombosis in the tibial-popliteal segment, even extending into the distal femoral vein at the adductor canal. In these cases, repair of the more proximal incompetent femoral valve affected by primary disease has been found to yield nearly as good long-term results as repair in a totally primary-diseased extremity, and better results than treatment of secondary reflux by other techniques (Fig. 20.6).

A second combination of reflux and obstruction is found in pure post-thrombotic disease when there are partial obstructions in the recanalized femoral and popliteal veins in addition to reflux due to destroyed valves in the same or adjacent femoral-popliteal veins of the extremity. These vein segments may cause severe symptoms because they are sources of both reflux and obstruction, and the other veins of the extremity may be poorly constituted to provide compensation. When the obstruction is severe, these patients will complain of venous claudication and external elastic compression may exacerbate rather than relieve their symptoms.

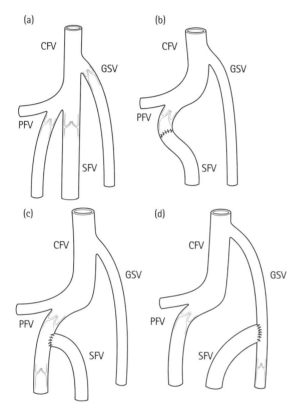

Figure 20.5 *Transposition procedure. (a) Usual location of valves in femoral veins. (b) End-to end anastomosis of diseased superficial femoral vein (SFV) to descending branch of profunda vein with competent proximal valve. (c) End-to-side anastomosis of diseased SFV to descending branch of profunda vein with competent proximal and distal valves. (d) End-to-side anastomosis of diseased SFV to great saphenous vein (GSV) with competent proximal and distal valves. CFV, common femoral vein; PFV, profunda femoris vein.*

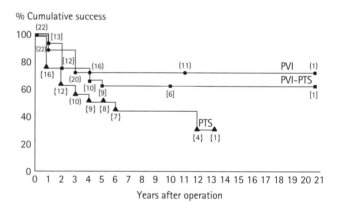

Figure 20.6 *Kaplan–Meier life table of cumulative success rate of venous reconstructions in patients with primary (PVI), post-thrombotic (PTS) and combination of primary and post-thrombotic diseases (PVI-PTS).*

Table 20.3 *Results of vein transposition*

Authors	Year reported	No. limbs	FU (months)	Good results (%)	Competence (%)
Johnson et al.[42]	1981	12	18	25	Not reported
Masuda and Kistner[17]	1994	14	120	40	10–14 partial competence
Perrin[29]	1997	13	60	54	5/12 competent (49 months)
Sottiurai[16]	1997	31	89	39	12/31 competent

FU, follow-up.

These extremities require great care in diagnosis and are best studied with combinations of detailed duplex scanning and complementary ascending and descending venography. Their diagnosis and surgical treatment is on a case-by-case basis, but surprisingly good results can be obtained with precise repairs by combinations of bypass utilizing transplanted vein-valve segments, transpositions, and even ligation of detrimental veins.

A third combination of reflux and obstruction occurs when proximal post-thrombotic obstruction exists in the iliac veins and is coupled with post-thrombotic or primary disease below the common inguinal ligament. Since the iliac obstruction will be described in another chapter, it is sufficient to say here that the first treatment would be directed to relief of the proximal obstruction. When symptoms persist after this has been done, additional repair of reflux or obstruction in the thigh or calf may be needed to restore function, and would follow the precepts described above.

COMPLICATIONS AND RISKS OF DEEP VEIN RECONSTRUCTION

Given the ability to operate in the deep venous system, it is important to recognize the risk these procedures entail. The time when it was considered unthinkable to operate in the deep veins because of the risk of thrombosis and embolism came to an end when the first reports of bypass appeared in the 1960s, and were further buried by the demonstration that reflux could be treated by intraluminal surgery with relative safety.

To date, there are no reports of significant mortality due to postoperative thromboembolic episodes after reconstructive venous surgery. Morbidity does occur secondary to postoperative thrombosis, especially in the post-thrombotic veins. Other morbidity due to delayed wound healing and postoperative infection is consistent with the magnitude of the various repairs. Some of the surgery is prolonged due to its complexity in abnormal diseased veins, but it is neither contaminated nor especially bloody. Transfusion requirements would be unusual.

The sources of morbidity are postoperative thrombosis, prolonged wound healing, and recurrence of the reflux or obstruction.

Post-operative thrombosis. This has been reported as a minor clinical occurrence in most of the series, but it was studied more carefully by Perrin[14] with postoperative venograms in asymptomatic patients after reconstruction. He found an incidence of 20.3 percent of focal venous defects in these venograms, but many of these were very small defects which disappeared spontaneously and were not of clinical significance. Reports of clinically significant postoperative thrombosis after valve repair in primary disease are unusual when heparin is used perioperatively. Reports of significant thrombosis after repair of secondary reflux are more frequent and have been reported to be 10–15 percent.[43]

Prolonged wound healing may be due to interruption of lymphatics in the femoral region with extensive deep vein

dissections or to wound hematomas related to the use of perioperative anticoagulants. Wound hematomas can be a difficult problem in cases that have persistent venous hypertension in the region of surgical dissection after the reconstruction.

PRESENT STATUS OF DEEP VEIN RECONSTRUCTION

The developments of the past 50 years prove that the deep veins can be operated upon with success. Due in large measure to the need for definitive diagnoses in the surgical patients, an increased clarity about the pathology and pathophysiology of chronic venous disease has emerged. With the growing use of the CEAP classification of chronic venous disease, there is a new appreciation of the interrelationships between etiology, anatomy, and pathophysiology. As this process continues, outcome analysis will develop and the indications for extended surgical repair will become more obvious.

The ultimate justification for deep venous surgery requires scientific proof that it improves upon the results achieved with less complicated treatment. Unfortunately, a problem exists in comparing the results of venous reconstruction with conventional best medical care because the medically managed cases in the literature are not adequately evaluated to determine the segmental distribution of their disease, the separation of primary from secondary disease, or of reflux from obstructive problems. Correlations between all of these factors are needed in the future.

For the present, the logical management of chronic venous disorders is to begin with external support, and add conventional superficial and perforator surgery to those who are still symptomatic after trying the non-surgical approach. For cases that still do not respond, or recur, definitive work-up of the venous system with imaging and physiological testing of pressures and volume will lead to options for deep venous reconstruction. In these cases, there are sufficient reports of repairs to anticipate the degree of risk and the likelihood of success in restoring the patient to a comfortable functional existence.

In the future, prospective testing of surgical and non-surgical methods can be performed in a comparative fashion to sharpen the focus on the indications for deep reconstruction in all forms of chronic venous disease.

REFERENCES

1. Homans J. The aetiology and treatment of varicose ulcers of the leg. *Surg Gynecol Obstet* 1917; **24**: 300–11.
2. Linton RR. The post-thrombotic ulceration of the lower extremity: its etiology and surgical treatment. *Ann Surg* 1953; **138**: 415–30.
3. Cockett FB. The pathology and treatment of venous ulcers of the leg. *Br J Surg* 1955; **43**: 260–78.
4. Bauer G. The etiology of leg ulcers and their treatment by resection of the popliteal vein. *J Int Chir* 1948; **8**: 937–61.

5. Warren R, Thayer TR. Transplantation of the saphenous vein for postphlebitic stasis. *Surgery* 1954; **35**: 867–76.

6. Eiseman B, Malette W. An operative technique for the construction of venous valves. *Surg Gynecol Obstet* 1953; **97**: 731–4.

7. Palma EC. Esperon R. Vein transplants and grafts in the surgical treatment of the post–phlebitic syndrome. *J Cardiovasc Surg* 1960; **1**: 94–107.

8. Dale WA. Crossover grafts for iliofemoral venous block. *Surgery* 1965; **57**: 608–12.

9. Husni EA. Venous reconstruction in postphlebitic disease. *Circulation* 1971; **43/44**(Suppl. 1): 147–50.

10. Gruss JD. Venous bypass for chronic venous insufficiency. In: Bergan JJ, Yao JST, eds. *Venous Disorders*. Philadelphia: WB Saunders, 1991; 316–30.

11. Kistner RL. Surgical repair of the incompetent femoral vein valve. *Arch Surg* 1975; **110**: 1336–42.

12. Kistner RL, Ferris EB. Technique of surgical reconstruction of femoral vein valves. In: Bergan JJ, Yao JST, eds. *Operative Techniques in Vascular Surgery*. New York: Grune & Stratton, 1980; 299.

13. Taheri SA, Lazar L, Elias SM *et al*. Surgical treatment of postphlebitic syndrome with vein valve transplant. *Am J Surg* 1982; **144**: 221–4.

14. Perrin M. Reconstructive surgery for deep venous reflux. a report on 144 cases. *Cardiovasc Surg* 2000; **8**: 246–55.

15. Raju S. Results of deep vein reconstruction. *Vasc Surg* 1997; **31**: 281–6.

16. Sottiurai VS. Results of deep vein reconstruction. *Vasc Surg* 1997; **31**: 276–8.

17. Masuda EM, Kistner RL. Long-term results of venous valve reconstruction: a 4–21 year follow-up. *J Vasc Surg* 1994; **19**: 391–403.

18. DePalma RG, Kowallek DL. Venous ulceration: a cross-over study from nonoperative to operative treatment. *J Vasc Surg* 1996; **24**: 788–92.

19. Classification and grading of chronic venous disease in the lower limb: a consensus statement. *Vasc Surg* 1996; **30**: 5–11.

20. Porter JM, Moneta GL. International Consensus Committee on Chronic Venous Disease. Reporting standards in venous disease: an update. *J Vasc Surg* 1995; **21**: 635–45.

21. Kistner RL, Eklof B, Masuda EM. Diagnosis of chronic venous disease of the lower extremities: the 'CEAP' classification. *Mayo Clin Proc* 1996; **71**: 338–45.

22. Labropoulos N, Delis K, Nicolaides AN *et al*. The role of the distribution and anatomic extent of reflux in the development of signs and symptoms in chronic venous insufficiency. *J Vasc Surg* 1996; **23**: 504–10.

23. Lowell RC, Gloviczki P, Miller VM. In vitro evaluation of endothelial and smooth muscle function of primary varicose veins. *J Vasc Surg* 1992; **16**: 679–86.

24. Kistner RL. Valve reconstruction for primary valve insufficiency. In: Bergan JJ, Kistner RL, eds. *Atlas of Venous Surgery*. Philadelphia: WB Saunders, 1992; 125–33.

25. Raju S. Supravalvular incision for valve repair in primary valvular insufficiency. method of Raju. In: Bergan JJ, Kistner RL, eds. *Atlas of Venous Surgery*. Philadelphia: WB Saunders, 1992; 135–7.

26. Sottiurai VS. Supravalvular incision for valve repair in primary valvular insufficiency. Method of Sottiurai. In: Bergan JJ, Kistner RL, eds. *Atlas of Venous Surgery*. Philadelphia: WB Saunders, 1992; 137–45.

27. Eriksson I. Reconstructive surgery for deep vein valve incompetence in the lower limb. *Eur J Vasc Surg* 1990; **4**: 211–8.

28. Lurie F. Results of deep vein reconstruction. *Vasc Surg* 1997; **31**: 275–6.

29. Perrin MR. Results of deep vein reconstruction. *Vasc Surg* 1997; **31**: 273–5.

30. Raju S, Fredericks RK, Neglen PN, Bass JD. Durability of venous valve reconstruction techniques for 'primary' and postthrombotic reflux. *J Vasc Surg* 1996; **23**: 357–67.

31. Makarova NP, Lurie F, Hmelniker SM. Does surgical correction of the superficial femoral vein valve change the course of varicose disease? *J Vasc Surg* 2001; **33**: 361–8.

32. Jessup G, Lane RJ. Repair of incompetent venous valves: a new technique. *J Vasc Surg* 1988; **8**: 569–75.

33. Gloviczki P, Merrell SW, Bower TC. Femoral vein valve repair under direct vision without venotomy: a modified technique with angioscopy. *J Vasc Surg* 1991; **14**: 645–8.

34. Hoshino S, Satokawa H, Takase S *et al*. External valvuloplasty for primary valvular incompetence of the lower limbs using angioscopy. *Int J Angio* 1997; **6**: 137–41.

35. O'Donnell TF Jr. The role of angioscopic valve repair for primary valve incompetence (PVI). *Hawaii Med J* 2000; **59**: 266–8.

36. Eriksson I, Almgren B. Influence of the profunda femoris veins on venous hemodynamics of the limb. *J Vasc Surg* 1986; **4**: 390–5.

37. Eriksson I. Vein valve surgery for deep valvular incompetence. In: Eklof B, Gjores JE, Thulesius O, Bergqvist D, eds. *Controversies in the Management of Venous Disorders*. London: Butterworths, 1989; 267–79.

38. Nash T. Long-term results of vein valve transplants placed in the popliteal vein for intractable post-phlebitic venous ulcers and pre-ulcer skin changes. *J Cardiovasc Surg* 1988; **29**: 712–6.

39. O'Donnell TF, Mackey WC, Shepard AD, Callow AD. Clinical, hemodynamic and anatomic follow-up of direct venous reconstruction. *Arch Surg* 1987; **122**: 474–82.

40. Taheri SA. Vein valve transplantation. *Vasc Surg* 1997; **31**: 278–81.

41. Kistner RL. Transposition techniques. In: Bergan JJ, Kistner RL, eds. *Atlas of Venous Surgery*. Philadelphia: WB Saunders, 1992; 153–6.

42. Johnson ND, Queral LA, Flinn WR *et al*. Late objective assessment of venous valve surgery. *Arch Surg* 1981; **116**: 1461–6.

43. Eklof B, Kistner RL. Complications of management of venous disease and arteriovenous fistulae. In: Strandness DE, Van Breda A, eds. *Vascular Disease: Surgical and Interventional Therapy*. New York: Churchill Livingstone, 1994; 1199–219.

21

Treatment of venous obstruction

PETER NEGLÉN

INTRODUCTION

Leg ulcer due to chronic venous insufficiency (CVI) is known to have several contributing pathophysiological factors. In the macrocirculation, the role of incompetent valves in the deep or superficial system has been emphasized and treatment has been directed largely towards correction of reflux. Although well recognized, other aspects, e.g. obstruction to the outflow, a poor calf muscle pump, low compliance and geometrical changes of the flow channels, have for the most part been ignored. An obstructive component has been shown to be predominant in approximately one-third of post-thrombotic limbs. Reflux is found to be combined with obstruction in 55 percent of symptomatic patients with CVI.[1,2] This combination of reflux and obstruction is most detrimental. It leads to the highest levels of venous hypertension and the most severe symptoms, including development of leg ulcer, as compared with either alone.[3,4] Because of diagnostic difficulties and lack of appropriate surgical interventions, however, the treatment of outflow obstruction has been neglected throughout the years. Open surgery has been unattractive because the operation is rather extensive and often combined with a temporary or permanent arteriovenous fistula; it always necessitates life-long anticoagulation postoperatively; and it has uncertain long-term patency. Therefore, venous bypass surgery has been restricted to a minority of patients with severe disabling symptoms and markedly increased venous pressure levels. Endovascular treatment of venous outflow obstruction with venous balloon angioplasty and stent insertion was introduced in the mid-1990s. Since that time, interest has refocused on the role of venous outflow obstruction in patients with chronic venous insufficiency and leg ulcers. Balloon dilation and stenting of the iliac vein has now largely replaced bypass surgery and the mid-term results indicate that the procedure is a safe and efficient alternative for a larger group of patients. Venous stenting has also led to a renewed interest in the nature and pathophysiology of venous obstruction *per se*, and in tests for detection of hemodynamically significant lesions. There is cautious optimism that iliac venous stent placement will be a useful modality in the management of patients with CVI and leg ulcer in the future. Several issues regarding diagnosis, indication for treatment and methods of outcome assessment, however, remain unresolved.

VENOUS OUTFLOW OBSTRUCTION

The majority of lower extremity outflow obstructions are observed following acute deep vein thrombosis (DVT) with subsequent absent or poor venous recanalization. It appears that proximal obstruction of the venous outflow, especially the iliac vein, is more symptomatic than lower segmental blockage.[5–7] The collateral formation is relatively poor around an iliofemoral obstruction, contrary to blockage of the femoro-popliteal vein. Collateralization is facilitated in the latter segment owing to the presence of double veins, direct connection to the profunda vein, sapheno-saphenous connection and deep muscular tributaries in the thigh. Following proximal DVT, only 20–30 percent of iliac veins completely recanalize spontaneously, while the remaining veins recanalize partially and develop varying degrees of collateralization (Fig. 21.1).[8,9] Although post-thrombotic obstruction is most frequent, an iliac vein obstruction may be 'primary' or non-thrombotic in nature (May–Thurner syndrome[10] or iliac vein compression

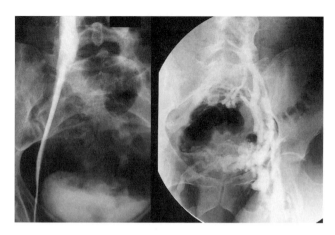

Figure 21.1   *Transfemoral phlebogram showing typical post-thrombotic iliofemoral vein segments, long uniform non-collateralizing stenosis (left) and occluded iliac vein with marked collateralization (right).*

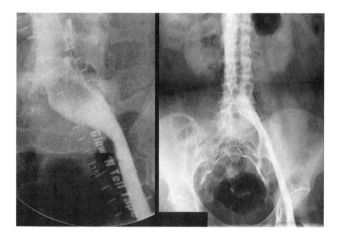

Figure 21.2   *Transfemoral phlebogram showing non-thrombotic lesion of the left common iliac vein (iliac vein compression syndrome) with pancaking (left) and translucent area at the iliocaval junction with transpelvic collaterals (right).*

syndrome[11]). This etiology appears to be a more common cause of venous obstruction than previously thought. In a group of 126 patients with active or healed leg ulcer and venous outflow obstruction treated with venous stenting, we found that 38/126 (30 percent) had non-thrombotic blockage (defined as absent history of DVT with no venographic or ultrasound findings indicating previous DVT). The majority of these limbs (34/38, 89 percent) also had primary deep or superficial reflux. Typically, a short stenosis of the proximal common iliac vein is observed. It is usually caused by compression of the vein by the right common iliac artery with secondary band or web formation (Fig. 21.2).[12] Of the limbs with 'primary' disease, however, 15 percent have been shown to have more extensive lesions involving both common and external iliac veins.[13] These limbs may have had a subclinical isolated iliac vein thrombosis, which was initiated at the vessel crossing and then propagated distally into the external iliac

vein. Conversely, limbs with obvious post-thrombotic disease may have had an underlying iliac vein compression, resulting in a clinical iliofemoral vein thrombosis.[14] Whatever the chain of events, it should serve to remind us that patients with leg ulcer and absent history and findings of previous DVT may have iliac vein obstruction, even in the presence of primary venous reflux.

HEMODYNAMIC TESTS

Unfortunately, there are no reliable tests to measure a hemodynamically significant stenosis. In fact, it is not known what degree of narrowing constitutes a 'critical stenosis' in the venous system. This lack of 'gold standard' is the major obstacle to assessing the importance of chronic outflow obstruction, directing treatment, and measuring outcome of treatment. The concept of a significant obstruction being a stenosis of >70–80 percent is derived from observations on the arterial system. This is probably not applicable for the venous system since there are many fundamental differences. When two obstructions are present in series, the resistance to flow will be dictated by the more severe stenosis.[15] A stenosis of the major arteries does not reduce blood flow significantly until it meets and exceeds the level of the high peripheral vascular resistance. Contrarily, antegrade flow through the iliac vein empties into the low resistance of the inferior vena cava (IVC). An iliac vein stenosis has to override only a low 'peripheral resistance', and may, therefore, in itself constitute a significant stenosis to a lesser degree. The geometrical form of an obstruction may change the pattern of blood flow. A slit-like narrowing of the lumen of a vein, even with no alteration in the cross-sectional area, may increase resistance to flow. This may perhaps explain why a relatively minor degree of compression may affect blood flow in the left iliac vein. Contrary to the arterial circulation, low pressure, low velocity, and large blood volume characterize the venous circulation. In such a system, the venous pressure is not only a function of resistance to the flow, but is also dependent upon the flow velocity and magnitude of volume flow. In fact, it is not known how much the resting flow must be increased to reach the physiological level necessary to detect a hemodynamically significant venous stenosis. This has important implications for the development of tests to evaluate outflow obstruction. We have attempted to increase the venous flow in the supine position by inducing hyperemia after ischemic occlusion with cuff, ankle exercise or intra-arterial injection of papaverin, and in the erect position by toe stands.[16,17] None of these methods appears to provide reproducible flow increases and they have not been helpful in delineating borderline obstructions.

Non-invasive duplex Doppler and plethysmography have been helpful in the diagnosis of acute complete obstruction. In chronic venous obstruction, however, ultrasound investigation and outflow fractions obtained by air and strain gauge plethysmography have been shown to be unreliable in measuring hemodynamically important obstruction. Outflow

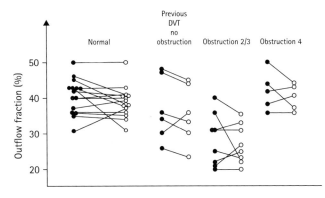

Figure 21.3 *Individual plethysmographic outflow fraction values with (○) and without (●) induced hyperemia in limbs with different degrees of outflow obstruction using Raju's venous pressure-based classification (0–4, where 4 is most severe). There is great overlapping among all groups, indicating the poor accuracy of outflow fraction measurements. DVT, deep vein thrombosis. (Adapted from Neglén and Raju[18] with permission from Society for Vascular Surgery and the American Association for Vascular Surgery.)*

fraction measurement is commonly used, but it is important to understand that, although abnormal findings may indicate outflow obstruction, significant blockage may be present with normal findings (Fig. 21.3).[18–20] This measurement may be of limited use in serial tests of the same patient in research, but cannot be used to detect significant outflow obstruction in a single measurement of a limb. Thus, no accurate, discriminative non-invasive test is available.

Invasive pressure measurements, i.e. hand/foot pressure differential and reactive hyperemia pressure, increase, and indirect resistance calculations appear better than non-invasive studies.[21–23] These studies require thigh cuff compression with high inflation pressure, which is sometimes painful and uncomfortable, and the calculations use volume measurements acquired by plethysmography, encompassing that method's inadequacy. Although invasive pressure measurements appear to be more specific, they are also relatively insensitive and do not define the level of obstruction.[18] Arm/foot venous pressures may be abnormal despite impressive collateralization.[21] Collaterals are probably often poor substitutes for the original vein, owing to their tortuosity and incompetent valves. The mechanism and inducement of collateral formation are unclear. The development of collaterals is commonly seen as a compensatory feature, which neutralizes the outflow obstruction by bypassing, but should perhaps instead be considered an indicator of an obstruction, in which an attempt is being made to compensate the obstructed outflow.

Venous pressures may also be obtained during phlebographic evaluation or at surgery. Pull-through pressure differential of venous obstruction or femoral pressure increase on exercise and following hyperemia is much lower than in the arterial system.[24–26] Because of the low central pressure of the venous system, only small pressure increases at rest may indicate significant obstruction. In addition, the contralateral veins converge beyond the iliac stenosis, which may also mitigate any pressure gradient at rest. At present, the accepted view is that a significant obstruction exists with a supine pull-through gradient greater than 2–3 mmHg at rest, or with a gradient compared with the contralateral femoral pressure in excess of 2–5 mmHg as measured in supine position. The prevailing rule is that femoral venous pressure increase on exercise should be at least 5 mmHg to warrant intervention. However, these suggested pressure levels to detect significance are set arbitrarily. In a supine position, especially during surgery, it is difficult to increase the venous outflow sufficiently to detect a hemodynamic obstruction. The difficulty does not arise when pressure gradients are high, but rather when the pressures are near normal.

Although a positive hemodynamic test may indicate hemodynamic significance, a normal test does not exclude it. Thus, it is presently impossible to detect potentially important borderline obstructions even with invasive pressure measurements.

MORPHOLOGICAL INVESTIGATIONS

In lieu of reliable hemodynamic tests, the diagnosis of outflow obstruction must be made by morphological investigations. Although a positive non-invasive or invasive test may support proceeding with phlebography, a negative test should not exclude it. If history and clinical signs and symptoms suggest outflow obstruction, certainly in patients with severe CVI and leg ulcer, morphological studies should be performed. A high index of suspicion must be maintained. Ascending or antegrade transfemoral phlebography is the time-honored method for imaging the morphology of the venous outflow tract, showing the site of obstruction and the presence of collaterals (Figs 21.1 and 21.2). To properly delineate the iliocaval vein, it is important to take images in multiple planes, including lateral views. Important lesions at the iliocaval junction will otherwise be missed. The most frequently used single-plane, anterior–posterior transfemoral phlebography has shown to be inadequate.[27] Although proximal obstruction appears to be hemodynamically more severe, a distal obstruction may still constitute a major hemodynamic outflow obstruction. The anatomic location, the extent and degree of an obstructive lesion, and the number and size of collateral vessels seen on phlebography are unfortunately not reliable guides to hemodynamic severity.[23]

Intravascular ultrasound (IVUS) has been utilized increasingly in diagnosis and treatment of femoro-iliocaval obstruction.[27–29] It has been shown to detect lesions that were not obvious on single-plane transfemoral phlebography. Injection of contrast dye can hide details, e.g. intraluminal webs and frozen valves, which are revealed by IVUS (Fig. 21.4). The ultrasound can differentiate axial collateral formation in near proximity to the post-thrombotic original vein from intraluminal trabeculation. An external compression and the resulting deformity of the venous lumen can be directly visualized (Fig. 21.5). Most importantly, IVUS appears superior

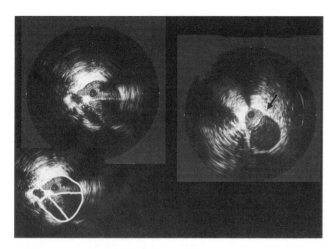

Figure 21.4 *Intraluminal details visualized by intravascular ultrasound (IVUS). Post-thrombotic trabeculation (left, trabeculae and vein wall artificially enhanced in lower image) and intraluminal web (right, arrow). (Reproduced from Neglén and Raju[27] with permission from Society for Vascular Surgery and the American Association for Vascular Surgery.)*

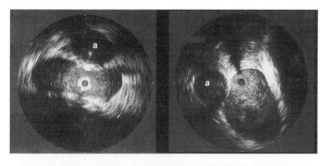
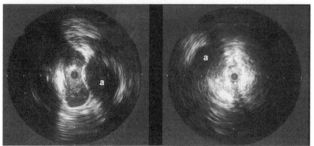

Figure 21.5 *Intravascular ultrasound (IVUS) images showing different degrees of outside compression by the left common iliac vein as it is crossed by the right common iliac artery (a). The position of the iliac artery depends upon the orientation of the catheter (black circle inside the vein) and does not necessarily reflect anatomical topography. (Reproduced from Neglén and Raju[27] with permission from Society for Vascular Surgery and the American Association for Vascular Surgery.)*

to standard single-plane phlebography for estimating the morphological degree and extent of iliac vein stenosis. A phlebogram may show only a 'pancaking' of the common iliac vein or a translucent area with no clearly delineated

stenosis. With IVUS, the actual lumen can be visualized and measured accurately by planimetry using machine software. The preoperative transfemoral single-plane phlebogram was actually considered 'normal' in 19 percent of post-thrombotic and 28 percent of non-thrombotic limbs, which were shown to have more than 50 percent obstruction on IVUS.[13] On average, the transfemoral phlebogram significantly underestimated the degree of stenosis by one-third. Phlebography was shown to be less accurate in detecting obstruction of greater than 70 percent compared with IVUS. Thus, IVUS appears superior to single-plane phlebography in providing adequate morphological information. The accuracy of transfemoral phlebography may improve if multiple side views are obtained. Multiple views are, however, not currently performed in standard practice. To our knowledge, no study comparing IVUS and multi-plane phlebography exists. It appears that IVUS is presently the best available method for determination of morphologically significant obstruction. In lieu of adequate hemodynamic tests, patients with significant signs and symptoms of CVI should have a transfemoral phlebography, or preferably an IVUS, performed in addition to routine non-invasive reflux investigations. Arbitrarily, we consider performing venous stenting in limbs with iliocaval vein stenosis >50 percent reduction of the luminal cross-cut area as measured by IVUS, especially if pre- or intraoperative pressure gradients indicate hemodynamic significance.

TREATMENT

Prior to the introduction of percutaneous endovascular venous stenting, open surgery was the only alternative treatment to conservative management. The common problem with bypass grafting is that of relatively poor long-term patency. The reasons for this are several. The grafts tend to clot because:

- the area of insertion has low-velocity flow
- external compression of the low-pressure bypass may occur
- the graft material is inherently thrombogenetic
- poor distal inflow due to extensive disease may exist
- frequent hypercoagulability of patients with recurrent thrombosis is observed.

The best clinical results have been shown with large-diameter polytetrafluoroethylene (PTFE) grafts (10 mm) with external support (ringed), adjunct use of an arteriovenous fistula and meticulous perioperative anticoagulation. The arteriovenous fistula is left in place as long as no side-effects are encountered. The anticoagulation is usually lifelong to keep the bypass open. If the graft suddenly occludes with a functioning fistula, symptoms usually exacerbate and the fistula must be disconnected. The operations most frequently performed are femoro-femoral crossover or unilateral iliocaval bypass for iliac vein occlusion, and sapheno-popliteal bypass for isolated femoropopliteal obstruction. For short, non-occlusive vein

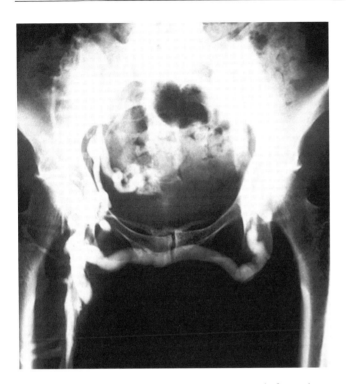

Figure 21.6 *Phlebogram showing an autogenous vein femoral crossover bypass of good caliber (Palma procedure).*

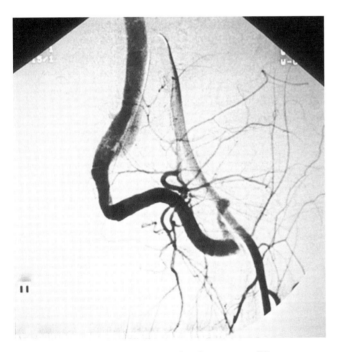

Figure 21.7 *Arterio-phlebogram showing contrast filling through a constructed arteriovenous fistulae into a ringed polytetrafluoroethylene (PTFE) femoro-iliac left-to-right bypass graft.*

stenosis (iliac vein compression syndrome), right iliac artery transposition and iliac vein patch angioplasty have been used.[30]

The crossover bypass has been reported to be durable with good symptom relief and a so-called 'clinical' and phlebographic patency ranging from 44 to 100 percent with

a follow-up of 5 years (Fig. 21.6).[31–38] Most series have small numbers of patients with inconsistent clinical and phlebographic follow-up. Clinical improvement is unfortunately not necessarily related to graft patency. The autogenous vein is the least thrombogenic bypass with best patency. Despite remaining patent, however, the saphenous grafts often give poor symptom relief owing to their small cross-cut area and relatively large resistance to flow. It has been shown that at least a 4.5-mm-diameter vein is necessary to adequately relieve the iliac vein outflow obstruction.[39] This is the reason for the recommended size of a 10 mm PTFE graft for femoral crossover bypass (Fig. 21.7).

Saphenopopliteal vein bypass has been performed only in extremely selected limbs with chronic segmental occlusion confined to the femoropopliteal vein segment. It can be performed only in limbs with a patent, non-varicose great saphenous vein with competent valves and a patent tibial inflow tract (essentially normal calf views on phlebography). In the few reported series of patients,[31,36,40] results are not impressive, with clinical success and patency rates of 31–58 and 56–67 percent, respectively, at 1–5 years' follow-up.

Owing to the invasiveness and magnitude of the above operations, continuous anticoagulation with its inherent risk of complications, and uncertain long-term results, open surgery has been offered only to patients with the most severe post-thrombotic symptoms. Strict criteria for selection, including severe disabling symptoms and markedly increased venous pressure levels, have been used. This has restricted the surgical treatment of limbs with suspected significant outflow obstruction to a minority of patients with chronic venous insufficiency.

ENDOVASCULAR SURGERY

The procedure involving percutaneous iliac venous balloon dilation and insertion of a stent has made it possible to correct pelvic and caval vein obstruction more safely with a less invasive alternative. Therefore, this procedure can be offered to a larger group of patients (Figs 21.8 and 21.9). Venous stenting has been used in the successful treatment of the following:

- remaining iliac vein stenosis after thrombolysis of acute deep vein thrombosis
- complete occlusion or partial obstruction in chronic post-thrombotic disease
- non-thrombotic chronic iliac vein compression syndrome
- malignant venous obstruction
- stenoses of other etiology.

There are few sizable series with acceptable follow-up reported in the literature and the majority of these have not differentiated between etiologies.

O'Sullivan *et al.*[41] reported a 1-year patency of 79 percent in a retrospective analysis of 39 patients. Only half of the patients were treated for chronic symptoms; the remainder presented

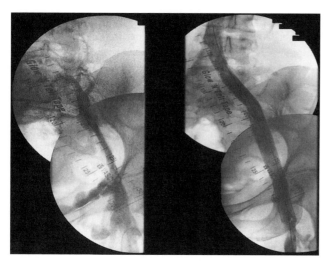

Figure 21.8 *Intraoperative transfemoral ascending phlebogram prior to balloon dilation and stenting in a patient with chronic thrombotic obstruction and filling of transpelvic collateral circulation (left). Repeat phlebogram following insertion of two overlapping stents placed well into the inferior vena cava (IVC) and covering the entire left iliac vein. There is an uninterrupted flow through the iliac vein to the IVC. No collateral circulation is visualized (right).*

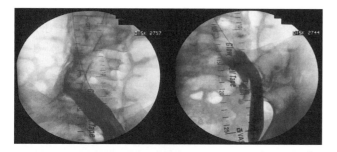

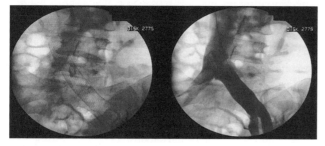

Figure 21.9 *Intraoperative transfemoral ascending phlebogram before (above) and after (below) balloon dilation and insertion of stent in a patient with non-thrombotic disease (iliac vein compression syndrome). The pre-stent translucent common iliac vein with poorly delineated stenosis is a typical finding.*

with acute DVT and were treated after successful thrombolysis. Excluding initial technical failures, the stented patients had a 1-year patency of 94 and 92 percent in the respective groups. The clinical results were excellent in the stented limbs.

A similar group of 18 patients were reported by Hurst et al.[20] Twelve limbs were treated for chronic obstruction. The primary patency rates at 12 and 18 months were 79 and 79 percent, respectively. Most patients (72 percent) had resolution or substantial improvement of leg swelling and pain. However, five remaining patients continued to have pain despite resolved swelling and widely patent stents on phlebogram.

Similarly, Binkert et al.[42] reported a 100 percent patency at an average follow-up time of 3 years in eight patients (in four limbs following surgical thrombectomy) with resolution or substantial improvement of symptoms in most patients.

In another group of patients, Nazarian et al.[43] reported a 1-year primary assisted patency rate of 66 percent of 29 iliac obstructions.[43] The lower patency rate may be explained by the selection of patients (13/29 had complete occlusion and 16/29 were caused by malignancy). Interestingly, few occlusions occurred after 6 months and the patency rate remained the same at 1- and 4-year follow-up. The same group has also reported overall 1-year primary and secondary patency rates of 50 and 81 percent, respectively, in a mixed population, including 56 patients with iliac obstruction caused by malignancy, trauma, pregnancy and postoperative stenosis.[44]

Our own experience includes more than 500 stented pelvic and caval veins in patients with chronic non-malignant occlusions with no pretreatment of acute DVT.[13,45,46] Our initial experience in 1996/1997 with stenting of 29 limbs resulted in substantial technical modifications.[45] These limbs have therefore been excluded from future analysis. The complication rate related to the endovascular intervention is minimal and comprises mostly cannulation site hematoma, but a small number of acquired arteriovenous fistulae when the canulation site is distal on the thigh has been observed and a few cases of retroperitoneal hematoma requiring blood transfusions have been described.[20,45] The utilization of ultrasound-guided canulation and closure of the canulation site with collagen plugs has largely abolished these problems. The mortality has been zero.

The follow-up of these patients is ongoing and final long-term results have not yet been acquired. Analysis of 455 limbs which underwent iliac vein stent deployment for correction of chronic iliac vein stenosis between December 1997 and July 2001 has, however, provided mid-term results.[46,47] The following is a summary of the available results. Patency rates as defined by reporting standards of the Society of Vascular Surgery/International Society of Cardiovascular Surgery (SVS/ISCVS),[48] frequency of in-stent restenosis, clinical results assessing pain, swelling, and ulcer healing, and limited quality-of-life data are available. The obstructive lesion was considered post-thrombotic when the patient had a known history of DVT or when post-thrombotic changes were found on phlebography or ultrasound at any level of the lower extremity (54 percent of limbs). The remaining limbs were considered non-thrombotic ('primary'). Cumulative primary and assisted-primary/secondary patency rates as per transfemoral phlebogram in 307 limbs at 3 years were 72 and 92 percent, respectively (Fig. 21.10). The stented limbs with 'primary' disease appeared to fare significantly better than those with

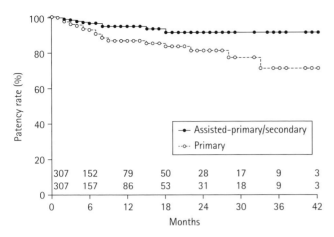

Figure 21.10 *Cumulative primary, assisted-primary and secondary patency rates of all stented limbs (n = 307). The lower numbers represent total limbs at risk for each time interval.*

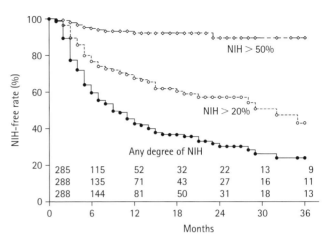

Figure 21.12 *Cumulative neointimal hyperplasia (NIH)-free rates for all limbs with any degree of NIH, and moderate (NIH > 20 percent) and severe (NIH > 50 percent) in-stent restenosis. The lower numbers represent total limbs at risk for each time interval.*

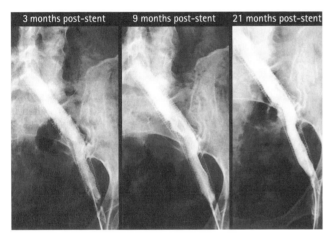

Figure 21.11 *In-stent restenosis 3–21 months after iliac vein stent insertion. Although observed already at 3 months, there seems to be no progress of the neointimal hyperplasia.*

post-thrombotic obstruction (primary and assisted-primary/secondary cumulative patency rates of 84 and 100 percent, and 73 and 86 percent at 30 months, respectively).[13,47] It appears that balloon dilation and stenting of an iliac vein obstruction is a safe, minimally invasive method with low complication rate, no mortality and acceptable patency in the mid-term.

Venous stent patency is, in general, dependent on many factors, including anatomic site, etiology of obstruction, concomitant venous disease and magnitude of inflow, presence of thrombophilia, and development of intimal hyperplasia (Fig. 21.11). Although some degree of neointimal hyperplasia is common (only 24 percent were completely hyperplasia-free after 3 years), severe in-stent restenosis, i.e., >50 percent diameter decrease on phlebography, is rare (only present in 11 percent at 3 years) (Fig. 21.12). It appears that severe in-stent restenosis (>50 percent stenosis) occurs in iliac venous stents at an annual rate of approximately 3 percent overall. The stented post-thrombotic obstructions have a higher annual rate

(6 percent) than non-thrombotic (1 percent). The rate of hyperplasia formation appears to level out after 12–18 months, after which the rate of hyperplasia development decreases substantially. Several factors, which may potentially influence the development of intra-stent hyperplasia, were analysed. A higher rate of in-stent restenosis occurs with treatment of thrombotic obstructions when the right limb is stented, in the presence of thrombophilia, and when long stents are inserted, especially when extended below the inguinal ligament. The gender of the patient, the original degree of stenosis or obtained luminal cross-cut area after stenting did not influence hyperplasia formation. The results suggested that in-stent restenosis may precede occlusion of stents in a small number of limbs, although other factors also contribute. All 11 limbs that subsequently occluded in this study were post-thrombotic with stent lengths >13 cm, and seven of the 11 limbs had stent placement below the inguinal ligament. At the time of the original balloon venoplasty and stenting, the iliac veins were completely occluded or had tight, non-yielding stenoses. Thus, these limbs appear to have the most extensive post-thrombotic disease and an additional cause of late occlusion may be recurrent attacks of thrombosis.

As alluded to above, the reports describing patency rates indicate clinical improvement in most patients (>90 percent).[41,42] Hurst *et al.*[20] showed resolution or substantial improvement in 72 percent of limbs. Since patients with chronic venous insufficiency may complain of varying symptoms, from mild swelling and diffuse discomfort to disabling pain, stasis dermatitis and ulcerations, we have not limited the clinical assessment to ulcer healing. The degree of swelling was also assessed by physical examination (grade 0, none; grade 1, pitting, not obvious; grade 2, ankle edema; grade 3, obvious swelling involving the limb), and the level of pain was measured by the visual analogue scale method.[49] The patient indicates the level of pain on a visual analogue scale (0–10) with the markings and numbers hidden to the patient but visible to the examiner. Recently, a number of quality-of-life questionnaires, validated for assessment of chronic venous insufficiency, have been introduced to assess the overall benefit of the interventions.[50] In this prospective evaluation of stented patients with iliac vein obstruction,[13,45,46] we found that the incidence of ulcer healing after iliac vein balloon dilation and stent placement in 41 limbs with active ulcer was 68 percent, and that the cumulative ulcer recurrence-free rate at 2 years was 62 percent.[46] During the observation period, no subsequent reflux procedure was performed in limbs when the ulcer stayed healed, despite frequently remaining reflux in these limbs. Median swelling and pain severity scores decreased significantly (grades 2 to 1 and 4 to 0, respectively). The rates of limbs completely free of any objective swelling increased significantly from 12 to 47 percent, and limbs completely free of any pain increased from 17 to 71 percent. The improvement of pain and swelling was significant in both ulcerated and non-ulcerated limbs, indicating that the ulcer was not the only cause of pain and swelling. The pre-intervention level of pain was similar in both groups, highlighting the important contribution of non-ulcer pain and swelling in limbs with iliac vein obstruction. Interestingly, patients with recurrence of obstruction also had recurrence of symptoms after a symptom-free period. These observations suggest that outflow obstruction is a more important and frequent component of CVI than previously recognized. Using a quality-of-life questionnaire assessing subjective pain, sleep disturbance, morale and social activities, routine and strenuous physical activities, the patients indicated significant improvement in all major categories after venous stenting. Thus, the clinical outcome is favourable in the mid-term. The results clearly indicate a significant symptom relief after dilation and stenting of iliac vein obstruction, even in the presence of remaining reflux.

Endovascular technique

Angioplasty with stenting of the venous system should be considered a different procedure from that in the arterial system. The detailed technique is described elsewhere.[13,41,45] Although venous balloon dilation and insertion of stents is a minimally invasive procedure, some important aspects should be emphasized:

- Stenting is advised in all cases. It has been shown that simple balloon dilation leads to early restenosis, and an immediate recoil of the iliac vein has been observed intraoperatively in the majority of limbs.[51–53]
- Use ultrasound to guide canulation of the femoral vein. This measure has largely eliminated access complications.
- IVUS is invaluable, both as a diagnostic tool and as an intraoperative tool to direct placement of the stent.
- Place the stent well into the IVC in stenosis close to the confluence of the common iliac veins. Otherwise the stent often appears to be 'squeezed' distally and a proximal restenosis may develop.[45] Although this IVC

placement raises concern for risk of occlusion of the contralateral limb, the stent does not appear to significantly impair the flow from the contralateral limb resulting in thrombosis. The few cases of contralateral limb DVT observed appear to be caused by recurrent attacks of thrombosis.

- Use of 'kissing' balloon technique at the confluence of the common iliac veins or insertion of bilateral stents is not necessary.
- A large stent (14–16 mm diameter) is recommended. The vein, unlike the artery, appears to accept extensive dilation without clinical rupture. To date, no clinical rupture of the vein has been reported, even when a total occlusion is recanalized and dilated up to 14–16 mm width.
- Re-dilate the stent after insertion to achieve a good wall apposition as evaluated by IVUS.
- Cover the entire obstruction as outlined by the IVUS investigation to decrease the risk of restenosis. Short skip areas between two stents should be avoided. The occlusion rate does not appear to be related to the length of stent or metal load *per se*, but to incomplete treatment or other factors.

The perioperative thrombosis prophylaxis was standardized in all patients. The patient received 2500 units of dalteparin subcutaneously preoperatively. During the procedure, 5000 units heparin and 30 mg ketorolac were administered intravenously. All patients were admitted for less than 23 h. Postoperatively, a foot compression device was applied, dalteparin (2500 units) was administered subcutaneously twice daily, and a ketorolac injection was repeated in the morning before discharge. Low-dose aspirin (81 mg p.o.) daily was started immediately postoperatively and continued. Most patients did not have additional anticoagulation. Only patients already on warfarin preoperatively were anticoagulated postoperatively. These were a minority of patients with prior recurrent DVT and/or thrombophilia, which made lifelong anticoagulation necessary. Warfarin was not routinely discontinued prior to surgery. If it had been, dalteparin (5000 units) was injected subcutaneously during the days warfarin had been discontinued.

SUMMARY

Interest in venous outflow obstruction is increasing with the emergence of practical treatment alternatives. The lack of accurate, objective non-invasive or invasive tests for evaluation of hemodynamically significant obstruction makes the selection of patients difficult. At present, patients must be selected on the basis of clinical signs and symptoms with a high index of suspicion, and final diagnosis and treatment must be based on morphological investigations. Transfemoral phlebography (multi-plane, if possible) or, preferably, IVUS should probably be utilized more generously in the work-up of patients with significant signs and symptoms of CVI, especially in patients with leg ulcer.

Mid-term evaluation indicates that venous balloon angioplasty and stenting is a safe, relatively simple and efficient method for the treatment of iliocaval vein obstruction. An immediate or late failure of the procedure does not preclude later open surgery to correct the obstruction. Associated reflux may be controlled subsequently when necessary. Open bypass surgery should probably be reserved for those patients in whom stenting initially could not be performed for technical reasons, late failures which cannot be adequately disobliterated, and long total occlusions, which appear to have a poorer result.

Although venous stenting appears to be a promising treatment, some caveats are necessary. The technology is relatively recent; thus the follow-up period is limited. The long-term effects of stents in the venous system are not fully known. Monitoring for several more years is required to assess the efficacy and safety of this therapeutic modality in venous disease. In addition, further research on understanding the nature of venous obstruction and development of reliable methods to test hemodynamic consequences are sorely needed.

REFERENCES

1. Johnson BF, Manzo RA, Bergelin RO *et al.* Relationship between changes in the deep venous system and the development of the post–thrombotic syndrome after an acute episode of lower limb deep vein thrombosis: a one- to six-year follow-up. *J Vasc Surg* 1995; **21**: 307–12.

2. Johnson BF, Manzo RA, Bergelin RO *et al.* The site of residual abnormalities in the leg veins in long-term follow-up after deep vein thrombosis and their relationship to the development of the post–thrombotic syndrome. *Int Angiol* 1996; **15**: 14–9.

3. Nicolaides AN, Hussein MK, Szendro G *et al.* The relation of venous ulceration with ambulatory venous pressure measurements. *J Vasc Surg* 1993; **17**: 414–9.

4. Nicolaides AN, Summer DS. *Investigation of Patients with Deep Vein Thrombosis and Chronic Venous Insufficiency.* Los Angeles: Medical-Orion, 1991.

5. May R. Anatomy. In: May R, Nissl R, eds. *Surgery of the Veins of the Leg and Pelvis.* Stuttgart, Germany: Georg Thieme Verlag, 1979; 1–36.

6. Mavor GE, Galloway JM. Collaterals of the deep venous circulation of the lower limb. *Surg Gynaecol Obstet* 1967; **125**: 561–71.

7. Kosinski C. Observations on the superficial venous system of the lower extermity. *J Anat* 1926; **60**: 131–42.

8. Mavor GE, Galloway JM. Iliofemoral venous thrombosis: pathological considerations and surgical management. *Br J Surg* 1969; **56**: 45–59.

9. Plate G, Åkesson H, Einarsson E *et al.* Long-term results of venous thrombectomy combined with a temporary arterio-venous fistula. *Eur J Vasc Surg* 1990; **4**: 483–9.

10. May R, Thurner J. The cause of the predominantly sinistral occurrence of thrombosis of the pelvic veins. *Angiology* 1957; **8**: 419–28.

11. Cockett FB, Thomas ML. The iliac compression syndrome. *Br J Surg* 1965; **52**: 816–21.

12. Negus D, Fletcher EWL, Cockett FB, Thomas ML. Compression and band formation at the mouth of the left common iliac vein. *Br J Surg* 1968; **55**: 369–74.

13. Neglén P, Berry MA, Raju S. Endovascular surgery in the treatment of chronic primary and post-thrombotic iliac vein obstruction. *Eur J Vasc Endovasc Surg* 2000; **20**: 560–71.

14. Cockett FB, Lea Thomas M, Negus D. Iliac vein compression – its relation to iliofemoral thrombosis and the post–thrombotic syndrome. *Br J Surg* 1967; **2**: 14–9.

15. The effect of geometry on the arterial blood flow. In: Strandness DE, Sumner DS. *Hemodynamics for Surgeons.* New York: Grune & Stratton, 1975; 96–119.

16. Raju S. New approaches to the diagnosis and treatment of venous obstruction. *J Vasc Surg* 1986; **4**: 42–54.

17. Illig KA, Ouriel K, Deweese JA *et al.* Increasing the sensitivity of the diagnosis of chronic venous obstruction. (Letter to the editor.) *J Vasc Surg* 1995; **24**: 176–8.

18. Neglén P, Raju S. Detection of outflow obstruction in chronic venous insufficiency. *J Vasc Surg* 1993; **17**: 583–9.

19. Labropoulos N, Volteas N *et al.* The role of venous outflow obstruction in patients with chronic venous dysfunction. *Arch Surg* 1997; **132**: 46–51.

20. Hurst DR, Forauer AR, Bloom JR *et al.* Diagnosis and endovascular treatment of iliocaval compression syndrome. *J Vasc Surg* 2001; **34**: 106–13.

21. Raju S. A pressure-based technique for the detection of acute and chronic venous obstruction. *Phlebology* 1988; **3**: 207–16.

22. Nicolaides AN. Outflow obstruction. In: Nicolaides AN, Sumner DS, eds. *Investigations of Patients with Deep Vein Thrombosis and Chronic Venous Insufficiency.* London: Medical-Orion, 1991; 56–62.

23. Raju S, Fredericks R. Venous obstruction: an analysis of one hundred thirty-seven cases with hemodynamic, venographic, and clinical correlations. *J Vasc Surg* 1991; **14**: 305–13.

24. Negus D, Cockett FB. Femoral vein pressures in post-phlebitic iliac vein obstruction. *Br J Surg* 1967; **54**: 522–5.

25. Rigas A, Vomvoyannis A, Giannoulis K *et al.* Measurement of the femoral vein pressure on edema of the lower extremity. *J Cardiovasc Surg* 1971; **12**: 411–6.

26. Albrechtsson U, Einarsson E, Eklöf B. Femoral vein pressure measurements for evaluation of venous function in patients with post-thrombotic iliac veins. *Cardiovasc Intervent Radiol* 1981; **4**: 43–50.

27. Neglén P, Raju S. Intravascular ultrasound scan evaluation of the obstructed vein. *J Vasc Surg* 2002; **35**: 694–700.

28. Satokawa H, Hoshino S, Iwaya F *et al.* Intravascular imaging methods for venous disorders. *In J Angiol* 2000; **9**: 117–21.

29. Forauer AR, Gemmete JJ, Dasika NL *et al.* Intravascular ultrasound in the diagnosis and treatment of iliac vein compression (May–Thurner) syndrome. *J Vasc Interven Radiol* 2002; **13**: 523–37.

30. Taheri SA, Taheri PA, Schultz RO *et al.* Iliocaval compression syndrome. *Contemp Surg* 1992; **40**: 9–15.

31. Husni EA. Clinical experience with femoropopliteal venous reconstruction. In: Bergan JJ, Yao JST, eds. *Venous Problems.* Chicago: Yearbook Medical Publishers, 1978; 485–91.

32. Hutschenreiter S, Vollmar J, Leoprecht H *et al.* Rekonstruktive Eingriffe am Venensystem; Spatergebnisse unter Kritischer Bewertung funtioneller und gefassmorphologischet Kriterien. *Chirurgie* 1979; **50**: 555–63.

33. Halliday P, Harris J, May J. Femoro-femoral crossover grafts (Palma operation): a long-term follow-up study. In: Bergan JJ, Yao JST, eds. *Surgery of the Veins.* Orlando: Grune & Stratton, 1985; 241–54.

34. O'Donell TF Jr, Mackey WC, Shepard AD, Callow AD. Clinical, hemodynamic and anatomic follow-up of direct venous reconstruction. *Arch Surg* 1987; **122**: 474–82.

35. Danza R, Navarro T, Baldozan J. Reconstructive surgery in chronic venous obstruction of the lower limbs. *J Cardiovasc Surg* 1991; **32**: 98–103.

36. Aburahma AF, Robinson PA, Boland JP. Clinical, hemodynamic and anatomic predictors of long-term outcome of lower extremities venovenous bypasses. *J Vasc Surg* 1991; **19**: 635–44.

37. Gruss JD. Venous bypass for chronic venous insufficiency. In: Bergan JJ, Yao JST, eds. *Venous Disorders*. Philadelphia: WB Saunders, 1991; 316–30.

38. Corey JJ, Gloviczki P, Cherry KJ Jr *et al*. Surgical reconstruction of iliofemoral veins and the inferior vena cava for nonmalignant occlusive disease. *J Vasc Surg* 2001; **33**: 320–8.

39. Lalka SG, Lash JM, Unthank JL *et al*. Inadequacy of saphenous vein grafts for cross-femoral venous bypass. *J Vasc Surg* 1991; **13**: 622–30.

40. Frileux C, Pillot-Bienayme P, Gillot C. Bypass of segmental obliteration of ilio-femoral venous axis by transposition of saphenous vein. *J Cardiovasc Surg* 1972; **13**: 409–14.

41. O'Sullivan GJ, Semba CP, Bittner CA *et al*. Endovascular management of iliac vein compression (May–Thurner) syndrome. *J Vasc Interv Radiol* 2000; **11**: 823–36.

42. Binkert CA, Schoch E, Stuckmann G *et al*. Treatment of pelvic venous spur (May–Thurner syndrome) with self-expanding metallic endoprostheses. *Cardiovasc Intervent Radiol* 1998; **21**: 22–6.

43. Nazarian GK, Austin WR, Wegryn SA *et al*. Venous recanalization by metallic stents after failure of balloon angioplasty or surgery: four-year experience. *Cardiovasc Intervent Radiol* 1996; **19**: 227–33.

44. Nazarian GK, Bjarnason H, Dietz CA Jr *et al*. Iliofemoral venous stenosis: effectiveness of treatment with metallic endovascular stents. *Radiology* 1996; **200**: 193–9.

45. Neglén P, Raju S. Balloon dilation and stenting of chronic iliac vein obstruction. Technical aspects and early clinical outcome. *J Endovasc Ther* 2000; **7**: 79–91.

46. Raju S, Owen S Jr, Neglén P. The clinical impact of iliac venous stents in the management of chronic venous insufficiency. *J Vasc Surg* 2002; **35**: 8–15.

47. Neglén P, Raju S. In-stent recurrent stenosis in stents placed in the lower extremity venous outflow tract. *J Vasc Surg* 2004; **39**: 181–8.

48. Porter JM, Moneta GL. Reporting standards in venous disease: an update. International Consensus Committee on Chronic Venous Disease. *J Vasc Surg* 1995; **21**: 635–45.

49. Scott J, Huskisson EC. Graphic presentation of pain. *Pain* 1976; **2**: 175–84.

50. Launois R, Rebpi-Marty J, Henry B. Construction and validation of a quality of life questionnaire in chronic lower limb venous insufficiency (CIVIQ). *Qual Life Res* 1996; **5**: 539–54.

51. Neglén P, Al-Hassan HKH, Endrys J *et al*. Iliofemoral venous thrombectomy followed by percutaneous closure of the temporary arteriovenous fistula. *Surgery* 1991; **110**: 493–9.

52. Wisselink W, Money SR, Becker MO *et al*. Comparison of operative reconstruction and percutaneous balloon dilatation for central venous obstruction. *Am J Surg* 1993; **166**: 200–5.

53. Marzo KP, Schwartz R, Glanz S. Early restenosis following percutaneous transluminal balloon angioplasty for the treatment of the superior vena caval syndrome due to pacemaker-induced stenosis. *Cathet Cardiovasc Diagn* 1995; **36**: 128–31.

22

The treatment of ischemic ulceration

PETER R. TAYLOR, DAVID NEGUS

Ischemic ulcers may result from small-vessel disease, atherosclerotic occlusion of the main limb arteries, or a combination of both. Vasculitic ulcers are described in Chapter 8 (p. 68).

Many patients with ischemic ulceration arrive in the clinic with a letter requesting treatment of an intractable 'venous ulcer' and with tight bandages conscientiously applied by a district nurse. It is obviously important that these are removed and replaced by light crepe bandages. An appropriately tactful letter then has to be composed to the general practitioner and his hardworking nurses to avoid repetition of tight compression.

It is important to differentiate between critical limb ischemia and subcritical limb ischemia. Patients with critical limb ischemia usually have extensive tissue loss, multi-level arterial disease and ankle pressures that are 40 mmHg or less, and have a high rate of amputation of greater than 50 percent at 1 year. Adjunctive techniques in these patients are probably of little value, and arterial reconstruction, with both endovascular techniques and surgery is the treatment of choice. There is a group of patients with subcritical limb ischemia with limited tissue loss, single-level arterial disease, with pressures of 50 mmHg or above who have a low rate of amputation (<50 percent at 12 months) and who are likely to benefit both from adjunctive techniques and from arterial procedures, both endovascular and surgical. The measurement of ankle pressures is therefore paramount in the initial assessment of patients presenting with ulceration.

The first line of investigation is duplex scanning of the arteries to the limb. This non-invasive test can identify occlusions and stenoses and allows any subsequent intervention to be planned. Those suitable for angioplasty can be dealt with radiologically, while the others can be treated by other modalities. The mainstay of investigation continues to be arteriography, but magnetic resonance angiography has also proved to be useful in detecting patent distal vessels suitable for bypass. Magnetic resonance imaging is also useful to identify the extent of any tissue gangrene. As many of these patients are very old and unfit for direct arterial surgery, it is often more sensible to try to obtain ulcer healing by conservative measures before proceeding to invasive investigations.

Patients with a palpable popliteal pulse, even those sufficiently young and fit for surgical treatment, are unlikely to be suitable for direct arterial surgery but may respond favourably to chemical lumbar sympathectomy or prostanoid treatment followed by skin grafting. However, improvements in distal bypass grafting, with the use of vein cuffs, have improved the results in these cases.

It is often thought that the presence of one ankle pulse indicates adequate blood supply to the foot and ankle so that any ulceration is unlikely to be ischemic in origin. This is a dangerous assumption and the authors have experience of three patients who presented with supramalleolar ulceration, apparently of venous origin. In each case, only one ankle or foot pulse could be felt or detected by Doppler ultrasound, and examination and further investigation showed no evidence of venous disorder. These patients' ulcers all healed following chemical lumbar sympathectomy.

CONSERVATIVE TREATMENT

Bed rest, dressings and antibiotics

Bed rest and good nursing in hospital, with daily dressings and appropriate antibiotics for infected ulcers, will often effect remarkable improvement, particularly in the elderly and those on low income and in poor housing. Dressings should consist of one layer of non-adhesive dry dressing covered by absorbent cotton gauze and kept in place by a lightly applied crepe bandage. Hydrocolloid dressings, such as Granuflex (Convatec, Uxbridge, UK), are a suitable and comfortable alternative. Elevating the head of the bed may assist blood flow to the foot, but in the elderly this can result in unacceptable edema and require a return to the horizontal position. Appropriate antibiotics should be prescribed after obtaining a swab result. Warm conditions and good food undoubtedly assist healing. Cigarette smoking must be stopped.

Drug treatment

Several drugs have been tried to improve leg ulceration. Previously, vasodilators were tried but proved useless. More recently, drugs affecting the microcirculation have been prescribed. These compounds reduce cell aggregation and adhesion, and may cause vasodilatation of the microcirculation. In a small placebo-controlled trial in critical limb ischemia, naftidrofuryl did no better than the placebo.[1] Pentoxifylline has been shown to have only a small effect on rest pain when it was investigated in placebo-controlled trials.[2,3] L-Arginine is the precursor of nitric oxide which inhibits platelet aggregation and causes vasodilatation; however, no long-term effect has yet been proven with infusions of this compound.[4] Finally gene therapy may, in future, prove to be useful in patients with ulceration. A clinical study of nine patients using gene transfer of vascular endothelium showed new collaterals developing with healing of ischemic ulcers in four out of seven limbs; however, this technique awaits confirmation in large clinical trials.[5]

THE PROSTANOIDS

The effectiveness of prostacyclin (epoprostenol, Flolan; GlaxoSmithKline, Uxbridge, UK) in the treatment of ischemic ulcers was first demonstrated by Szczeklik et al.[6] in 1979. In this series, prostacyclin was given by femoral artery cannulation. In a double-blind controlled trial, 14 patients were randomized to receive a 72-h intra-arterial infusion of prostacyclin dissolved in glycine buffer and 16 control patients received glycine buffer alone. The starting dose of prostacyclin was 2.5 ng/kg per min, increasing over 3 h to 5 ng/kg per min. Patients were assessed before treatment and at 24 h, and 4 and 6 weeks after infusion. By the sixth week, seven out of 21 initial ulcers were healed in the prostacyclin-treated group, whereas in the placebo group the number of ulcers had increased from 29 to 30. At the beginning of the trial, there was no difference in mean ulcer area between the two groups, but at its end the area was significantly smaller in the prostacyclin group. By the sixth week the mean ulcer area decreased in the prostacyclin group but not in the placebo group. Prentice et al.[7] have demonstrated the effectiveness of intravenous prostacyclin in patients with severe arterial disease

causing ischemic rest pain. Prostacyclin (PGI_2) is a strong vasodilator and antiplatelet agent which prevents the activation of platelets and their interaction with white blood cells. It also inhibits the release of platelet-derived growth factor and therefore has a negative effect on myointimal hyperplasia. The relatively short half-life of only 2–3 min has limited the use of prostacyclin in the clinical setting. Iloprost (Schering, Berlin, Germany) is a stable synthetic prostacyclin analogue which has a prolonged half-life of 30 min. A meta-analysis of randomized clinical series comparing iloprost and placebo in the treatment of 705 patients with critical limb ischemia with Fontaine stages III and IV disease has been published.[8] There was a significant decrease in amputation rate with iloprost (35 percent compared with 55 percent in the placebo group), and patients were significantly more likely to be alive with both legs at 6 months with iloprost.

The complications of prostanoid therapy are hypotension and flushing. It is our policy to start the infusion at 6 ng/kg per min and then cautiously increase by steps up to a maximum of 10 ng/kg per min.[7] Hourly blood pressure measurements are recorded and the nursing staff are particularly asked to look out for flushing. Should either hypotension or flushing occur, the infusion pump is immediately turned down. In a 5-year experience of this form of treatment, we have not encountered any serious complications, although a few patients are completely unable to tolerate intravenous prostanoid therapy. Most patients have been relieved of rest pain and many ulcers have reduced in size, although no precise follow-up figures are available at present. It is now our policy to give infusions intermittently, for 12 in each 24 h, for a total of 4 or 5 days. If there is no improvement in rest pain after the first 24 h, the infusion is stopped. If there is definite improvement in rest pain and some diminution in ulcer size at the end of 5 days' treatment, skin grafting is performed on the next available operating list. A further course of prostanoid is started at operation and continued for the first 3 or 4 postoperative days in order to help the graft to take.

There are no definite guidelines to indicate which ischemic ulcers are likely to respond to prostanoid therapy, although our experience in treating patients with severe ischemic rest pain has indicated that those with diabetes and those with an ankle:brachial pulse pressure index of less than 0.3 are unlikely to respond.[9] These contraindications are, of course, the same as those for lumbar sympathectomy, as might be expected from the similarity of action of the two vasodilator methods. It seems reasonable to try the effect of a short course of intravenous prostanoid on all patients with ischemic ulceration whose arteries are unsuitable for surgical reconstruction (apart, of course, from those mentioned above), or where the patient has failed to produce an adequate response. Theoretically, prostanoid should produce no further improvement in a patient who has undergone lumbar sympathectomy, but in practice we have sometimes found it useful. Treatment with prostanoids such as PGI_2 and iloprost can make a definite but modest improvement in patients with ulceration, but their effect cannot be predicted and their use is often reserved for those who are unfit or unsuitable for surgical reconstruction.

Lumbar sympathectomy

Lumbar sympathectomy has been demonstrated to produce a 10 percent increase in capillary skin blood flow[10] and, in one series, was demonstrated to relieve ischemic rest pain in 83 percent of 36 patients and to heal 50 percent of 52 trophic lesions.[11] However, some very poor results have also been recorded in the literature.[12]

Chemical lumbar sympathectomy, by the injection of phenol in water around the lumbar sympathetic chain, with the help of image intensifier radiography, is less traumatic than the operative procedure and it has been suggested that its effects are more durable than those obtained by surgical denervation.[13] Chemical sympathectomy has the additional advantage of avoiding the need for admission to hospital. Sympathectomy is usually ineffectual in patients with an ankle:brachial index less than 0.3. It is also usually ineffectual in patients with diabetes. It is most important to establish that the ulcer is truly ischemic before recommending sympathectomy. Linton[14] described 'serious post-sympathectomy complications' in some patients with the post-thrombotic syndrome who were treated by lumbar sympathectomy.

Spinal cord stimulation

Electrical stimulation of the posterior parts of the spinal cord was shown to have beneficial effects in patients with ulceration and rest pain in 1976.[15] The exact mechanism for the beneficial effect of spinal cord stimulation is still unknown, but there are many hypotheses, including the activation of fibres which in turn block the stimuli from pain pathways, the inhibition of sympathetic impulses to peripheral vessels and finally the release of vasoactive substances resulting in vasodilatation. The Dutch multicentre randomized controlled trial of 120 patients with non-reconstructable critical limb ischemia showed that, although spinal cord stimulation was associated with higher rates of limb salvage, this was not significantly different from the control group, and there was no difference in ulcer healing.[16] Further analysis showed that spinal cord stimulation was much more expensive due to the cost of the stimulator and its implantation compared with the control group.

This technique is only indicated in patients with no arterial reconstructive option, and expertise is essential for successful implantation.

ARTERIAL RECONSTRUCTION OF THE LOWER LIMB

Patients with lower limb ulceration and weak or absent leg pulses should be investigated by arteriography. This can now be performed as an outpatient procedure, using a 3 Fr gauge catheter (cross-sectional diameter 1 mm), using digital subtraction angiography. The films should then be reviewed by a team of surgeons and radiologists to decide on the best course of action. Many arterial lesions are suitable for radiological intervention, either alone or in conjunction with a surgical procedure. This team approach is paramount in the treatment of arterial problems. Radiologists may be more willing to undertake balloon angioplasty of unfavourable lesions (e.g. long occlusions in distal vessels) if they can be assured that these are salvage procedures, and that surgery would be undertaken if they fail.

Operative technique: general principles

Arteries are very unforgiving and poor operative technique may jeopardize the outcome of reconstructive surgery. It is imperative that there is adequate exposure of the relevant arteries. The body should be dissected from the artery to avoid damaging it during mobilization. Intravenous heparin should be given before the application of arterial clamps, which should be well away from the extent of the subsequent arteriotomy. When suturing, the needle should be passed from the inside to the outside of the artery along the curve of the needle. If calcified plaques are encountered, the surgeon should be beware of performing an endarterectomy, as this can sometimes lead to a very aggressive neointimal hyperplasia which may rapidly cause graft occlusion. By juggling the needle, a soft part of the arterial wall can usually be found. Strong taper-pointed needles can be passed through many plaques without fracturing the intima. All arterial anastomoses should be performed to evert the edges. It is important not to damage the arterial wall by crushing it with dissecting forceps. These can be used either to hold the adventitia only, to open up the arteriotomy, or both blades can be passed into the artery and opened up to display the lumen of the artery. If vein is used as a graft, very small bites should be taken with the needle inserted about 2 mm from the edge so as not to narrow the anastomosis. Vein is much stronger than diseased artery in its ability to hold sutures. It is also important that large quantities of venous adventitia are not included in the suture line as this can also distort the graft and lead to narrowing.

Accuracy is of paramount importance at both the heel and toe of any arterial anastomosis, and by using the parachute technique all sutures at the heel may be placed under direct vision. Some surgeons also place interrupted sutures at the toe of the anastomosis in order to achieve accurate placement and also because of theoretical advantages in terms of compliance.

Infection is a much-feared complication following prosthetic graft insertion. All grafts should be kept in their packaging until just before use. All patients should be given prophylactic antibiotics, and the authors always cover the skin with a Steridrape (3M, Bracknell, UK) to reduce the chances of contamination by skin organisms.

Vein should always be used as the first choice of conduit below the inguinal ligament. If vein is not available, the choice of graft is one of personal preference. Polytetrafluoroethylene (PTFE) with or without a vein cuff is the authors' choice. The human umbilical vein graft is an alternative, as are the newer polyurethane grafts. Above the inguinal ligament, Dacron for grafts of 10 mm or greater in diameter and PTFE for grafts of 8 mm or less are recommended.

The main risk to the patient during operations to increase the amount of arterial inflow to the leg is death from myocardial ischemia. Left ventricular function should be assessed by a cardiologist before surgery if the condition of the leg allows sufficient time for this.

Aortic occlusion

The aorta usually occludes just below the level of the renal arteries. If the patient is fit with good left ventricular function, the best solution is to perform an aortic endarterectomy. The authors use a transperitoneal approach to the aorta via a midline incision. The aorta is dissected on each side at the level of the renal vein so that a vertical clamp (such as a Glover's endarterectomy clamp) can be applied from front to back. After heparin is given, the clamp is positioned just below the renal arteries but not closed. The aorta is opened via a longitudinal arteriotomy and a plane established between the friable atheromatous debris on the inside and the aortic wall outside. This plane is continued circumferentially and the atheroma removed. The plane of dissection is then developed proximally towards the renal arteries. Great care must be taken not to send any debris into the renal arteries; usually the loosened atheroma is expelled like a champagne cork followed by a gush of blood. The clamp is quickly closed to regain control. Some surgeons like to control the aorta proximal to the renal arteries during this phase of the dissection, in order to prevent debris entering the renal arteries – this can more easily be achieved by a retroperitoneal approach to the suprarenal aorta. When good proximal flow has been achieved, all the remaining loose debris is removed from the aorta using a small wet swab to abrade the luminal surface together with saline flushed from a syringe. Usually the common iliac arteries are also occluded and therefore a bypass graft has to be inserted from the aortic arteriotomy to patent distal arteries. It is important to perfuse at least one internal iliac artery in order to prevent colonic ischemia. If there is a patent iliac artery, either common iliac or external iliac, this should be used in preference to the femoral arteries. Dissection of the groin, although quick and easy to perform, is associated with a much higher incidence of graft infection. The distal anastomoses may therefore be end-to-end to the junction of the internal and external iliac arteries, end-to-side to the external iliac arteries, or end-to-side to either the common or profunda femoral arteries (Fig. 22.1). If the whole operation is performed within the abdomen, no drains should be used, and great care should be taken to cover the graft with peritoneum

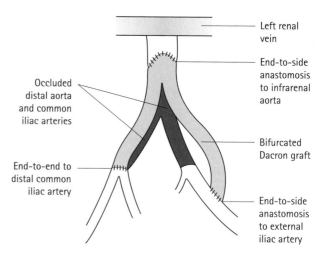

Figure 22.1   *Aorto bi-iliac graft.*

Labels: Left renal vein; End-to-side anastomosis to infrarenal aorta; Occluded distal aorta and common iliac arteries; Bifurcated Dacron graft; End-to-end to distal common iliac artery; End-to-side anastomosis to external iliac artery

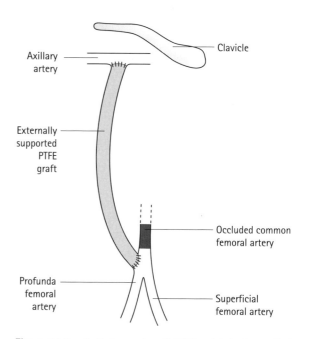

Figure 22.2   *Axillofemoral graft. PTFE, polytetrafluoroethylene.*

Labels: Clavicle; Axillary artery; Externally supported PTFE graft; Occluded common femoral artery; Profunda femoral artery; Superficial femoral artery

in order to reduce the chances of subsequent graft infection from adherence of bowel to the graft. Patency rates for aortic grafts are excellent, 80–90 percent being open at 5 years and 60–80 percent at 10 years.

If the patient is unfit, or very obese, an axillofemoral (Fig. 22.2) or axillobifemoral graft may be used in order to bypass an occluded aorta. The axillary artery is approached by making a horizontal incision 2 cm below the clavicle. The fibres of pectoralis major are split to reveal pectoralis minor. This is divided close to its insertion into the coracoid process of the scapula if required. Careful dissection will reveal the axillary vein and this is gently pushed inferiorly to show the axillary artery. Several branches can be controlled with large ties passed twice underneath the vessel to form a double loop around it. The femoral vessels can be approached either via a longitudinal incision placed over the artery or by a skin crease incision placed 2 cm above the groin crease. The latter heals well, but the longitudinal incision allows better access to the distal vessels when atheromatous disease is extensive.

Dissection of the distal profunda femoral artery frequently needs to be performed in arterial reconstructions and branches of the profunda veins may need to be divided in order to display an adequate length of artery. A tunnelling device is used to pass the graft beneath pectoralis major, keeping posteriorly as the rib margin is crossed, to lie medial to the anterior iliac crest. Passage of the tunneller from the axillary to the femoral wound will ensure that it lies below the pectoralis major and will avoid the potentially disastrous consequence of passing the tunneller beneath the costal margin.

Once the graft has been passed, and blood taken to preclot the graft if a knitted Dacron graft is used, heparin is given. We prefer to use either an externally supported PTFE graft or an externally supported impregnated knitted Dacron graft in order to decrease the chances of occlusion if the patient happens to fall asleep on the side of the graft, or if a tight belt is worn. In general, blood should not be let into the graft until all anastomoses have been completed, to minimize the risk of clot forming within the lumen. Good venting of both the forward and back flow is essential before the sutures are finally tied.

Suction drains are used for each anastomosis; the deeper layers are closed with absorbable suture material and the skin with an absorbable subcuticular suture.

Iliac occlusion

A unilateral iliac occlusion can be bypassed by one of the following:

An ipsilateral graft from either the aorta or common iliac artery, to the patent distal vessel, usually the common femoral artery or the profunda femoral artery.

An iliofemoral crossover graft (Fig. 22.3) This is commonly performed in association with balloon angioplasty of the proximal donor iliac artery. The external iliac artery on the donor side is approached retroperitoneally via a skin crease incision 2 cm above the inguinal ligament. The external and internal oblique muscles are split in line with their fibres, and the transversus abdominus muscle is divided laterally to avoid opening the peritoneum, which is more firmly adherent medially. An extraperitoneal plane is developed inferiorly to expose the external iliac artery lying medial to the psoas muscle. The artery is controlled by slings. The ureter is readily identified and preserved.

The common iliac artery can also be exposed via this approach, although it is wise to use a slightly higher skin incision. The femoral artery is dissected as previously described and a tunnel is developed anterior to the bladder behind the rectus abdominus muscles. The distal part of the tunnel is begun beneath the inguinal ligament and the graft is brought through using sponge-holding forceps. The author usually uses a 6 or 8 mm PTFE graft for this operation.

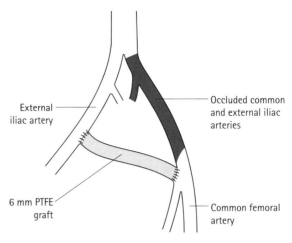

Figure 22.3 *Iliofemoral crossover graft. PTFE, polytetrafluoroethylene.*

The advantage of using the external iliac artery for the origin of the graft is that the femoral artery on that side may be used for further radiological interventions. A second potential advantage is the passage of the graft deep to the rectus muscles where it is protected from compression likely to precipitate thrombosis.

Femorofemoral graft The femoral arteries are exposed and a tunnel is developed anterior to the inguinal ligament crossing the pubic bone anterior to the rectus muscles. This is a very quick and easy approach, and despite the theoretical disadvantage of retrograde flow in the proximal segment of the graft, some authors claim a superior patency rate over the iliofemoral crossover graft.

Axillofemoral graft This has already been discussed in the section on 'Aortic occlusion'.

The patency rates for iliofemoral and femorofemoral crossover grafts vary from 60 percent to 82 percent at 5 years.

Femoral artery occlusion

COMMON FEMORAL ARTERY OCCLUSION

Usually the external iliac artery is patent, as is the profunda femoral artery. A long arteriotomy is performed and an endarterectomy of the occluded artery is covered by a vein patch.

SUPERFICIAL FEMORAL ARTERY OCCLUSION

The common femoral artery is exposed and a decision made as to the choice of graft. Some authors feel that, as the results of above-knee synthetic grafts are as good as vein grafts, the great saphenous vein should be preserved for more distal grafts or for coronary artery reconstruction. A synthetic graft must be used if no vein is available, such as when the saphenous vein has previously been stripped or if it is too small and there is no arm vein available.

Femoropopliteal bypass

THE SYNTHETIC GRAFT

A 6 mm PTFE graft is usually used. The distal incision should be made on the medial aspect of the lower third of the thigh, well anterior to the course of the long saphenous vein so as to avoid damage to it. The dissection is continued anterior to the sartorius muscle, and the popliteal fossa is opened. The artery is easily identified by following its branches back to the parent vessel. A direct anastomosis is performed between the graft and the artery and the proximal end of the graft is sutured to the common femoral artery.

Synthetic grafts should be avoided in the presence of ulceration or ischemic necrosis as there is a real risk of graft infection. If a suitable vein cannot be found, it is wise to excise the ulcer and necrotic tissue down to deep fascia and cover the defect with antiseptic dressings. Following a 3- or 4-day course of antibiotics, arterial grafting is carried out, still covered by antibiotics, and skin grafts are later applied to the excised area when an adequate blood supply has been restored.

VEIN GRAFTING

If saphenous vein is used, the upper incision should be placed over the vein and the great saphenous vein identified at its junction with the femoral vein. The incision is then continued distally under direct vision, over the course of the vein in order to minimize the chances of undermining the skin flaps. The vein is exposed to well below the site of the distal anastomosis to ensure adequate length. A decision is then made as to whether the vein is to be reversed or kept *in situ*. If the vein is the same diameter throughout its length, it is better to reverse it. If there is a significant size discrepancy, an *in situ* graft should be used.

The reversed saphenous vein graft

If reversed, all tributaries are ligated in continuity and divided. Care must be taken not to tie the branches too close to the vein, as this can lead to narrowing. Too great a length of tributary may allow thrombus to build up. Therefore, the tributary is usually ligated 1–2 mm from the vein wall. It is not usually critical to fully dissect the saphenofemoral junction when the vein is reversed.

The *in situ* saphenous vein graft

Complete and careful dissection of the saphenofemoral junction is imperative in an *in situ* bypass. All tributaries must be found and ligated. The first and last 5–10 cm of vein should have the tributaries ligated in continuity and divided in order to allow natural movement to facilitate the arterial anastomosis. After giving intravenous heparin, an arterial clamp is applied to the saphenofemoral junction deep enough on the main femoral vein to ensure the almost total preservation of the great saphenous vein. The junction is then divided, and the venotomy closed with continuous prolene. The most proximal valve is usually visible after the venotomy is lengthened, and this should be excised under direct vision. The vein is then anastomosed to the common femoral artery and blood is allowed into the graft. This expands the vein to the first competent valve. A valvulotome is then passed proximally to this valve; great care should be taken not to allow this to snag on the anastomotic suture. The valves are destroyed by the valvulotome, using the pressure of the arterial inflow to avoid too much damage to the vein wall as the instrument is gently maneuvered distally. Blood flow in the graft is then assessed and should be greater than 120 mL/min, and the distal anastomosis is then performed. It is wise to undertake some form of intraoperative monitoring. Flow within the graft can be assessed by Doppler ultrasonography, and on-table duplex scanning is becoming more popular. On-table angiography is routinely used in some centres for more distal grafts. If the *in situ* technique is used, Doppler ultrasound may identify significant patent side branches which should be ligated. It can also show areas of narrowing related to retained valve cusps which should be dealt with on the table.

Popliteal artery occlusion

Occlusion of the popliteal artery above the knee should be bypassed using a graft from the nearest normal proximal arterial segment. This may be the superficial femoral artery, but more frequently is the common femoral artery. Again, vein is the best conduit. If the great saphenous is available, there is usually a considerable size discrepancy between the vein at the groin and below the knee, so that the *in situ* technique is to be preferred. However, there is no proven difference in patency rates between reversed and *in situ* grafts, although technical errors may be reduced by reversing the vein. If the great saphenous vein has been used or is too small, then the small saphenous vein may well be usable. Failing this, arm vein can be used, although it is more fragile than leg vein. Composite grafts using vein from all these sources can be used in order to provide a vein of sufficient length to complete the graft. If no such vein is available, then a Miller cuff or a Taylor patch can be used to facilitate the distal anastomosis. These two techniques are of proven benefit when prosthetic bypass grafts are undertaken to single crural vessels or the popliteal artery below the knee.

The Miller cuff (Fig. 22.4)

The recipient artery is opened via a longitudinal arteriotomy in the usual fashion. A segment of vein harvested from the long saphenous, small saphenous or the arm is opened along its length. The vein is anastomosed to the artery starting at the midpoint of the arteriotomy, so completing a circle. The redundant vein is then excised, and the vein is anastomosed to itself to form a collar. The synthetic graft (usually PTFE) is then anastomosed to the vein. A modification of this technique, developed at St Mary's Hospital, starts the vein collar at the toe of the arteriotomy (Fig. 22.5). This allows a more graduated decrease in diameter at the distal end of the anastomosis, but there are no objective data proving its superiority.

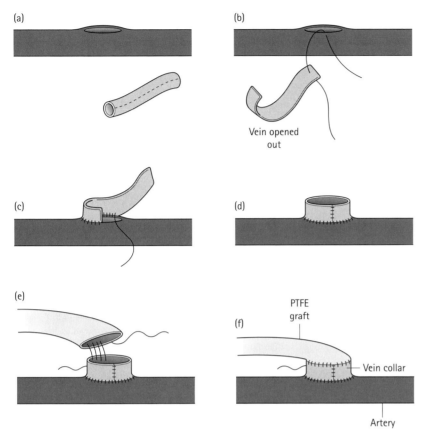

Vein opened
out

PTFE
graft

(f)

Vein collar

Artery

Figure 22.4   *The Miller cuff. (a) Longitudinal arteriotomy and longitudinal venotomy; (b) start of anastomosis of vein to arteriotomy; (c) the anastomosis is continued the full circumference of the arteriotomy; (d) the excess vein is excised and the edges of vein are sutured to form a collar; (e) the polytetrafluoroethylene (PTFE) graft is now sutured to the vein collar; (f) the completed anastomosis.*

The Taylor patch (Fig. 22.6)

A direct anastomosis is performed between the synthetic graft and the recipient artery starting at the heel, but leaving the toe of the anastomosis free. An arteriotomy is then performed distally along the artery for 3–5 cm, extending proximally for a similar length on the front of the synthetic graft. A diamond patch of vein is then sutured over the defect, using interrupted sutures at the toe of the anastomosis.

The results of femoropopliteal vein grafts show a patency of 65 percent at 5 years. The results above the knee are better, with 70 percent of vein grafts remaining patent at 5 years. The UK femoropopliteal bypass trial showed that, for prosthetic grafts, the 3-year patency was 65 percent for above-knee popliteal grafts and 35 percent for below-knee popliteal grafts.

Tibial and peroneal arterial occlusion (pulse-generated run-off)

Occlusions of the tibial and peroneal arteries may be suitable for bypass if a good segment of distal artery is patent. Pulse-generated run-off (PGR)[17] may be used to detect patent calf vessels which may not be shown by arteriography. PGR is performed by placing a cuff around the upper calf and this is then inflated rapidly with compressed air. A Doppler probe is placed over the distal posterior and anterior tibial and peroneal arteries, and the waveform assessed. No signal

indicates occlusion of the vessel. Patency is shown by the presence of a signal which may be monophasic or biphasic depending on the quality of the vessel. The status of the pedal arch can also be determined by this technique.

Often these vessels are more easily dissected in the lower third of the leg, where they lie superficially compared with the upper third of the leg. If all the tibial vessels are occluded, successful bypass grafts can be performed to the posterior tibial vessel below the ankle or to the dorsalis pedis artery on the dorsum of the foot. A patent pedal arch may improve the chances of a successful procedure, but is by no means essential. All anastomoses at this level need some form of intraoperative monitoring, with on-table arteriography being the current gold standard. It is essential that vein is used at this level, and due to the large size discrepancy, the author would use the *in situ* technique. If no vein is present, PTFE can be used in combination with either a Miller cuff or a Taylor patch.

The anterior tibial artery lies on the lateral aspect of the leg, and vein grafts commencing at the common femoral artery must be brought across the surface of the tibia through a tunnel beneath the skin. Some authors suggest that a bevel is made in the anterior aspect of the bone so that the graft is not compressed. A synthetic graft or a reversed or composite vein graft can be tunnelled via the lateral aspect of the thigh to the anterior tibial artery. The posterior and peroneal arteries can be approached from the medial aspect of the leg.

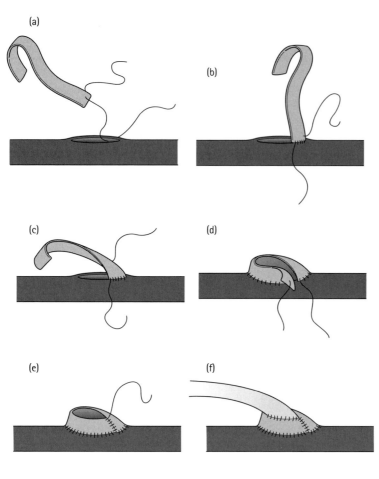

Figure 22.5 *The St Mary's Hospital modification of the Miller cuff. (a) The corner of the vein is sutured to the distal apex of the arteriotomy; (b) the end of the vein is sutured to the distal part of one wall of the arteriotomy; (c) the longitudinal part of the vein is now sutured from the apex proximally; (d) the anastomosis is continued for the full circumference; (e) the collar is formed by suturing the vein to itself; (f) the polytetrafluoroethylene (PTFE) graft is sutured to the modified vein collar.*

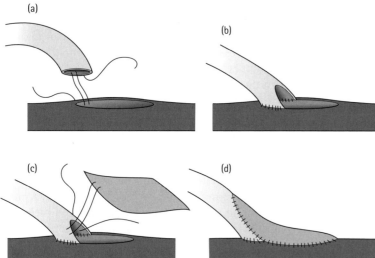

Figure 22.6 *The Taylor patch. (a) The polytetrafluoroethylene (PTFE) graft is sutured to the heel of the arteriotomy; (b) the anterior part of the graft is opened; (c) a diamond-shaped vein patch is sutured to both graft and artery; (d) the completed anastomosis.*

An alternative approach to the peroneal artery is to remove a portion of the fibula via a lateral approach.

The results for femorodistal grafts are much better if the vein is used, with patency rates of 80 percent at 3 years. Prosthetic grafts have a much lower patency rate, with some authors quoting only 35 percent of grafts patent at 3 years. Experts using the vein interposition techniques improve this to 45–65 percent patency at 3 years.

ULCERATION OF MIXED ARTERIAL AND VENOUS ORIGIN

The principles of treatment are, not unsurprisingly, exactly the same as those of treating ischemic ulcers and venous ulcers. Successful management does depend, however, on observing certain priorities. In general, it is important to treat the arterial lesion before attempting any venous surgery, as the incisions required for the latter are unlikely to heal in the absence of a good arterial supply. Caution must be observed in this respect, as direct arterial surgery is inadvisable in the presence of an infected ulcer and is absolutely contraindicated if any synthetic graft is required. Fortunately, many patients with mixed arterial and venous ulcers have a short arterial occlusion suitable for balloon angioplasty. If arterial reconstruction is necessary, it is most important to heal the ulcer before this is attempted; however, the firm compression required to control venous reflux is likely to exacerbate the ischemia and therefore lead to ulcer deterioration rather than healing.

These contradictory problems are best dealt with by making every attempt to improve the arterial circulation by non-surgical means before embarking on either arterial or venous surgery. Chemical lumbar sympathectomy alone may be sufficient, but if this is inadequate, a course of intravenous iloprost should be tried. This requires admission to hospital and therefore, at the same time as prostanoid treatment, the ulcer can be treated by light compression bandaging, cleaning and dressings, with appropriate antibiotic therapy. If, in spite of these measures, the ulcer is still incompletely healed and arteriograms have shown arterial occlusion requiring bypass surgery, the ulcer should be excised down to deep fascia 2 or 3 days before operation. Appropriate antibiotics are continued in high doses. Following successful restoration of arterial supply, firm compression bandaging can be applied and venous surgery undertaken in the usual way.

It is the authors' experience that, in many of these patients, arterial insufficiency is not severe and very often responds to conservative measures (chemical sympathectomy or prostacyclin), without involving the need for direct arterial surgery. The situation is then not as complicated as might at first appear.

REFERENCES

1. Greenhalgh RM. Naftddrofuryl for ischaemic rest pain: a controlled trial. *Br J Surg* 1981; **68**: 265–6.
2. Anonymous. Intravenous pentoxifylline for the treatment of chronic critical limb ischaemia. The European Study Group. *Eur J Vasc Endovasc Surg* 1995; **9**: 426–36.
3. The Norwegian Pentoxifylline Multicentre Trial Group. Efficacy and clinical tolerance of parenteral pentoxifylline in the treatment of chronic lower limb ischaemia. A placebo-controlled multicentre study. *Int Angiol* 1996; **15**: 75–80.
4. Bode-Boger SM, Boger RH, Alfke H *et al.* L-Arginine induces nitric oxide-dependent vasodilatation in patients with critical limb ischaemia. A randomized, controlled study. *Circulation* 1996; **93**: 85–90.
5. Baumgartner I, Pieczek A, Manor O *et al.* Constitutive expression of phVEGF165 afterbintramuscular gene transfer promotes collateral vessel development in patients with critical limb ischaemia. *Circulation* 1998; **97**: 1114–23.
6. Szczeklik A, Nizankowski R, Skawinski S *et al.* Successful therapy of advanced arteriosclerosis with prostacyclin. *Lancet* 1979; **i**: 1111–4.
7. Prentice CR M, Belch JJF, McKay A *et al.* Prostacyclin in severe arterial disease. In: Gryglewski RJ, Szczeklik A, McGill JC, eds. *Prostacyclin – Clinical Trials.* New York: Raven Press, 1985; 1–5.
8. Loosemore TM, Chalmers TC, Dormandy JA. A meta-analysis of randomized placebo control trials in Fontaine stages III and IV peripheral occlusive disease. *Int Angiol* 1994; **13**: 133–42.
9. Negus D, Irving JD, Friedgood A. Intra-arterial prostacyclin in the management of advanced atherosclerotic lower limb ischaemia. In: Gryglewski RJ, Szczeklik A, McGill JC *et al.*, eds. *Prostacyclin – Clinical Trials.* New York: Raven Press, 1985; 107–13.
10. Moore WS, Hall AD. Effects of lumbar sympathectomy on skin capillary blood flow in arterial occlusive disease. *J Surg Res* 1973; **14**: 151–7.
11. Bracale G. Is there a place for lumbar sympathectomy for critical ischaemia? In: Greenhalgh RM, Jamieson CW, Nicolaides AN, eds. *Limb Salvage and Amputation for Vascular Disease.* Philadelphia: Saunders, 1988; 241–55.
12. Fulton RL, Blakeley WR. Lumbar sympathectomy: a procedure of questionable value in the treatment of arteriosclerosis obliterans of the legs. *Am J Surg* 1968; **116**: 735–44.
13. Yao ST, Bergan JJ. Predictability of vascular reactivity relative to sympathetic ablations. *Arch Surg* 1973; **107**: 676–80.
14. Linton RR. The post-thrombotic ulceration of the lower extremities; its aetiology and surgical treatment. *Ann Surg* 1953; **138**: 415–30.
15. Cook AW, Oygar A, Baggenstos P *et al.* Vascular disease of the extremities. Electrical stimulation of spinal cord and posterior roots. *NY State J Med* 1976; **76**: 366–8.
16. Klomp HM, Spincemaille GH, Steyerberg EW *et al.* Design issues of a randomised controlled clinical trial on spinal cord stimulation in critical limb ischaemia. *Eur J Vasc Endovasc Surg* 1995; **10**: 478–85.
17. Beard JD, Scott DJA, Evans M *et al.* Pulse generated run-off: a new method of determining vessel patency. *Br J Surg* 1988; **75**: 361–3.

23

Venous surgery in ulcer management: a review

DAVID NEGUS, CHRISTINE J. MOFFATT, PETER J. FRANKS

Although it is logical to suppose that the control of venous hypertension, whether by surgery or injection sclerotherapy, will assist healing and prevent recurrence, the majority of venous ulcers continue to be treated by dressings and compression. This has resulted from the general perception that there is little objective evidence for the use of surgery in treating this common condition. In fact, there is now a significant amount of published work on the subject. Admittedly, most papers consist of retrospective reviews and some of these are flawed by small numbers or insufficient length of follow-up, but the number of studies has increased in recent years, although few are controlled.

HISTORICAL

According to Linton,[1] surgery for venous ulceration was first performed by Rémy in 1901,[2] but John Homans of Boston is generally acknowledged as being its originator. Homans[3] distinguished between 'varicose' and 'postphlebitic' ulceration and his paper includes the following description:

> The less noticeable the veins, the more malignant and resistant [to treatment] the accompanying ulcers and the more radical and thorough must be the curative operation. Large tortuous varicosities are gradually established, perforating vessels and collateral circulation are then usually competent, ulcers if present ride on veins and cure is usually easy. On the other hand, the varicosity of the small sclerosed [postphlebitic] vessel is rapidly established by inflammatory processes, collateral circulation is ineffective, perforating veins are almost invariably crippled, disturbances in the skin are widespread and severe, and cure is correspondingly difficult.

Homans described eight operations for the treatment of venous ulcers, all of which were initially successful, although two ulcers subsequently recurred.

No further studies were published until 1938, when Robert Linton[1] published his detailed studies on the anatomy of the calf perforating veins. He describes the operation for their ligation but does not include any results. He was followed by Cockett,[4] whose descriptions of the calf perforating veins have become so well known that they are often referred to as 'Cockett perforators'. Cockett also coined the term 'ankle blowout' for an incompetent perforating vein.

VARICOSE VEIN SURGERY

A recent meta-analysis of non-invasive diagnostic tests in patients with venous ulceration has shown that 45 percent of limbs suffer from superficial disease in isolation, with 12 percent suffering from deep vein disease alone and 43 percent suffering from a combination of both.[5] The high proportion of patients with superficial disease makes surgical correction of the superficial system appropriate.

Superficial surgery is usually interpreted as saphenous ligation and strip with perforator ligation, but in Dunn's series of 78 ulcerated patients treated surgically, 66 were treated by saphenous ligation and strip alone and only 11 required perforating vein ligation.[6] This study was also controlled, 107 limbs being randomized to surgery and 52 (33 percent) managed conservatively. Follow-up was from 1 to 5 years (median 3 years) and 68 limbs were reviewed. Surgery was followed by some improvement in healing rates [surgery 60 (88 percent), conservative 12 (52 percent)] and, more significantly, the recurrence rates were significantly smaller in those ulcers treated surgically [surgery 8 (11.8 percent) conservative 11 (48 percent)]. More recently, work has been undertaken to determine the outcome of patients with isolated superficial vein incompetence and normal deep veins. In a cohort of 122 limbs treated by superficial venous surgery, cumulative healing rates were 57 percent after 6 months and 82 percent after 18 months.[7] Of the 18 legs which failed to heal, re-examination showed that these were largely due to fixed ankle joints or osteoarthritis of the knee, both of which would have serious effects on the calf muscle pump.

PERFORATING VEIN LIGATION

Perforating vein ligation has been practiced since the pioneering work of Linton and Cockett. In 1990 Jamieson et al.[8] reported the results of superficial vein surgery in 112 patients (122 limbs) with venous ulceration refractory to conservative treatment. Diagnosis was by examination and venography was performed in 96 limbs. Long saphenous ligation and strip was performed on four limbs and subfascial ligation of perforators on 118. Compression hosiery was not worn postoperatively and at follow-up (mean 7.9 years, median 11) there was no ulcer recurrence in 82 percent.

Nachbur et al.'s[9] small series of 25 legs treated surgically for superficial venous incompetence resulted in 100 percent healing rate and 13 percent recurrence 2 years after surgery following saphenous stripping and perforator ligation, but surgery was less successful in 76 patients with deep vein incompetence and 'rebellious' ulcers, who were treated by wide and deep excision of the ulcer, and ligation of underlying perforators and surrounding varicose veins, with 59 percent ulcer healing at 2 years.

In a small series of 43 patients undergoing superficial and perforating vein ligation for recurrent venous ulceration, Bradbury et al.[10] reported nine recurrent ulcers at follow-up (mean 66 months, range 18–144), six with femoral vein incompetence and all with popliteal vein incompetence.

It should be understood that perforating vein ligation may not always be necessary to achieve ulcer healing in limbs with superficial and perforating vein incompetence but with normal deep veins. In a study which challenged convention, Darke and Penfold[11] reported a series of 53 patients with 54 ulcerated limbs, all of whom had saphenous and perforating vein incompetence but with normal deep veins. These were treated by saphenous ligation and strip, without perforating vein interruption, and 91 percent remained healed at a mean follow-up period of 3–4 years (see Ch. 4, p. 28).

A more recent but similar study[12] has confirmed the effectiveness of varicose vein surgery in limbs with normal deep veins and the failure of ulcers to heal following surgery to the superficial veins in those with deep venous reflux.

SUBFASCIAL ENDOSCOPIC PERFORATOR SURGERY

Subfascial endoscopic perforator surgery (SEPS) was introduced in the1980s. This procedure avoids the poor healing which often complicated the previously popular Cockett operation and has revived interest in perforating vein occlusion in the treatment of venous ulcers.

Recent studies have indicated that the technique leads to few serious complications[13,14] and a shorter hospital stay than the open operation.[15] A randomized study comparing the results of open surgery for perforator ligation with SEPS has shown no difference in operating time or in results; 21 months postoperatively, all ulcers were healed in both groups.[16]

A retrospective series from the Mayo Clinic[17] reported the results of SEPS in 49 consecutive patients (57 limbs), of whom 20 (35 percent) had a history of venous ulceration and 22 had active ulcers at the time of operation. These were followed up for a mean 17 ± 2 months and all the active ulcers were healed in an average 99 ± 37 months. There were five recurrent ulcers, all in post-thrombotic limbs and a 57 percent recurrence rate in seven patients with a history of deep vein thrombosis and venous obstruction as well as reflux.

The relatively poor results of SEPS in preventing ulcer recurrence in the presence of deep venous incompetence is also reported by Nelzen[13] in a series of 149 limbs; follow-up was a median 32 months (range 14–57 months), at which time ulcers were open in 33 percent of those with deep vein incompetence and 13 percent with superficial incompetence alone.

Every series of venous ulcer treatment by perforator ligation, whether by open or endoscopic operation, describes poor results in limbs with deep venous incompetence, and the North American registry (NASEPS) has indicated that, on average, 28 percent of patients recur within 2 years of the procedure.[18]

DEEP VEIN INCOMPETENCE

Reconstructive operations

The disappointing results of saphenous and perforating vein ligation in healing ulcers related to deep venous incompetence has stimulated a few vascular surgeons on both sides of the Atlantic to develop reconstructive operations to restore deep venous competence.

In an early retrospective study of valve reconstruction in 107 limbs, Raju and Fredericks[19] found that complete healing occurred in 84 percent of ulcerated limbs 1 year after deep vein reconstruction, but this was not sustained, with only 63 percent remaining healed after 2 years.[19]

In 1982, Ferris and Kistner[20] reported the results of venous valve surgery. Out of a total of 46 cases, 80 percent had clinical outcomes classified as good to excellent, where an excellent outcome was defined as one in which the patient remains free of the symptoms of swelling, aching, induration and ulceration, and a good result was defined as a patient who is asymptomatic but requires full- or part-time elastic support. Fifteen of 17 descending venograms performed 2–13 years postoperatively showed correction of valve reflux Postoperative ankle venous pressure tests were better in those who had both perforator and deep veins repaired than those with only deep vein repair.

More recently, Sottiurai[21] reported a series of 76 limbs in 46 patients with recurrent ulcers refractory to conservative treatment. All had deep vein and perforating vein incompetence shown on venography. Thirty-three patients were treated by perforator ligation with saphenous vein stripping (PLSVS) and 43 by PLSVS and by a variety of methods for deep venous reconstruction [valvuloplasty 21 (28 percent), venous transposition 14 (18 percent), venous valve transplantation 8 (11 percent)]. Eighty percent of those undergoing PLSVS alone wore elastic stockings postoperatively, as did between 19 and 25 percent of those having deep venous surgery. Follow-up was at a mean 37 months (range 10–73 months) when ulcers persisted in 56 percent (19 of 33) of the PLSVS group and in 20 percent of the deep venous reconstruction group.

In 1995 Perrin et al.[22] reported the results of valvuloplasty in 11 limbs with a combination of primary deep vein incompetence and post-thrombotic syndrome; at an average follow-up of 43 months, there were two non-healing ulcers and two recurrences.

The results of vein segment transposition, without perforator interruption, have not been satisfactory. In a series of 12 operations reported in 1981,[23] all had initial good results but nine developed recurrent ulcers after 1 year. This study was designed to see if it is necessary to ligate perforators or whether proximal valve transposition alone is sufficient: the answer was that the perforators should be treated.

Ulcer treatment by superficial and perforating vein surgery and compression

In a study of 92 ulcerated limbs treated by ligation of calf perforators, saphenous ligation and stripping, 84 percent remained healed after a mean follow-up of 6 years.[24] Patients with deep vein incompetence wore knee-length compression hosiery permanently following surgery and there was no significant difference in long-term healing between those with deep vein incompetence and those with superficial venous incompetence and normal deep veins.

Another small series of 10 patients with 11 ulcers, all with both superficial and deep venous incompetence, were treated by saphenous and perforator ablation.[25] Postoperative compression hosiery was worn by five patients; six wore none. At follow-up (mean 16.4 months) all ulcers were healed. The number of patients is too small and the length of follow-up too short to allow any firm conclusions.

SUBMALLEOLAR SAPHENOUS INTERRUPTION

A small study[26] has demonstrated that ligation of the great saphenous vein on the dorsum of the foot (submalleolar saphenous interruption) achieved successful healing of four out of five ulcers which recurred after saphenous and perforator ligation and compression. This simple procedure prevents the transmission of high venous pressures from the deep veins to the corona phlebectatica (see Ch. 4, p. 31) and has recently been included in a prospective study by DePalma and Kowallek.[27]

This involved a cohort of 11 males (aged 49–69 years) whose venous ulcers were initially treated by dressings and compression (Unna's boot) for 3 years. In this period, there were 44 occurrences of ulceration (three to eight per individual), with an average time to heal of 13 weeks. At the end of this 3-year period, duplex scans and venograms were performed. These showed superficial venous incompetence, perforating vein incompetence, deep vein incompetence and two cases of deep vein obstruction. Ten patients were treated surgically (one with caval thrombosis was excluded); saphenous strip, with perforator and submalleolar saphenous interruption, was performed in seven, superficial femoral vein valvuloplasty in one and a Palma crossover graft in one. All patients wore graduated compression stockings postoperatively and nine of the 10 ulcers were healed 2 years after the completion of treatment.

This study has gone some way to confirming the value of submalleolar saphenous interruption; further confirmation is needed. If such confirmation is achieved, this procedure, with great saphenous ligation and strip and SEPS, could provide a simple and rapid form of surgical treatment.

RANDOMIZED STUDIES

Dunn et al.'s[6] randomized study (107 limbs treated surgically, 52 conservatively) was undertaken before the introduction of SEPS and 'open' ligation of perforating veins was performed. More recently, a randomized controlled study from the Netherlands[28] compared the results in 97 patients treated conservatively (ambulatory compression therapy) with those of 103 treated surgically (ambulatory compression therapy with SEPS and, in selected cases, surgery of the superficial system) with an average follow-up of 29 (surgical) and 26 (conservative) months. Patients with recurrent ulceration and those with a medial ulcer had an active ulcer for a significantly shorter period of time during follow-up in the surgical group (38 and 22 percent) than those in the conservative group (67 and 57 percent).

Others have had more difficulty in organizing randomized controlled trials; Davies et al.[29] were unable to recruit sufficient patients. They found that, out of a total of 759 patients assessed across 17 clinics, some 446 were immediately non-eligible because 'they did not have surgically correctable disease'. It seems probable that most, if not all, of these patients were suffering from deep venous insufficiency and that the assessing surgeons did not consider that this constituted operability (A. H. Davies, personal communication). It is to be hoped that others will not be deterred from organizing controlled trials as a result of this unfortunate experience.

A definitive trial on the use of superficial vein surgery in patients with open and healed venous ulcers has recently been published.[30] Five-hundred patients with isolated superficial vein incompetence or superficial incompetence with deep vein incompetence were randomised to receive compression therapy alone or compression therapy in combination with superficial vein surgery. At the start of the trial 341 had open ulcers and were treated with high-compression bandaging, whereas the remaining 159 had healed ulcers and were prescribed compression hosiery. Patients whose ulcers healed during the trial were also analysed for recurrence. The trial showed that healing rates were similar between groups at 65 percent in both groups after 24 weeks. However, ulcer recurrence rates were substantially reduced in the patients randomised to surgery at 12% versus 28% after 1 year of follow up ($P < 0.0001$). The trial has proven the benefits of surgery in reducing venous ulcer recurrence rates but failed to find a benefit in ulcer healing.

FOAM INJECTION SCLEROTHERAPY

Cabrera et al.[31] have recently reported the results of a series of 116 patients with 151 venous ulcers, which were treated by the ultrasound-guided injection of polidoconol microfoam (UIPM). The microfoam was injected under ultrasound guidance into the original source of reflux, the saphenous or perforator veins, or both. Sclerotherapy sessions were given every 2–4 weeks at the beginning of the treatment and reduced in frequency as the patient improved. No major complications were encountered. There were no cases of DVT, pulmonary embolism or neurological lesions. There were 10 recurrent ulcers; the 24-month recurrence rate was 6.3 percent overall and 8.5 percent across all subgroups apart from elderly patients, the largest ulcers, ulcers of the longest duration and patients with deep vein incompetence. These results compare favourably with those of Darke and Penfold,[11] using a significantly less invasive technique.

Cabrera's method has been modified by Bergan and Pascarella,[32] who inject the foam under ultrasound guidance by butterfly needle into varices proximal to the severely affected area, and then, by elevating the distal limb 45°, the foam is guided into the tangle of vein and venules under the most profoundly damaged tissue. They have now treated 91 limbs of 66 patients, of whom 34 had venous ulcers and 57 painfully disabling lipodermatosclerosis or unstable healed ulcers. Active ulcers are treated provided that there is no infection. Favourable results have been seen regularly within 10–14 days of treatment and there have been no serious complications.

Bergan's series included a crossover group of patients who were treated successfully by foam sclerotherapy after failing conventional treatment.

It is not impossible that foam sclerotherapy will eventually overtake surgery as the most favoured option for the treatment of venous ulcers.

REFERENCES

1. Linton RR. Post-thrombotic ulceration of the lower extremity; its aetiology and surgical. Management. *Ann Surg* 1938; **107**: 582–93.
2. Rémy C. Traité des varices des membres inférieurs et de leur traitment chirurgical. Paris: Vigot fréres, 1901.
3. Homans. J. The operative treatment of varicose veins and ulcers, based on a classification of these lesions. *Surg Gynecol Obstset* 1916; **22**: 143–58.
4. Cockett FB, Elgin Jones DE. The ankle blowout syndrome. A new approach to the venous ulcer problem. *Lancet* 1953; **i**: 17–23.
5. Tassiopoulos AK, Golts E, Oh DS, Labropoulos N. Current concepts in chronic venous ulceration. *Eur J Vasc Endovasc Surg* 2000; **20**: 227–32.
6. Dunn JM, Cosford EJ, Kernik VF, Campbell WB. Surgical treatment for venous ulcers: is it worthwhile? *Ann R Coll Surg Eng* 1995; **77**: 421–4.
7. Bello M, Scriven M, Hartshorne T et al. Role of superficial venous surgery in the treatment of venous ulceration. *Br J Surg* 1999; **86**: 755–9.
8. Jamieson WG, De Rose G, Harris KA. Management of venous stasis ulcer: long-term follow-up. *Can J Surg* 1990; **33**: 222–3.
9. Nachbur B, Blanchard M, Rothlisberger H. Chirurgische therapie des ulcus cruris. *Wien Med Wochenschr* 1994; **144**: 264–8.
10. Bradbury AW, Stonebridge PA, Callam MJ et al. Foot volume try and duplex ultrasonography after saphenous and subfascial perforating vein ligation for recurrent venous ulceration. *Br J Surg* 1993; **80**: 845–8.
11. Darke G, Penfold C. Venous ulceration and saphenous ligation. *Eur J Vasc Surg* 1992; **6**: 4–9.
12. Scriven JM, Hartshorne T, Thrush AJ et al. Role of saphenous vein surgery in the treatment of venous ulceration. *Br J Surg* 1998; **85**: 781–4.
13. Nelzen O. Prospective study of safety, patient satisfaction and leg ulcer healing following saphenous and subfascial endoscopic perforator surgery. *Br J Surg* 2000; **87**: 86–91.
14. Gloviczki P. Subfascial endoscopic perforator surgery: indications and results. *Vascular Med* 1999; **4**: 173–80.
15. Stuart WP, Adam DJ, Bradbury AW, Ruckley CV. Subfascial endoscopic perforator surgery is associated with significantly less morbidity and shorter hospital stay than open operation [Linton's procedure]. *Br J Surg* 1997; **84**: 1364–5.
16. Pierik EGJM, van Urk H, Hop WCJ, Wittens CHA. Endoscopic versus open subfascial division of incompetent perforating veins in the treatment of venous leg ulceration: a randomised trial. *J Vasc Surg* 1997; **26**: 1049–54.
17. Rhodes JM, Gloviczki P, Canton LG et al. Factors affecting clinical outcome following endoscopic perforator vein ablation. *Am J Surg* 1998; **176**: 162–7.
18. Gloviczki P, Bergan JJ, Rhodes JM et al. Mid-term results of endovascular perforator vein interruption for chronic venous

insufficiency: lessons learnt from the North American Study Group. *J Vasc Surg* 1999; **29**: 489–502.

19. Raju S, Frederricks R. Valve reconstruction procedures for non-obstructive venous insufficiency rationale, techniques and results in 107 procedures with two to eight year follow-up. *J Vasc Surg* 1998; **7**: 301–10.

20. Ferris TJ, Kistner RL. Femoral vein reconstruction in the management of chronic venous insufficiency. *Arch Surg* 1982; **117**: 1571–9.

21. Sottiurai VS. Surgical correction of recurrent venous ulcer. *J Cardiovasc Surg Torino* 1991; **32**: 104–9.

22. Perrin M, Calvignac JL, Hiltbrand B, Bayon JM. Surgical results on recurrent leg ulcers in primary deep vein insufficiency treated by valve repair. In: Negus D, Jantet G, Coleridge Smith PD, eds. *Phlebology '95*. London: Springer-Verlag, 1995; 969–70.

23. Johnson ND, Queral LA, Flinn WR. Late objective assessment of venous valve surgery. *Arch Surg* 1981; **116**: 1461–6.

24. Holme TC, Negus D. The treatment of venous ulceration by surgery and elastic compression hosiery; a long term review. *Phlebology* 1990; **5**: 125–8.

25. Padberg FT, Pappas PJ, Araki CT et al. Hemodynamic and clinical improvement after superficial vein ablation in primary combined venous insufficiency with ulceration. *J Vasc Surg* 1996; **24**: 711–8.

26. Negus D. The distal long saphenous vein in recurrent venous ulceration: a preliminary report. In: Raymond-Martimbeau P, Prescott R, Zummo M, eds. *Phlébologie '92*. Montrouge, France: John Libbey Eurotext, 1992; 1291–3.

27. DePalma RG, Kowallck L D. Venous ulceration: a cross-over study from nonoperative to operative treatment. *J Vasc Surg* 1996; **24**: 788–92.

28. Wittens CHA, van Gent WB, Hop WCJ. Conservative versus surgical treatment of venous leg ulcers [Dutch SEPS trial] (Abstr). *Phlebology* 2004; **19**: 157.

29. Davies AH, Hawdon AJ, Greenhalgh RMM, Thompson S. On behalf of the USABLE trial participants. *Phlebology* 2004; **19**: 137–42.

30. Barwell JR, Davies CE, Deacon J et al. Comparison of surgery and compression with compression alone in chronic venous ulceration (ESCHAR study): randomised controlled trial. *Lancet* 2004: **363**: 1854–59.

31. Cabrera J, Redondo P, Becerra A et al. Ultrasound guided injection of polidocanol microfoam in the management of venous leg ulcers. *Arch Dermatol* 2004; **140**: 667–73.

32. Bergan JJ, Pascarella I. Severe chronic venous insufficiency, primary treatment with sclerofoam. *Semin Vasc Surg* 2005; **18**: 49–56.

24

Recurrent ulceration: prevention, diagnosis and treatment

DAVID NEGUS, PHILIP D. COLERIDGE SMITH

PREVENTION

Patients with healed ulceration of the legs, whether venous or arterial in origin, are liable to develop breakdown and recurrent ulcers. Previously ulcerated skin is never as stable as normal skin and it is important to prevent even minor trauma. Recurrence has been reported in one-quarter of patients with healed venous leg ulcers within the first year.[1] This is clearly an important economic problem but remains one that is difficult to address successfully. The use of compression hosiery is effective in preventing recurrence of ulceration following healing. This applies whether healing was achieved using compression alone or following surgical treatment for superficial and perforating vein incompetence. Class 2 or 3 below-knee compression stockings are effective in reducing recurrence. However, many elderly patients find considerable difficulty in applying stockings or find them uncomfortable. It has been found that patients who are unwilling or unable to comply with advice to wear compression hosiery are at greatest risk of further leg ulceration.[1] This problem will continue to be a significant drawback to the use of one of the most effective measures in healing and preventing the recurrence of venous leg ulcers. Various devices are now available which simplify the application of compression stockings (see Ch. 25, p. 230) but these are only used on a limited scale.

A further problem is that some patients have very limited mobility because of other medical conditions, including arthritis, previous stroke and cardiopulmonary disease. These patients are also at considerable risk of experiencing problems with the healing of ulcers and maintaining these ulcers in a healed state.[2] They often sit with the feet dependent for long periods, resulting in raised venous pressure in the lower limbs. This is a well known factor encouraging the development of leg ulcers. Where possible, patients with venous leg ulcers should sit with their feet elevated to minimize the venous pressure at the ankle.

Patients with leg ulcers in whom there is considerable superficial venous reflux may benefit from superficial venous surgery. This has been shown to speed leg ulcer healing as well as to prevent recurrence.[3] This treatment should be considered in all patients who present with recurrent ulceration who are fit enough and willing to undergo surgical treatment.

The skin at the ankle remains fragile in many patients with healed venous ulcers, and even extremes of heat and cold may be sufficient to trigger the recurrence of ulceration. One of us (DN) has experience of a patient who suffered bilateral recurrence of venous leg ulceration following exposure of the fragile skin to extreme cold. The ulcers healed successfully with conventional dressings and compression bandaging and she was advised to wear warm boots during cold weather.

Patients with healed ischemic ulcers must similarly be careful to avoid trauma and, unfortunately, these patients, who are often elderly and whose eyesight may be poor, have a tendency to bump into things, particularly supermarket trolleys. On a few occasions, the author has advised such patients to buy hockey shin-pads from their local sports shop and to wear these when they go shopping. The heels of bedridden patients with lower limb ischemia must be protected from pressure by sheepskin or (less expensively) by water-filled surgical rubber gloves under the ankles.

INVESTIGATION AND TREATMENT

When a patient presents again in an ulcer clinic, months or sometimes years after appropriate venous or arterial surgery has achieved initial ulcer healing, there is a natural tendency to consider the situation hopeless and to continue conservative treatment with dressings or bandages as the only feasible form of management in the future. While this approach may be correct in the very elderly or debilitated patient, who is clearly not fit for any further active treatment, such a pessimistic view should be resisted in the majority of patients presenting with recurrent ulceration. A positive approach must be taken to examination and investigations, with a view to finding out the underlying cause of the recurrent ulcer.

The recurrent venous ulcer: exclude ischemia

In investigating a recurrent venous ulcer, it should be remembered that many elderly patients, whose initial ulcer was venous in origin, may have developed atherosclerotic ischemia of the foot and ankle skin in the years since the original venous ulcer healed. It is therefore most important to check that ankle pulses are present and to measure pulse pressures with Doppler ultrasound. Provided that there is no evidence of ischemia, attention can then be paid to diagnosing the venous abnormality responsible for recurrence. It is not unusual for further perforating veins to become incompetent following ligation of those which were incompetent at the first operation, particularly in patients with deep venous incompetence. Recurrent or primary superficial venous reflux may be found which is the cause of further ulceration. Careful examination and investigations will often demonstrate a correctable lesion which can be effectively dealt with by further surgery or injection sclerotherapy. Duplex ultrasound examination is essential in the investigation of recurrent venous ulceration, and the investigation and treatment of these patients should only be undertaken where this is available – usually a department of vascular surgery.

Recurrent varicose veins

The most common reason for recurrent great saphenous incompetence is failure to perform a flush saphenofemoral ligation with ligation and division of all tributaries.[4] Failure to perform (limited) stripping of the great saphenous vein is also followed by high recurrence rates,[5] usually related to the persistence of one or more incompetent thigh perforating veins (Fig. 24.1). Stripping of the great saphenous vein is likely to reduce the need for further surgery to treat recurrent varices.[6] Despite a systematic approach to surgical management, including stripping the saphenous vein, many patients still experience recurrence of varices.[7,8] This reflects the nature of varicose veins which may reappear as a consequence of technical failures to control venous reflux as well as progression

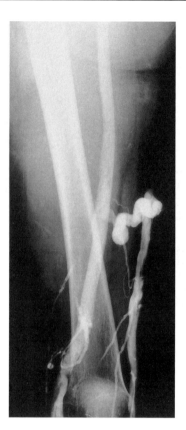

Figure 24.1 *Varicogram demonstrating a large, incompetent mid-thigh perforating vein.*

of venous disease, i.e. appearance of varicose veins in previously normal veins. Technical failures include incorrectly performed operations, e.g. incorrectly identifying the anatomy at the saphenofemoral junction and not ligating the junction correctly. Even when ligation has been correctly performed, some junctions develop further convoluted recurrences which communicate with new varicose veins. This phenomenon is probably due to the growth of new veins, often referred to as 'neovascularization'. This tendency can be reduced but not eliminated by stripping the saphenous vein. Various strategies have been investigated to eliminate neovascularization, including introducing a silicone barrier between the ligated junction and superficial veins.[9] None is totally effective and surgeons have to admit that varicose vein surgery does not offer a permanent cure in every patient.

EXAMINATION AND INVESTIGATIONS

Recurrent varicose veins may be quite obvious, particularly in thin subjects, and simple examination, with the help of a hand-held Doppler ultrasound probe, is then sufficient to diagnose the venous 'leak points' responsible for recurrence.[10] Where possible, a duplex scan should be arranged by an experienced operator using a high-resolution ultrasound machine. This investigation should provide a detailed map of the sources of recurrent varices allowing a systematic approach to be planned

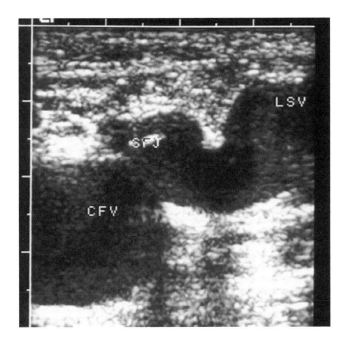

Figure 24.2 *Duplex ultrasound examination of the saphenofemoral junction following previous surgery. A large recurrence is shown which fills recurrent varices.*

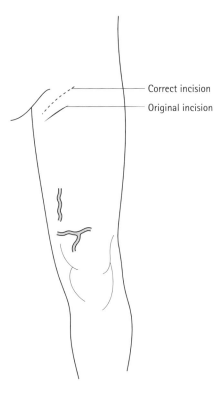

Figure 24.3 *The scar of a low groin incision in a patient with recurrent great saphenous incompetence indicates that the saphenofemoral junction was not ligated by the previous operation and recurrence results from persistent tributaries at reoperation. Through a correctly placed high incision, no scar tissue will be encountered and the saphenofemoral junction can be ligated without difficulty.*

for surgical treatment. (Fig. 24.2) The investigator should search for the source of varices, including junction recurrence, residual saphenous trunks and perforating veins. The location of residual saphenous trunks and perforating veins can be marked on the skin to facilitate their treatment by surgery. Varicography has been used to demonstrate the connections of recurrent superficial veins with the deep system. This remains an effective technique but is very little used these days.

THE SURGERY OF RECURRENT VENOUS ULCERATION

Most frequently, good results can be obtained by relatively simple surgery to the superficial and perforating veins, followed by class 2 knee-length compression stockings in those patients with deep venous incompetence, and more complex reconstructive surgery to the deep veins is not often indicated.

Great saphenous recurrence

Very often, the scar of a low incision (Fig. 24.3) indicates that the great saphenous vein has been ligated well below the saphenofemoral junction (the original Trendelenburg operation) and recurrent venous incompetence is the result of persisting saphenofemoral incompetence and communication between patent groin tributaries and the more distal great saphenous vein. In this situation, the operation is a simple one as the origin of the saphenofemoral junction will be free

of scar tissue. If, however, the scar of the original incision is in its proper place, high in the groin and extending laterally from the origin of adductor longus, the surgeon must expect to encounter more difficulty, due to dense scar tissue. This operation can be very difficult indeed for the inexperienced, and should never be undertaken for the first time without supervision. If the scar tissue is not too dense, as sometimes happens, a normal approach to the saphenofemoral junction may be possible, controlling numerous varicose tributaries by diathermy, coagulation or ligation as these are found during the dissection. If, however, very dense scar tissue is found, the wise operator will use the technique described by Li.[11] Through a standard groin incision, dissection is aimed directly down on to the femoral artery, whose pulsation can usually be felt without difficulty. The operator must be careful not to stray lateral to the artery, where branches of the femoral nerve may be damaged. Tributaries of the saphenofemoral junction are likely to be encountered and are divided and controlled (Fig. 24.4a).

After opening the femoral sheath, the femoral artery is exposed and the dissection then proceeds medially to the femoral vein. Proximal dissection along its lateral border will soon lead to the saphenofemoral junction, which is then approached from below. There is no need for complicated

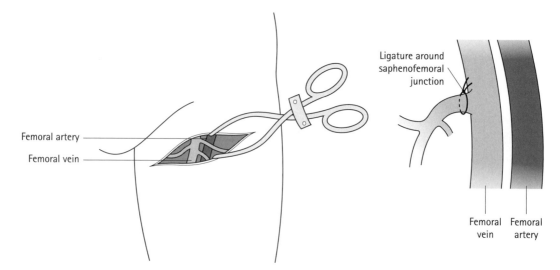

Figure 24.4 *(a) The femoral artery is exposed and dissection medially exposes the femoral vein, deep to the deep fascia and to scar tissue. (b) Dissection is continued proximally along the femoral vein until the saphenofemoral junction is reached. This is ligated in continuity with an unabsorbable ligature.*

dissection of all its branches; it is sufficient simply to pass a non-absorbable ligature round the termination of the saphenous vein into the femoral vein by means of an aneurysm needle or a large round-bodied needle (Fig. 24.4b). The ligature is then tied and effectively cuts off all communication between the great saphenous vein and its tributaries and the common femoral vein. It is highly desirable to divide the saphenofemoral junction following ligation to minimize the risk of further neovascularization. The recurrent varices should be separated from the saphenofemoral junction as far as possible. The authors recognize that it is not always possible to remove all recurrent varices from the femoral region, and excessively zealous dissection may risk damage to the lymphatics lying medially to the femoral vein. This can lead to a lymphatic leak, lymphocele or even lymphedema!

Residual great saphenous vein

For many years it was common practice to ligate the saphenofemoral junction on the assumption that this would prevent reflux in the great saphenous vein, which was not stripped. Unfortunately, this is not the case[12] and reflux in the residual vein often leads to the development of recurrent varicose veins. This operation also increased the risks of saphenofemoral recurrence. The management of this pattern of recurrence includes re-ligation of any recurrence at the saphenofemoral junction with stripping of the residual vein. Preoperatively the anatomy of the recurrence should be studied using duplex ultrasonography and the position of the saphenous trunk marked on the leg. If re-exploration of the groin has been undertaken, it may be possible to identify the proximal part of the saphenous trunk in the femoral triangle. Stripping can then be undertaken in a conventional manner. The

authors' preference is to use the Oesch pin-stripper, which can usually be guided down residual saphenous trunks (Plates 24.1 and 24.2).

In patients where there is no need to re-explore the groin, the saphenous vein can be easily located via an incision in the skin crease at the knee. The vein usually lies fairly close to the skin at this point, although it is still contained in its fascial compartment in most patients. It is not normally in close proximity to the saphenous nerve as the vein crosses the knee. An Oesch pin-stripper can then be passed proximally along the vein and easily retrieved through a tiny incision near the groin. This allows the residual vein to be stripped from the knee to the groin. If necessary, the saphenous vein in the calf can also be stripped from the knee, although the saphenous nerve may be damaged if care is not taken during this procedure.

The surgery of recurrent small saphenous incompetence

INVESTIGATION

Exposure of the saphenopopliteal junction in recurrent small saphenous incompetence is made difficult by scar tissue from the previous dissection and its precise localization is of the utmost importance. It is essential to undertake an imaging procedure to establish the anatomy of a recurrence in this region. The most effective way of doing this is to undertake duplex ultrasonography. In preference, this should be done by the surgeon or demonstrated to the surgeon by a technologist. An alternative is to use varicography, in which contrast medium is injected into one of the posterior calf varices but does not give a direct indication of the relationship of the

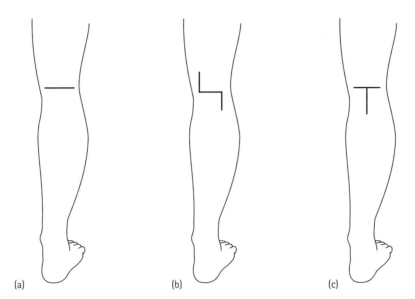

Figure 24.5   *Z or T incisions increase exposure in the surgery of recurrent saphenopopliteal incompetence: (a) popliteal incision; (b) Z incision; (c) T incision.*

recurrence to the soft tissues. Simple hand-held Doppler ultrasonography can be used but is less accurate and gives no anatomical information. It is regarded as insufficient to be used alone as a method of preoperative assessment. The level of the saphenopopliteal junction above the knee joint, or above the popliteal skin crease, must be recorded precisely, as an error of even 1 or 2 cm can result in difficulties in dissection, especially if the incision is placed too high. Duplex ultrasonography will usually indicate the surgical approach that will be least complex. The location of the vein and the recurrent saphenopopliteal junction can be marked on the skin before operation (Plate 24.3).

THE OPERATION

The operation is essentially the same as that for primary saphenopopliteal ligation in the treatment of small saphenous incompetence, but the presence of scar tissue makes it wise to increase the exposure. Usually this can be achieved via a slightly longer transverse incision than usual. This provides the best cosmetic result. If essential, the transverse incision can be converted to a T or a Z incision (Fig. 24.5) and is rarely needed these days if preoperative assessment is correctly performed. The muscle fascia should be divided. It is common practice to divide the fascia longitudinally in order to obtain better access to the popliteal fossa. Dissection is continued through scar tissue and the sciatic nerve and branches are identified at an early stage in the operation to minimize the risk of neurological injury. The varicose tributaries of the saphenopopliteal junction are ligated and divided as these are encountered. The popliteal vein should be identified positively and flush ligation of the saphenopopliteal junction performed. This will usually mean retraction of the overlying popliteal and common peroneal nerves, which must be

undertaken with the utmost gentleness to avoid a postoperative neuropraxia.

This is probably the most difficult dissection in superficial vein surgery and should never be undertaken by those with inadequate experience.

Recurrent varices on the posterior, medial or lateral surface of the calf may result from gastrocnemius vein incompetence. This can be identified by duplex scan or varicography and the responsible vein is divided at operation, taking care not to damage the adjacent popliteal nerve.

In cases of recurrent saphenopopliteal reflux, it is the authors' experience that many patients have residual small saphenous veins which are incompetent and fill calf varices. No publication has attempted to show whether small saphenous vein stripping is effective in preventing recurrence of varices, as has been done with the great saphenous vein. However, it is likely that stripping this vein will help in reducing recurrence of varices. Where this vein remains following previous surgery, it is often the source of filling of recurrent calf varices and should be stripped at operations for saphenopopliteal recurrence. This can be done easily at operations for primary varices, but is more difficult where a previous operation has been done. If the vein can be identified in the popliteal fossa then it can be removed by inverting stripping to the ankle using an Oesch pin-stripper. If this proves to be infeasible, the distal small saphenous vein can be dissected near the ankle and the pin-stripper passed proximally. Inverting stripping does not damage the sural nerve accompanying the vein if care is taken with dissection of the point at which the stripper is passed into the vein. The authors have routinely used this technique to remove the small saphenous vein for more than 10 years and have encountered very few cases of sural nerve neuropraxia.

The surgery of incompetent perforating veins in recurrent venous ulceration

Unlike surgery in the groin, this is usually straightforward. Mid-thigh perforators are identified by duplex scan or varicography (see Fig. 24.1). Duplex ultrasonography allows the exact location of the perforating vein to be marked on the skin to facilitate correct placing of the skin incision. The perforating vein is approached and ligated through a vertical incision. Calf perforating veins in patients with recurrent ulceration are likely to lie under lipodermatosclerotic skin and it is important to avoid this by using a subfascial endoscopic approach. Traditionally, incompetent medial calf perforating veins were ligated using an open approach though a vertical incision, described originally by Linton. Such operations were commonly associated with delayed healing of the incision made through liposclerotic skin. More recently, an endoscopic technique has been employed which avoids incisions in liposclerotic skin. This achieves a much shorter stay in hospital and does not prejudice the long-term outcome.[13] The only problem which remains is to define exactly which patients will benefit from such operations. This remains a matter of uncertainty at present.

Ligation of the distal great saphenous vein in the treatment of recurrent ulceration

In patients with recurrent ulceration and deep venous incompetence, who have previously been treated by saphenous

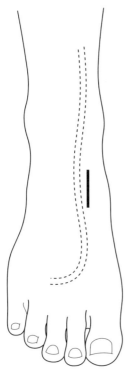

Figure 24.6 *The incision for distal long saphenous ligation in patients with ulceration and deep vein incompetence.*

ligation and stripping and perforating vein ligation, and in whom no saphenous reflux or perforating vein incompetence can be demonstrated, it is worth measuring resting and exercising pressures (see Ch. 4, p. 31) in the great saphenous vein distal to the medial malleolus and, if temporary occlusion reduces the peak systolic pressures produced by calf muscle contraction, ligating the distal great saphenous vein will often achieve ulcer healing (Fig. 24.6).

DEEP VENOUS RECONSTRUCTIVE SURGERY

Only when all other venous surgery has been exhausted without effective ulcer healing should duplex scan or descending venography be performed to confirm deep venous reflux. Deep venous reconstructive surgery is described by Kistner *et al.* in Chapter 20.

THE INVESTIGATION AND TREATMENT OF RECURRENT ISCHEMIC ULCERATION

Recurrent ischemic ulceration may result from occlusion of the original bypass graft or from further atherosclerotic stenosis or occlusions in the leg arteries. The method of choice for the investigation of lower limb arterial disease is now duplex ultrasonography, which will reveal exactly where the arterial occlusion lies and indicate the severity of any stenosis. Intravenous digital subtraction angiography is used to obtain detailed images of vessels, usually as part of an interventional procedure. Treatment by balloon angioplasty may be possible, and a few ischemic ulcers may heal following chemical lumbar sympathectomy, but arterial bypass surgery is likely to be necessary (see Ch. 22).

In many of these elderly patients, no suitable vessel can be found for bypass surgery and amputation is then necessary.

Amputation for ischemic ulceration: delayed primary wound closure

Most patients with ischemic ulcers have severely diseased femoral as well as distal vessels, and below-knee amputations are unlikely to heal. Mid-thigh amputation is therefore more usual. Ischemic ulcers are all infected to a greater or lesser extent and whether the amputation is above or below the knee, the incisions will necessarily cut through lymph trunks which contain bacteria originating from the ulcer. If primary closure is performed, these will multiply and lead to wound infection, which is likely to require revision of the amputation stump.

It is therefore wiser to adopt the principle of delayed primary closure; appropriate antibiotic therapy is given pre- and postoperatively and, following amputation, the skin edges are approximated loosely over gauze packs soaked in Flavine emulsion. These are removed after 48 hours and formal closure of the muscles, deep fascia and skin is then undertaken. With this regimen, it is unusual for postoperative infection to develop and most amputation stumps heal satisfactorily.

The same principle is applied to digital or forefoot amputations, although these should not usually be attempted in the presence of main vessel atherosclerosis, and local toe or foot amputation is usually only appropriate for ischemic ulceration resulting from diabetic microangiography. Occasionally, healing can be obtained in patients with occlusions of the main arteries following a course of intravenous prostacyclin, but only in those with ankle pulse pressures above 50 mmHg.[14]

ALLERGIC ULCERATION

If no other cause for recurrence can be found, consider the possibility of allergy to compression stockings, usually a rubber allergy, and change these to stockings containing Lycra or other synthetic material. Systematic testing for sensitivity for common allergens can be performed if this diagnosis is suspected.

CONCLUSIONS

No method of treatment of leg ulcers has ever achieved 100 percent success, whatever the underlying cause. The surgeon with a busy leg ulcer clinic is therefore bound to meet many disappointments. Many patients can benefit from modern methods of investigation and treatment, and in cases where patients with recurrent ulceration would be fit enough to undergo surgical treatment, full investigation should be undertaken in the hope that a surgically remediable problem can be identified. Assiduous use of firm compression bandaging and stockings will benefit the many patients unsuitable for surgical intervention.

REFERENCES

1. Franks PJ, Oldroyd MI, Dickson D *et al*. Risk factors for leg ulcer recurrence: a randomized trial of two types of compression stocking. *Age Ageing* 1995; **24**: 490–4.

2. Franks PJ, Bosanquet N, Connolly M *et al*. Venous ulcer healing: effect of socioeconomic factors in London. *J Epidemiol Community Health* 1995; **49**: 385–8.

3. The ESCHAR ulcer study: a randomised controlled trial assessing venous surgery in 500 leg ulcers. Belfast: Vascular Surgical Society of Great Britain and Ireland, 2002.

4. Brown DB, Irvine RW, Forrest H. Long term results of 'high ligation' for varicose veins. *Scott Med J* 1961; **6**: 322–6.

5. Sarin S, Scurr JH, Coleridge Smith PD. Assessment of stripping the long saphenous vein in the treatment of primary varicose veins. *Br J Surg* 1992; **79**: 889–93.

6. Dwerryhouse S, Davies B, Harradine K, Earnshaw JJ. Stripping the long saphenous vein reduces the rate of reoperation for recurrent varicose veins: five-year results of a randomized trial. *J Vasc Surg* 1999; **29**: 589–92.

7. van Rij AM, Jiang P, Solomon C *et al*. Recurrence after varicose vein surgery: a prospective long-term clinical study with duplex ultrasound scanning and air plethysmography. *J Vasc Surg* 2003; **38**: 935–43.

8. Fischer R, Linde N, Duff C *et al*. Late recurrent saphenofemoral junction reflux after ligation and stripping of the greater saphenous vein. *J Vasc Surg* 2001; **34**: 236–40.

9. De Maeseneer MG, Giuliani DR, Van Schil PE, De Hert SG. Can interposition of a silicone implant after sapheno-femoral ligation prevent recurrent varicose veins? *Eur J Vasc Endovasc Surg*, 2002; **24**: 445–9.

10. Bradbury AW, Stonebridge PA, Ruckley CV, Beggs I. Recurrent varicose veins: correlation between pre-operative clinical and hand-held Doppler ultrasonographic examination, and anatomical findings at surgery. *Br J Surg* 1993; **80**: 849–51.

11. Li AKC. A technique for re-exploration of the sapheno-femoral junction for recurrent varicose veins. *Br J Surg* 1975; **62**: 745–6.

12. McMullin GM, Coleridge Smith PD, Scurr JH. Objective assessment of high ligation without stripping the long saphenous vein. *Br J Surg* 1991; **78**: 1139–42.

13. Sybrandy JE, van Gent WB, Pierik EG, Wittens CH. Endoscopic versus open subfascial division of incompetent perforating veins in the treatment of venous leg ulceration: long-term follow-up. *J Vasc Surg* 2001; **33**: 1028–32.

14. Negus D, Irving JD, Friedgood A. Intra-arterial Prostacyclin compared to Praxilene in the management of advanced atherosclerotic lower limb ischaemia. In: Gryglewski RJ, Szczeklik A, McGiff JC, eds. *Prostacyclin, Clinical Trials*. New York: Raven Press, 1985; 111.

25

Compression hosiery: compression measurements and fitting

ROBERT GARDINER, DAVID NEGUS

Compression hosiery is used to control edema from any cause, to compress varicose veins and to prevent venous thrombosis. This account will concentrate on its role in the prevention and treatment of venous ulceration. It is important that those doctors responsible for running ulcer clinics have some knowledge of elastic hosiery construction and compression

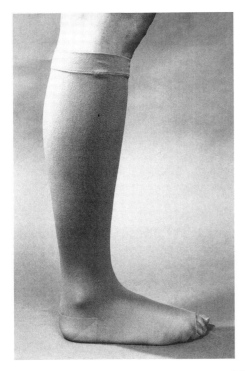

Figure 25.1 *Class 2, knee-length compression stocking (Medi UK, Hereford, UK).*

values and of the various products available, as this aspect of management is as important as accurate diagnosis and treatment.

There have been a number of important developments in the design and manufacture of elastic compression hosiery in recent years. Modern garments are better fitted, more comfortable and more effective than those that were available 15 or 20 years ago (Fig. 25.1). Most modern elastic hosiery is of two-way stretch construction, using Lycra for the elastic fibres, although a few manufacturers still use natural rubber. In 1985, a British Standard (BS6612:1985)[1] was introduced. This was prepared by the Textile and Clothing Standards Committee, which included physicians, surgeons and hosiery manufacturers. The major requirements of the British Standard have been incorporated in the drug tariff, which was revised in 1988, which now makes it possible for doctors and surgeons to prescribe effective, comfortable and attractive stockings without difficulty.

STOCKING PRESSURES AND TESTING METHODS

The British Standard allows manufacturers to assign a standard compression value (in mmHg) to each garment, after it has been washed and conditioned for at least 16 hours in a standard atmosphere. Compression must be graduated up the stocking, from a maximum at the ankle to a minimum at the thigh; the greater the compression at the ankle, the steeper this decrease must be. The standard also specifies the stiffness and durability of garments and requires them to be marked with size, compression value, washing instructions, the manufacturer's label and 'BS 6612:1985'. Stockings in the Drug

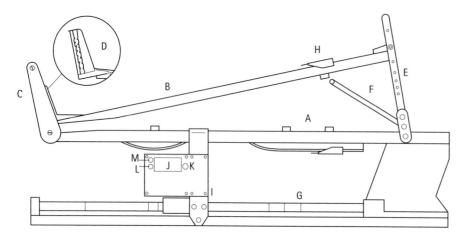

Figure 25.2 *The HATRA stocking tester. A, fixed lower bar; B, movable top bar; C, fixed outer foot; D, movable inner foot with adjustment holes; E, upper adjustment bar; F, raising bar; G, traverse rail; H, suspender clip; I, measurement head; J, digital display; K, operating switch button; L, zero adjustment; M, scale adjustment (Segar Design, Nottingham, UK).*

Tariff are graded into three classes according to the compression they exert at the ankle: class 1, light (14–17 mmHg); class 2, medium (18–24 mmHg); and class 3, strong (25–35 mmHg).

Unfortunately, there is still some confusion about measuring stocking pressures as accepted methods vary from one country to another. While all British-made stockings are expected to comply with the Drug Tariff specification and British Standard, with pressures measured by the Hosiery and Allied Trades Retail Association (HATRA) device, there are many excellent brands of stockings available in the UK which are manufactured in Europe, mainly in Germany or Switzerland. German and Swiss stockings are tested by the Hohenstein (HOSY) method, in which the stocking is stretched and tension measured using a computerized system. Details of the HATRA method are given below and the results provided by this and the HOSY method are compared. Some stockings are also imported from the USA, particularly by the Kendall Company, and the pressures of these are measured by yet another device, the Instron Tester, a modified tensiometer, which measures the tension in a section of stocking held between two movable T-pins. Stockings tested only by the HOSY method have been available for use in hospitals for several years and continue to be so.

These testing devices are all independent of the actual leg on which the stocking is to be fitted. There are devices now available which measure the actual pressure exerted by a compression stocking on the human leg. The first of these was developed by Dr Sigg of Switzerland over 40 years ago. This consisted of a small balloon connected to an aneroid manometer. The balloon is slid under the stocking and the subsequent pressure noted on the manometer. Unfortunately, the shape of the balloon distorts the radius of curvature of the leg and therefore does not measure the pressure accurately. An improvement on this device is the Borgnis medical stocking tester, which consists of a thin plastic sleeve inserted between the stocking and the leg. Electrodes are printed into the walls of the sleeve and compressed air is pumped into the sleeve by a small pump. As soon as the pressure produced by

the compressed air inside the sleeve overcomes the pressure of the stocking compressing the sleeve against the leg, the proximal pair of electrodes (where the pressure should be least) are forced apart. This breaks an electrical circuit, which automatically stops the pump and simultaneously records the pressure within the sleeve. The pressure is noted and the pump restarted; the pressure increases and, provided that the stocking is correctly graduated, the next more distal pair of electrodes are then forced apart, stopping the machine and recording the pressure again. This process is continued until all the electrodes in the sleeve have been forced apart and a record of pressures at 10 cm intervals along the leg is then obtained. Care must be taken that the sleeve is not placed over any bony points, which will provide a false reading. This is a simple device and useful for the clinician, who can check that his patients are being fitted correctly by surgical fitters. The disadvantage is that pressures are measured at fixed points and that the device cannot be left on the leg under a stocking or bandage for any length of time in order to enable serial measurements to be carried out. An improvement on the Borgnis tester is the Oxford Pressure Monitor marketed by Talley Medical Ltd. The sensors can be placed independently over areas of specific interest and the small plastic sleeves can be retained under compression hosiery for hours or days in order to allow repeat measurements.

HATRA and HOSY pressure measurement

The HATRA tester consists of a 'leg former' (Fig. 25.2), on which the stocking is placed and then stretched by pulling out a movable bar. A measuring head is then applied to the stretched stocking to obtain the fabric tension at the desired position. The HATRA tester thus requires the stocking to be stretched so that it is in a similar energy state to that when it is applied to the leg. The HOSY tester measures the tension between numerous points marked on a stocking stretched over an expandable leg former by means of a computerized device.

Drug tariff	Class 1	Class 2		Class 3		
HATRA test	15 mmHg	20 mmHg	25 mmHg	30 mmHg	35 mmHg	
HOSY test	18–21 mmHg		23–32 mmHg	34–46 mmHg		50 mmHg
	Continental class 1	Continental class 2		Continental class 3		

Ankle compression →

Figure 25.3 *The Drug Tariff classification of stocking pressures with HATRA and HOSY measurements (see text). Note that the latter are consistently higher in each class.*

Figure 25.3 shows the relationship between Drug Tariff compression classes and HOSY compression classes; although test methods differ, this shows that the HOSY garments are manufactured to ankle pressure consistently higher than Drug Tariff.

EFFECT ON THE VENOUS PUMP

In the following paragraphs, stocking pressures are those measured by the HATRA method, except where otherwise indicated.

Struckmann[2] has demonstrated that venous muscle pump function (assessed by ambulatory calf volume strain gauge plethysmography) in patients with saphenous and perforating vein incompetence is improved by class 2 and 3 graduated compression stockings exerting pressures of between 20 and 40 mmHg (Borgnis MST-Salzmann, Switzerland) at the ankle. Class 3, 'strong' stockings, providing compression of 25–35 mmHg, have been demonstrated to be effective in improving calf muscle pump function in patients with post-thrombotic deep venous reflux.[3] In practice, class 2 compression stockings (18–24 mmHg) seem to be equally effective, possibly because of better compliance. The precise compression required remains controversial, but it is generally agreed that the hosiery need exert less compression than that theoretically expected from measurements of the ankle venous pressures in patients with superficial or deep venous pathology. During walking, venous pressure at the ankle is about 25 mmHg in normal subjects, 40 mmHg in patients with superficial varicose veins and 60 mmHg in those with post-thrombotic deep vein incompetence. However, hosiery pressures lower than these are effective in controlling edema and 'heaviness' of the leg and this appears to be for two reasons. First, by Laplace's formula for tubes ($P = T/R$, where P is the pressure in dyn/cm^2, T is the tension in dyn/cm, and R is the radius of curvature of the surface being compressed), the pressure exerted on an individual superficial vein with its small radius will be greater than that exerted on the limb as a whole.[4] Second, the plasma protein osmotic pressure of 25 mmHg opposes tissue fluid formation and edema.

PRACTICAL APPLICATIONS

Class 1 (UK), light (14–17 mmHg) stockings are recommended for simple varicose veins. In fact, simple varicose veins can often be controlled perfectly adequately by lighter hosiery providing only 5–10 mmHg compression. This is due to the Laplace relationship. Most women now prefer to wear tights and, if prescribed on an FP10, these will not be reimbursed by the Family Health Services Authority. Present prescribing regulations treat each leg of a pair of tights prescribed in hospital as a separate prescription item; the present (2005) prescription charge is £6.50; the total cost to the patient is therefore £6.50 × 2 = £13.00, which is greater than the retail price of most support tights with low compression values. In the venous ulcer clinic, the most commonly prescribed stockings are class 2 (UK) (medium) graduated compression stockings, exerting pressures of 18–24 mmHg (HATRA) at the ankle. These include Duomed (Medi UK, England), Venosan (Salzmann, Switzerland), and Kendall Class 2 (Tyco, USA).

Mediven Plus (Medi, UK), Venosan 2002 (Salzmann, Switzerland) and Sigvaris 503 (Ganzoni, Switzerland) are HOSY class 2 stockings. Knee-length compression stockings are usually perfectly adequate and are much preferred by men. A number of manufacturers now produce colored class 2 compression socks – black and brown – which are much preferred for normal daily wear. These stockings should be prescribed for patients who have had acute deep vein thrombosis and are likely to develop post-thrombotic incompetence of the deep and perforating veins, leading eventually to ulceration. There is no scientific evidence that application of such stockings does, in fact, delay the onset of ulceration, but post-thrombotic heaviness and edema are well controlled by class 2 stockings and the authors' impression is that the more severe symptoms and signs of the post-thrombotic syndrome, liposclerosis and ulceration, do seem to be delayed.

A number of surgeons recommend the use of class 2 compression stockings, applied over appropriate non-adherent dressings, in ulcer healing. There is no doubt that stockings maintain their pressure better than bandages, but the disadvantage is that exudate from an ulcer will seep through dressings and stain overlying bandages or stockings. Both can be washed, but bandages can be replaced more cheaply than stockings and for that reason bandages are used in most ulcer clinics. Others may find class 2 compression stockings preferable and, as bandages have to be replaced more frequently than stockings, there is probably little difference in the overall cost of healing an ulcer.

In the authors' series of 77 patients with 109 ulcerated legs, patients with evidence of deep venous incompetence were fitted with knee-length class 2 compression stockings, following ligation of incompetent perforating and saphenous veins (see p. 31). This regimen has given satisfactory results. Only very few patients, with very large legs or very severe venous disorders, require class 3 compression stockings. The Sigvaris 504 stockings (Ganzoni) (HOSY class 3) have proved very satisfactory. Great care must be taken to exclude any arterial insufficiency before prescribing either class 2 or class 3 stockings.

STOCKING APPLICATION

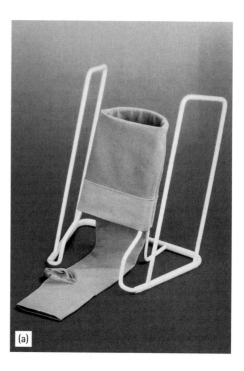

Medium compression or strong stockings (class 2 or 3) are often difficult to apply, particularly for the elderly. Patients with arthritis of the hands may find stocking application quite impossible. In practice, we have found that most patients can get help from a relative or neighbour. However, there are a number of tricks and devices that will help. Most Continental stocking manufacturers provide a nylon or silk sock to help the stocking slide over the foot. Rubber washing-up gloves are of considerable help in obtaining a good grip of the top of the stocking and even elderly patients who thought they would be unable to manage find that they can exert sufficient strength with the help of these. Finally, an ingenious device has been developed in Germany and is marketed by Medi UK Ltd. This is called the Medi Valet and consists of a plastic-covered steel frame (Fig. 25.4) over which the stocking is stretched. The patient slips the foot and ankle into the opened stocking. The frame is then pulled up the leg, allowing the stocking to slip off in the correct position. Other manufacturers (Crendenhill, Kendal and Sigvaris) now offer similar devices.

One final tip about applying stockings is most useful if, as happens quite frequently, a stocking is a little too long for the patient's leg. The natural tendency then is for the patient to pull hard on the stocking, so as to remove wrinkles in the lower leg and ankle, and then fold over the stocking top so that it lies just below the patella. Folding over the top of the stocking is liable to result in excessive pressure just below the knee with a consequent tourniquet effect, which negates the whole point of a graduated elastic stocking. To avoid this problem, the stocking top should be pulled up so that it lies in its natural position just below the patella. If the stocking is a little too long, this will result in wrinkles in the lower leg. Any large wrinkle should be picked up between finger and thumb so that it is converted into two or three smaller wrinkles. These are then rubbed briskly with the hand and, due to the elasticity of the material, they will gradually iron out so that the stocking lies flat and at normal tension. This trick is most useful in practice and we have met few surgical appliance officers, doctors or nurses who were aware of it. A number of manufacturers now provide stockings with a choice of leg length, and made-to-measure stockings are also available.

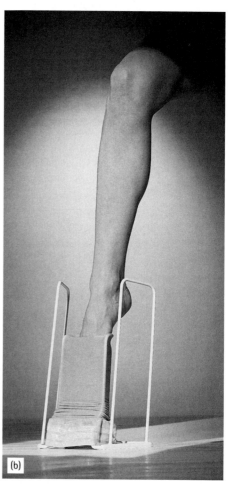

Figure 25.4 *The Medi Valet. (a) Stocking in place over frame; (b) insertion of the foot. The frame and stocking is then pulled up over the lower leg.*

CONSTRUCTION AND DURABILITY

Until the Drug Tariff was revised in 1988, only rubber elastic threads were permitted in the construction of approved compression hosiery. However, rubber is more susceptible to damage by heat, oil and medicaments and a number of patients become sensitized and develop allergic dermatitis. The revised Drug Tariff specification permits the use of Lycra. Most stockings currently available are now of synthetic construction. With wear and tear and regular washing, they maintain their elasticity for about 3 months. It is our policy to prescribe a pair of stockings to any patient with ulceration of one leg. The stockings are interchangeable between legs and they can therefore be worn alternately, one being washed and dried while the other is in use. In this way, a pair should last for 6 months. It is most important that they are renewed after this time.

REFERENCES

1. British Standards Institution. *BS 6612 Specification for Graduated Compression Hosiery.* Milton Keynes: British Standards Institution, 1985.
2. Struckmann J. Compression stockings and their effect on the venous pump – a comparative study. *Phlebology* 1986; **1**: 37–45.
3. Cornwall JV, Dor E, Lewis JD. To graduate or not? The effect of compression garments on venous refilling time. In: Negus D, Jantet G, eds. *Phlebology '85.* London: Libbey, 1986; 676–8.
4. Fentem PH, Goddard N, Gooden PA. The pressure exerted on superficial veins by support hosiery. *J Physiol* 1976; **263**: 151–2.

26

Pharmacological treatment in venous leg ulcers

PHILIP D. COLERIDGE SMITH

INTRODUCTION

Venous ulceration and the skin changes which precede ulceration are best managed by careful objective evaluation of the venous system of the lower limb followed by compression bandaging or stockings and surgical treatment where appropriate. Systemic drugs and topical applications are widely used in the management of leg ulceration but what should we use and when? Surgical intervention is appropriate where leg ulceration is attributable mainly to superficial venous incompetence alone in a patient fit enough for this procedure. In some studies, this would apply to as many as half the patients presenting with venous ulceration.[1,2] A number of studies show that healing usually progresses well in such patients and recurrent ulceration is not a common problem.[3] A relatively small proportion of patients are suitable for deep vein reconstructive procedures; many are excluded because of age and infirmity or medical unfitness for major surgery. In general, such patients are best managed by compression treatment alone. Unfortunately, whilst compression treatment can usually achieve healing if high enough levels of compression are used, recurrence is a common problem, with an annual recurrence rate of 25 percent per year.[4] Perhaps drugs can speed healing or prevent recurrence? Many clinical studies have been published over the years. Examination of them is informative and revealing!

The question is, which mechanisms of leg ulceration should be addressed and therefore which drugs should be used? The factor which initiates leg ulceration is incompetence of venous valves leading to venous hypertension. No drug has been shown to restore valvular competence or reduce venous reflux. It may be possible to modify the consequences. Bacterial infection can be influenced by antibiotics. Dietary supplements (such as zinc) can be added to make up for deficiency in diet. In 1982, Browse and Burnand[5] published a medical hypothesis suggesting that pericapillary fibrin cuffs observed microscopically in histological sections of skin led to hypoxia of the tissues and ulceration. This led to the use of pro-fibrinolytic treatments to manage leg ulcers. More recently, a role of inflammatory mechanisms has been suggested.[6] These too can be influenced by a number of groups of drugs.

ANTIBIOTICS

'Virtually every antibiotic that has ever been produced has been used to treat venous ulcers but there is very little evidence that they help healing unless the ulcer is contaminated by a single pathogenic organism'.[7] The reliability of this assertion by Browse et al. has not been revised by subsequent research. A detailed review of the use of chronic wounds has been published recently and this finds no support for the routine use of antibiotics in the management of venous leg ulcers.[8] Naturally, clinical infection of an ulcer must be treated, but this is best done by local ulcer toilet, unless cellulitis or septicemia supervene. In these circumstances, intravenous antibiotics are usually indicated.

VITAMINS, ZINC AND DIETARY DEFICIENCY

The finding by Greaves and Skillen[9] that leg ulceration was healed after a 4-month course of 220 mg zinc sulfate three times daily[9] led to interest in dietary supplements. In a double-blind trial of oral zinc in 38 patients with venous ulcers,[10] no advantage of oral zinc supplements was found. This has been confirmed by other authors.[11,12]

Adequate nutrition is as essential for leg ulcer healing as it is for wound healing of other types. A group of authors in the USA found deficiencies of vitamins A and E, the carotenes and zinc in patients being treated for venous leg ulcers.[13] They speculated that this reflected compromised nutritional status which might influence leg ulcer healing rates. It was found in a further study that the dietary intake of protein, vitamin C and zinc may be inadequate in elderly patients with leg ulcers.[14] This has led to a renewal of the suggestion that dietary supplements should be given to elderly patients with leg ulcers;[15] however, a broader approach than single vitamin supplements was used.

FIBRINOLYTIC THERAPY

The fibrin cuff hypothesis of Browse and Burnand[5] led to more research into the changes of fibrinolytic mechanisms in patients with venous disease. The modulation of coagulation and fibrinolysis has been studied in patients with venous disease and in control subjects.[16] There was an increase of systemic levels of plasminogen activator inhibitor 1 (PAI-1) activity and tissue plasminogen activator (tPA) with inpatients with more severe venous disease. In the group with active ulceration, there was an elevation of fragments $1 + 2$ (F1 + 2). These data suggest increased fibrinolytic activity and fibrin turnover but do not indicate the role of these factors in venous disease.

Stacey et al.[17] has examined the leg skin of patients with venous disease to assess the role of pericapillary fibrin deposition in patients with venous disease. He studied 19 patients with healed unilateral venous ulceration and no history of venous disease in the other leg. Pericapillary fibrin distribution was studied by skin biopsy and immunofluorescence microscopy. Pericapillary fibrin deposits were observed in the dermis in 16 of the biopsies of the gaiter region and in eight of the biopsies from the thigh. There was no correlation with euglobulin clot lysis time. The authors conclude that pericapillary fibrin deposition is an early sign of the development of skin changes in patients with venous disease.

Therapeutic manipulation of the fibrinolytic system has been attempted in a number of clinical trials in patients with venous disease. A double-blind trial in 60 patients was performed to evaluate the efficacy of this drug.[18] Stanozolol combined with compression stockings caused a reduction of liposclerotic skin area of 28 percent over 6 months. However, when the separate contributions of the two treatment elements (compression and stanozolol) were calculated using multivariate analysis of variance, the effect attributable to stanozolol alone was not statistically significant.

Fibrinolytic treatment for venous ulceration has been evaluated in one trial of 75 patients.[19] Patients were allocated to receive either stanozolol or placebo for up to 420 days, with conventional compression treatment in all cases. In an interim report, the authors found complete healing in 26 out of 40 ulcers in the stanozolol group and 27 out of 44 in the placebo group, indicating no benefit from active over placebo treatment. Stanozolol has now been withdrawn from use in the UK for the treatment of patients with venous disease.

In a recent study, tPA has been added as a topical treatment to leg ulcers as an ointment.[20] The authors assessed the presence of pericapillary fibrin on skin biopsies before and after the treatment but found no difference. However, despite this, three out of six ulcers studied healed during the 12 weeks of the investigation.

Dermatan sulfate (DS) is a glycosaminoglycan which selectively catalyses the inactivation of thrombin by heparin cofactor II without interacting with antithrombin III. It does not interact with other coagulation factors and, unlike heparin, is able to inactivate thrombin bound to fibrin or to the surface of an injured vessel. Two DS-containing compounds, sulodexide and, in particular, mesoglycan, have been clinically studied in a number of trials and found to be effective in the treatment of venous and arterial leg diseases.

Sulodexide, a highly purified glycosaminoglycan with pro-fibrinolytic properties, has also been used to treat patients with venous leg ulcers.[21] A total of 235 patients were randomized to receive sulodexide or placebo for 3 months. The authors reported improved healing in the active treatment group compared with placebo. No further detailed work on this compound has been published.

DRUGS WHICH MODIFY LEUKOCYTE METABOLISM

The discovery of the involvement of leukocytes in the development of venous ulceration has opened new avenues of investigation in this area.[6] A number of drugs which modify white cell activation have been evaluated in patients with venous ulceration, with interesting results.

Prostaglandin E₁

Prostaglandin E_1 (PGE_1) has a number of profound effects on the microcirculation, including reduction of white cell activation, platelet aggregation inhibition, small vessel vasodilatation and reduction of vessel wall cholesterol levels.[22] It has been evaluated in the treatment of various aspects of arterial disease; less work has been done on its use in venous ulceration. An early trial of the use of intravenous PGE_1 in ulcers of both arterial and venous etiology reported improvement in four out of five venous ulcers on PGE_1 as opposed to four out of seven on placebo – hardly a dramatic result.[23] A further trial yielded more impressive findings.[24] Forty-four patients with proven venous ulceration took part in a double-blind placebo-controlled trial. Each received an infusion of PGE_1 (or placebo) over 3 hours daily for 6 weeks, in addition to standard dressings and compression bandaging. Those on PGE_1 showed a significant improvement in such parameters as edema reduction, symptoms and 'ulcer score', based on depth, diameter, etc. Perhaps more importantly, eight out of 20 patients on active treatment healed their ulcers completely within the trial period, whereas only two out of 22 controls did so.

The reason for the different outcomes in these two trials probably relates to the dose of PGE_1 given. In Beitner et al.'s study,[23] only two infusions were given. These consisted of 360 μg of PGE_1 in 3 L of isotonic saline over 72 h, a month apart. In the second trial, 60 μg were given over 3 h every day for 6 weeks – a total dose 3.5 times than that in the earlier study. Although this rather intensive way of treating ulcers is not, at first sight, attractive, the cost of such treatment must be weighed against the large cost of the outpatient care of unhealed ulcers.

Unfortunately, no further studies have been published and the regular use of PGE_1 in the management of leg ulceration has proceeded no further.

Prostacyclin analogues

Iloprost (Schering, Berlin, Germany), a synthetic prostacyclin analogue, has been used with success in the treatment of arterial and diabetic ulcers.[25] The mechanism of action of prostacyclin includes increased fibrinolytic activity;[26] the drug also has profound effects on leukocyte activity by reducing aggregation and adherence to endothelium,[27,28] in addition to its better known effects on platelet behavior.[29] However, a study in which this was applied topically to venous ulcers was disappointing.[30] The trial design was a randomized, double-blind, placebo-controlled study in 11 centres in Germany with 49 patients allocated to placebo, 49 patients to 0.0005 percent Iloprost, and 50 patients to 0.002 percent Iloprost. The study solutions were applied twice weekly for a period of 8 weeks on the ulcer edge and ulcer surrounding. This study failed to show any statistically significant reduction in the ulcer size as a result of the Iloprost treatment compared with placebo. Perhaps this was true failure of efficacy of this drug, or perhaps the drug delivery system did not achieve therapeutic levels in the tissues. No further data have been published concerning Iloprost in the management of venous disease and it is not in common use in the management of leg ulceration.

Pentoxifylline

A Cochrane review addressed the use of pentoxifylline in the management of venous leg ulcers.[31] The authors of this review identified eight clinical trials which could be analysed. They found that overall pentoxifylline led to improved venous ulcer healing with a relative risk of 1.41 [95 percent confidence interval (CI) 1.19–1.66] overall and, when used in combination with compression, of 1.30 (95 percent CI 1.10–1.54) compared with placebo. They concluded that this drug is an effective adjunct to compression bandaging when used to treat venous ulcers.

Aspirin

The use of aspirin has been reported in a small number of patients undergoing treatment for leg ulceration.[32] The authors describe a measurable effect of aspirin on the rate of ulcer healing. However, this study includes 20 patients of whom only four healed their ulcers after 4 months' treatment. These are extremely preliminary data on which to base any conclusions concerning treatment of patients. One paper proposes that abnormalities in coagulation measurements (fibrinogen, factor VIII related antigen, von Willebrand antigen and PAI-1), which are perturbed in patients with venous disease, may be modified by the therapeutic use of aspirin.[33] Currently, the mode of action of aspirin and the extent of its efficacy in the management of venous ulceration remain to be shown. No further paper has been published since 1995 which addresses the efficacy of aspirin in venous leg ulceration, so the actual effect of aspirin on leg ulceration has never been reliably established.

Ifetroban

The effect of the oral thromboxane A2 receptor antagonist Ifetroban (250 mg daily) on healing of chronic lower-extremity venous stasis ulcers has been studied. This drug has a profound inhibitory effect on platelet activation and therefore could be a commercially viable successor to aspirin should efficacy be shown. In a prospective, randomized, double-blind, placebo-controlled multicentre study,[34] 165 patients were randomized to Ifetroban ($n = 83$) versus placebo ($n = 82$) for a period of 12 weeks. Both groups were treated with sustained graduated compression and hydrocolloid dressings for the ulcers. Complete ulcer healing was achieved after 12 weeks in 55 percent of patients receiving Ifetroban and in 54 percent of those taking a placebo with no significant differences; 84 percent of ulcers in both groups achieved greater than 50 percent area reduction in size. This was a well conducted study with a clear primary end-point (complete ulcer healing in a patient). The findings strongly refute the suggestion that platelet inhibition will lead to leg ulcer healing.

VENOACTIVE DRUGS IN LEG ULCERATION

Far less has been written about the efficacy of this group in the management of leg ulceration than in the management of the symptoms of varicose veins. Interest in this field has increased in recent years and a few studies have been published.

A study on the effect of rutosides on symptoms in 112 patients with venous insufficiency included four with ulceration. All four took rutosides for 8 weeks; only one showed any evidence of improvement.[35] Other studies have shown no evidence that hydroxyrutosides improve venous ulcer healing or prevent its recurrence. In 138 patients with recently healed venous ulcers, Wright et al.[36] compared the efficacy of below the knee elastic stockings combined with hydroxyrutosides (Paroven 500 mg b.d.) or placebo. The recurrence rates at 12 months were 23 percent with hydroxyrutosides and 22 percent with placebo. After 18 months the figures were 34 and 32 percent, respectively. These results show no evidence that hydroxyrutosides prevent ulcer recurrence when combined with elastic compression. It is clear that rutosides have a measurable effect on edema in patients with venous disease. Unfortunately they do not have any effect on preventing venous leg ulcer recurrence. A possible extension of this conclusion is that treatment of edema alone (where rutosides have efficacy) is insufficient to treat leg ulceration. Some additional factor must be influenced in order to speed ulcer healing (in which rutosides have not been tested) or to prevent recurrence of ulceration.

A pilot study in 25 patients with venous ulceration or skin changes at the ankle was performed in India.[37] Patients all received calcium dobesilate 500 mg twice a day for 8 weeks. Symptoms of venous disease improved and ulcers decreased in size. This uncontrolled study provides no suggestion of activity of this drug in the management of venous ulceration.

FLAVONOIDS

The effect of Daflon 500 mg (Servier, Paris, France) in a venous ulcer healing study has been reported.[38] Patients were randomized to receive Daflon 500 mg or placebo combined with standard compression bandaging during an 8-week follow-up period. In 91 patients with an ulcer diameter of 10 cm or less, 14 out of 44 (32 percent) patients receiving Daflon 500 mg compared with six of 47 (13 percent) receiving placebo healed their ulcers ($P = 0.028$, χ^2) after 8 weeks' treatment (Fig. 26.1). The time to achieve healing was shorter in the Daflon 500 mg group than in the placebo group ($P = 0.037$) (Fig. 26.2). This is the only member of the 'edema protective' drug group which has been shown to modify ulcer healing. Despite the fact that the study was relatively small and the duration of treatment was short (8 weeks), the results are encouraging. A further study conducted in Poland compared a series of patients treated with either conventional treatment plus Daflon 500 mg or conventional treatment alone.[39] More ulcers healed in the Daflon-treated group compared with the conventional treatment alone group. However, this study was conducted in an open way so that both patients and doctors were aware of the treatment being given. Most recently a third study by Roztócil et al.[40] has demonstrated the influence of Daflon 500 on ulcer healing. This was a controlled trial, conducted in 17 different centres, comparing Daflon 500 treatment with compression therapy against compression therapy alone in patients with ulcers of diameter ≥ 2 cm to ≤ 10 cm.

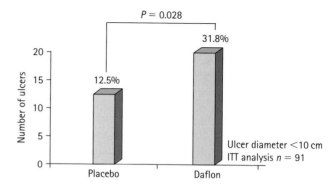

Figure 26.1 *Number of ulcers healed in randomized clinical trial of Daflon versus placebo after 8 weeks' treatment.[38]*

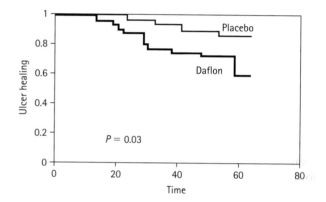

Figure 26.2 *Rate of ulcer healing in Daflon treatment and placebo groups in a randomized clinical trial.[38]*

Significantly more ulcers healed ($P = 0.004$) and there was greater ulcer area reduction ($P = 0.012$) in the Daflon 500 group. This occurred from as early as 8 weeks. In addition, the rate of healing for large ulcers was twofold higher in the Daflon 500 group ($P = 0.008$) and the percentage of large ulcers healed before 24 weeks was significantly higher ($P = 0.008$). In fact, Daflon 500, in addition to conventional treatment compared with conventional therapy alone, reduced the ulcer 'complete' healing time by 29 days (Daflon 500 group + conventional therapy, 137 days; conventional therapy alone, 166 days). The results of a meta-analysis of five randomized controlled studies using Daflon 500 in venous leg ulcer healing were recently presented at the UIP Meeting (August 27–31, 2003; San Diego, CA, USA). This meta-analysis confirmed that venous ulcer healing is accelerated by adding Daflon 500 to conventional treatment.

A pilot study has been conducted using Daflon 500 mg.[41] Twenty patients with chronic venous disease (CEAP clinical stage 2–4) were treated for 60 days with Daflon 500 mg twice daily taken orally. There was no placebo control group in this pilot study. Blood samples before and after the treatment were collected from a foot vein. Plasma levels of the soluble endothelial adhesion molecules sVCAM-1, sICAM-1, sP-selectin and sE-selectin were determined. In addition, the endothelial-derived von Willebrand factor (vWF), the neutrophil secondary granule enzyme lactoferrin and vascular endothelial growth factor (VEGF) levels were determined using a standard sandwich enzyme-linked immunosorbent assay (ELISA) method. In addition, the neutrophil and monocyte surface adhesion molecules CD11b and L-selectin (CD62L) were assessed by a flow cytometric technique.

The expression of the leukocyte adhesion molecule CD62L was substantially decreased on monocytes and neutrophils by Daflon 500 treatment; however, CD11b expression was not modified. This finding suggests that leukocyte L-selectin interaction with endothelial selectins responsible for the initial stages of adhesion may be modulated by Daflon 500 treatment, reducing the likelihood of leukocyte adhesion and presumably acting as an anti-inflammatory mechanism.

Significant downregulation of plasma levels of sVCAM-1 and sICAM-1 activity following therapy was observed, indicating that endothelial damage which ensues in venous disease from chronic venous hypertension was mitigated by Daflon 500 treatment. In a model of venous hypertension achieved by formation of an arteriovenous fistula between the femoral vessels of the Wistar rats,[42] the results show that venous reflux developed which could be significantly inhibited by the administration of Daflon 500 (Takase et al., unpublished data). More detailed study is required to determine whether these measurable anti-inflammatory effects of flavonoids are central to the efficacy of flavonoids in the management of venous disease.

TOPICALLY APPLIED PREPARATIONS

A wide range of preparations is applied to venous leg ulcers in an attempt to heal them. A review of these would constitute a chapter in itself! A particular feature of patients with chronic venous disease of the leg and leg ulceration is their ability to become sensitized to many topically applied compounds. In most leg ulcer clinics, extreme care is used in topical applications since many commonly used drugs can produce skin sensitization. Antibiotics are common culprits. Aminoglycoside antibiotics, commonly present in preparations for topical use, may cause skin sensitization. They have no effect on the healing of venous leg ulcers and should never be used. Topical steroids are often invaluable in the management of skin eczema resulting from sensitivity to one of the many chemicals used in the treatment of leg ulcers. Sometimes sensitization occurs to one of the components of steroid creams and, occasionally, to the steroids themselves.

'Active' treatments which might be applied topically include antiseptics such as cadexomer iodine. Cadexomer iodine paste has been compared with hydrocolloid dressings and paraffin gauze dressings and has been found to lead to more rapid reduction in ulcer surface area.[43] However, this paper did not assess time to complete healing of ulcers and therefore falls short of modern levels of proof of efficacy. The use of local antiseptic agents might address the bacterial colonization of

ulcers, but since it seems unlikely that infection is the main cause of the continuation of a leg ulcer, the effect of this type of treatment might be limited.

The work of Knighton et al.[44] suggested to many that venous leg ulcer healing could be speeded by the use of growth factors derived from platelets. This has led to preparations of platelet growth factors being licenced in the USA for use in non-healing leg and foot ulcers in patients with diabetes.[45] However, there is evidence that this type of compound has no effect in venous leg ulcers.[46] Some authors have investigated granulocyte–macrophage colony-stimulating factor (GM-CSF) in the treatment of venous leg ulcers.[47] No large-scale leg ulcer healing study has been published showing an advantage of this type of treatment. A number of problems present themselves with this method of management. First, it makes the assumption that venous leg ulceration is the result of faulty healing as well as the mechanisms which resulted in leg ulceration in the first place. It presumably makes the assumption that levels of growth factors in healing ulcers are pathologically reduced. There is no published evidence to support this assumption. Studies that have investigated the levels of tissue growth factors in ulcers show no reduction of growth factors in ulcers, although there is some evidence of reduced receptors for transforming growth factor-β (TGF-β).[48] Interestingly, ulcer fluid appears to have an inhibitory effect on angiogenesis.[49] Finally, there are the logistics of delivering a drug to an ulcer at a dose which is sustained and effective. This is especially difficult since ulcer dressings may remain in place for several days. It seems highly improbable that such an approach will be effective in patients with venous leg ulcers.

CONCLUSIONS

In the management of leg ulceration, the following systemically administered drugs are ineffective at achieving healing of ulcers: aspirin, ifetroban, stanozolol, antibiotics and hydroxyrutosides. Topical growth factors have yet to be shown to have efficacy in this context. Pentoxifylline and Daflon 500 mg have some efficacy in achieving ulcer healing when given systemically. It is clear that the available pharmacological treatments for venous disease are less effective than compression treatments or surgery in achieving healing of ulcers and that drug treatments should usually be used as part of a regime of management rather than as an isolated treatment.

SUMMARY

Drugs are widely used in the management of chronic venous disease and leg ulceration. Compression and surgical treatment of incompetent superficial veins are the first-line measures which should be used to manage leg ulceration and skin changes. Antibiotics are useful where there is clinically obvious infection such as cellulitis, but are ineffective in speeding ulcer healing. Topical steroids are helpful in managing skin allergy but do not promote ulcer healing. The nutritional status of elderly patients with leg ulcers may be compromised and measures should be taken to maintain an adequate diet. Many topical drugs have been applied to leg ulcers but none has been shown to promote leg ulcer healing to a clinically useful extent.

Only two drugs have been found to promote leg ulcer healing in clinical trials. These include the methylxanthine pentoxifylline which promotes blood flow, downregulates leukocyte activation and enhances fibrinolytic mechanisms. The flavonoid drug Daflon 500 mg has also been found to promote leg ulcer healing in clinical trials. This drug has anti-edema effects as well as downregulating several inflammatory mechanisms which may be involved with the development of leg ulcers. These drugs may be used in combination with compression and surgery to superficial and perforating veins in the management of leg ulcers.

REFERENCES

1. Scriven JM, Hartshorne T, Thrush AJ et al. Role of saphenous vein surgery in the treatment of venous ulceration. Br J Surg 1998; 85(781): 4.

2. Shami SK, Sarin S, Cheatle TR et al. Venous ulcers and the superficial venous system. J Vasc Surg 1993; 17: 487–90.

3. Ghauri AS, Nyamekye I, Grabs AJ et al. Influence of a specialised leg ulcer service and venous surgery on the outcome of venous leg ulcers. Eur J Vasc Endovasc Surg 1998; 16: 238–44.

4. Franks PJ, Oldroyd MI, Dickson D et al. Risk factors for leg ulcer recurrence: a randomized trial of two types of compression stocking. Age Ageing 1995; 24: 490–4.

5. Browse NL, Burnand KG. The cause of venous ulceration. Lancet 1982; ii: 243–5.

6. Coleridge Smith PD, Thomas P et al. Causes of venous ulceration: a new hypothesis. Br Med J 1988; 296: 1726–7.

7. Browse NL, Burnand KG, Lea Thomas ML. Diseases of the Veins. London: Arnold, 1988.

8. O'Meara SM, Cullum NA, Majid M, Sheldon TA. Systematic review of antimicrobial agents used for chronic wounds. Br J Surg 2001; 88: 4–21.

9. Greaves MW, Skillen AW. Effects of long-continued ingestion of zinc sulphate in patients with venous leg ulceration. Lancet 1970; ii: 889–91.

10. Greaves MW, Ive FA. Double-blind trial of zinc sulphate in the treatment of chronic venous leg ulceration. Br J Derm 1972; 87: 632–4.

11. Myers MB, Cherry G. Zinc and the healing of chronic leg ulcers. Am J Surg 1970; 120: 77–81.

12. Phillips A, Davidson M, Greaves MW. Venous leg ulceration. evaluation of zinc treatment, serum zinc and rate of healing. Clin Exp Dermatol 1977; 2: 395–9.

13. Rojas AI, Phillips TJ. Patients with chronic leg ulcers show diminished levels of vitamins A and E, carotenes, and zinc. Dermatol Surg 1999; 25: 601–4.

14. Wipke-Tevis DD, Stotts NA. Nutrition, tissue oxygenation, and healing of venous leg ulcers. J Vasc Nurs 1998; 16: 48–56.

15. Wissing UE, Ek AC, Wengstrom Y et al. Can individualised nutritional support improve healing in therapy-resistant leg ulcers? J Wound Care 2002; 11: 15–20.

16. Blomgren L, Johansson G, Siegbahn A, Bergqvist D. Coagulation and fibrinolysis in chronic venous insufficiency. Vasa 2001; 30: 184–7.

17. Stacey MC, Burnand KG, Bhogal BS, Black MM. Pericapillary fibrin deposits and skin hypoxia precede the changes of lipodermatosclerosis in limbs at increased risk of developing a venous ulcer. Cardiovasc Surg 2000; 8: 372–80.

18. McMullin GM, Watkin GT, Coleridge Smith PD, Scurr JH. Efficacy of fibrinolytic enhancement in the treatment of venous insufficiency. Phlebology 1991; 6: 233–9.

19. Layer GT, Stacey MC, Burnand KG. Stanozolol and the treatment of venous ulceration – an interim report. Phlebology 1986; 1: 197–203.

20. Zeegelaar JE, Verheijen JH, Kerckhaert JA et al. Local treatment of venous ulcers with tissue type plasminogen activator containing ointment. Vasa 1997; 26: 81–4.

21. Coccheri S, Scondotto G, Agnelli G et al. Venous arm of the SUAVIS (Sulodexide Arterial Venous Italian Study) randomised, double blind, multicentre, placebo controlled study of sulodexide in the treatment of venous leg ulcers. Thromb Haemost 2002; 87: 947–52.

22. Sinzinger H, Virgolini I, Fitscha P. Pathomechanisms of atherosclerosis beneficially affected by prostaglandin E1 (PGE1) – an update. Vasa Suppl 1989; 28: 6–13.

23. Beitner H, Hamar H, Olsson AG, Thyresson N. Prostaglandin E1 treatment of leg ulcers caused by venous or arterial incompetence. Acta Dermatovenerol (Stockholm) 1980; 60: 425–30.

24. Rudofsky G. Intravenous prostaglandin E1 in the treatment of venous ulcers – a double-blind, placebo-controlled trial. Vasa Supplement 1989; 28: 39–43.

25. Muller B, Krais T, Sturzebacher S et al. Potential therapeutic mechanisms of stable prostacyclin (PGI2) mimetics in severe peripheral vascular disease. Biomed Biochim Acta 1988; 47: S40–4.

26. Musial J, Wilczynska M, Sladek K et al. Fibrinolytic activity of prostacyclin and Iloprost in patients with peripheral arterial disease. Prostaglandins 1986; 31: 61–70.

27. Belch JJ F, Saniabadi A, Dickson R et al. Effect of Iloprost (ZK 36374) on white cell behaviour. In: Gryglewski RJ, Stock G, eds. Prostacyclin and its Stable Analogue Iloprost. Berlin: Springer-Verlag, 1987; 97–102.

28. Muller B, Schmidtke M, Witt W. Adherence of leucocytes to electrically damaged venules in vivo. Eicosanoids 1988; 1: 13–7.

29. Sturzebecher CS, Losert W. Effects of Iloprost on platelet activation in vitro. In: Gryglewski RJ, Stock G, eds. Prostacyclin and its Stable Analogue Iloprost. Berlin: Springer-Verlag, 1987; 39–45.

30. Werner-Schlenzka H, Kuhlmann RK. Treatment of venous leg ulcers with topical Iloprost: a placebo controlled study. Vasa 1994; 23: 145–50.

31. Jull AB, Waters J, Arroll B. Pentoxifylline for treating venous leg ulcers (Cochrane Review). In: The Cochrane Library, Issue 4. Chichester, UK: John Wiley, 2003.

32. Layton AM, Ibbotson SH, Davies JA, Goodfield MJ. Randomised trial of oral aspirin for chronic venous leg ulcers. Lancet 1994; 34: 164–5.

33. Ibbotson SH, Layton AM, Davies JA, Goodfield MJ. The effect of aspirin on haemostatic activity in the treatment of chronic venous leg ulceration. Br J Dermatol 1995; 132: 422–6.

34. Lyon RT, Veith FJ, Bolton L, Machado F. Clinical benchmark for healing of chronic venous ulcers. Venous Ulcer Study Collaborators. Am J Surg 1998; 176: 172–5.

35. Pulvertaft TB. Paroven in the treatment of chronic venous insufficiency. Practitioner 1979; 223: 838–41.

36. Wright DD, Franks PJ, Blair SD *et al*. Oxerutins in the prevention of recurrence in chronic venous ulceration: randomised controlled trial. *Br J Surg* 1991; **78**: 1269–70.

37. Kaur C, Sarkar R, Kanwar AJ *et al*. An open trial of calcium dobesilate in patients with venous ulcers and stasis dermatitis. *Int J Dermatol* 2003; **42**: 147–52.

38. Guilhou JJ, Dereure O, Marzin L *et al*. Efficacy of Daflon 500 mg in venous leg ulcer healing: a double-blind, randomised, controlled versus placebo trial in 107 patients. *Angiology* 1997; **48**: 77–85.

39. Glinski W, Chodynicka B, Roszkiewicz J *et al*. The beneficial augmentative effect of micronized purified flavonoid fraction (MPFF) in the healing of leg ulcers. An open multicentre, controlled randomised study. *Phlebology* 1999; **14**: 151–7.

40. Roztócil K, Stvrtinová V, Strejæek J. Efficacy of a 6 month treatment with Daflon 500 mg in patients with venous leg ulcers associated with chronic venous insufficiency. *Int Angiol* 2003; **22**: 24–31.

41. Shoab SS, Porter J, Scurr JH, Coleridge Smith PD. Endothelial activation response to oral micronised flavonoid therapy in patients with chronic venous disease–a prospective study. *Eur J Vasc Endovasc Surg* 1999; **17**: 313–8.

42. Van Bemmelen SP. Venous valvular incompetence: an experimental study in the rat. *MD Thesis*. Amsterdam: University of Amsterdam, 1984.

43. Hansson C, Persson L-M, Stenquist B *et al*. The effects of cadexomer iodine paste in the treatment of venous leg ulcers compared with hydrocolloid dressing and paraffin gauze dressing. *Int J Derm* 1998; **37**: 390–6.

44. Knighton DR, Ciresi K, Fiegel VD *et al*. Stimulation of repair in chronic, nonhealing, cutaneous ulcers using platelet-derived wound healing formula. *Surg Gynecol Obstet* 1990; **170**: 56–60.

45. Steed DL, Webster MW, Ricotta JJ *et al*. Clinical evaluation of recombinant human platelet-derived growth factor for the treatment of lower extremity diabetic ulcers. *J Vasc Surg* 1995; **21**: 71–81.

46. Stacey MC, Mata SD, Trengove NJ, Mather CA. Randomised double-blind placebo controlled trial of topical autologous platelet lysate in venous ulcer healing. *Eur J Vasc Endovasc Surg* 2000; **20**: 296–301.

47. Marques da Costa R, Jesus FM, Aniceto C, Mendes M. Double-blind randomized placebo-controlled trial of the use of granulocyte-macrophage colony-stimulating factor in chronic leg ulcers. *Am J Surg* 1997; **173**: 165–8.

48. Cowin AJ, Hatzirodos N, Holding CA *et al*. Effect of healing on the expression of transforming growth factor beta(s) and their receptors in chronic venous leg ulcers. *J Invest Dermatol* 2001; **117**: 1282–9.

49. Drinkwater SL, Smith A, Sawyer BM, Burnand KG. Effect of venous ulcer exudates on angiogenesis *in vitro*. *Br J Surg* 2002; **89**: 709–13.

27

Topical agents to promote wound healing

PHILIP D. COLERIDGE SMITH

INTRODUCTION

Faced with a venous leg ulcer that fails to heal despite proper use of conventional treatments, it is an appealing thought that the topical application of a missing factor might lead to successful wound healing. The mechanisms which result in wound healing are complex and are coordinated by a complex system of chemical signalling mechanisms (cytokines) which are released by many of the cells involved in the healing process. These ensure that blood vessels grow into the region bringing fibroblasts to create the connective tissue and subsequently keratinocytes to form new skin. When healing is complete, the huge synthesis of new tissues must be switched off again. The many mechanisms involved are complex and might be manipulated by drugs or synthetic cytokines applied directly to the ulcer. In wound healing circles, cytokines which manipulate and regulate the growth of specific cell types are referred to as 'growth factors'.

GROWTH FACTORS INVOLVED IN WOUND HEALING

The growth factors referred to below all occur in a number different isoforms and therefore each type represents a 'family' of growth factors. In the summary here, each is referred to as if it were a single entity. The biological activity of each family is in general similar and this simplification is therefore justified for ease of understanding.

Platelet-derived growth factor

Platelet-derived growth factor (PDGF) is released by many different cell types in addition to platelets. These include fibroblasts, endothelial cells, macrophages and keratinocytes. Receptors for this growth factor are present on macrophages, polymorphonuclear cells and fibroblasts. When a cell binds PDGF this in turn triggers a number of intracellular events that achieve a number of different results. In the case of macrophages and polymorphonuclear cells this results in chemotaxis, therefore, the release of PDGF into a wound will attract these cells. The inflammatory cells deal with infection and foreign debris in a wound and are attracted by the growth factor which is released from the platelet plugs in vessels damaged in the creation of any wound. Macrophages attracted to the wound in turn release PDGF to attract fibroblasts. The fibroblasts are responsible for the formation of collagen and ground substance.

Transforming growth factor-beta

Transforming growth factor-beta (TGF-β) is released by platelets and macrophages. This process therefore occurs early in the healing of an acute wound as platelets granulate, and is sustained by the influx of macrophages as the wound begins to heal. This factor is chemotactic for neutrophils and macrophages, participating in the inflammatory phase of wound healing. Many cells possess receptors for TGF-β and can respond to its release. However, perhaps the most important cell type participating in wound healing which can respond is the fibroblast, which synthesizes greatly increased amounts of collagen and fibronectin in response. TGF-β also stimulates the expression of integrins on the surface of fibroblasts. These bind extracellular matrix, including collagen and fibronectin, and facilitate migration of these cells through the wound along the fibronectin scaffolding. TGF-β also stimulates the expression of integrins on the surface of keratinocytes which allows them to migrate across the wound in order to achieve healing.

Fibroblast growth factor

Fibroblast growth factor (FGF) is released by macrophages and fibroblasts. One isoform of FBG, basic FGF (b-FGF) is well characterized; it is chemotactic for fibroblasts and endothelial cells and this is a potent angiogenic factor. FGF stimulates fibroblasts to produce collagen, fibronectin and proteoglycan. These characteristics make FGF important in the formation of granulation tissue.

Epidermal growth factor

Epidermal growth factor (EGF) is released by platelets and macrophages. Many cells possess receptors for this growth factor which is chemotactic and mitogenic for keratinocytes, fibroblasts and endothelial cells. It also stimulates the production of intercellular matrix by fibroblasts. As well as stimulating epithelialization, this factor is responsible for stimulating the formation of granulation tissue.

Colony-stimulating factors

A range of colony-stimulating factors exist, including granulocyte–macrophage colony-stimulating factor (GM-CSF). These attract and stimulate leukocytes and macrophages in the chronic wound.

EVIDENCE FOR IMPAIRED WOUND HEALING IN PATIENTS WITH LEG ULCERS

The factors which lead to impaired wound healing in patients with leg ulcers are not entirely clear. It is generally accepted that ambulatory venous hypertension leads to a chronic inflammatory state in the skin and that this in turn leads to leg ulceration. Curiously, it has been found that there is considerable upregulation of healing processes in liposclerotic skin. Pappas et al.[1] found that activated leukocytes traverse perivascular cuffs in the skin of patients with lipodermatosclerosis. These release active TGF-β1, which binds to dermal fibroblasts which respond by synthesizing connective tissue proteins, including collagen.[1] The clinical consequence of this series of events is that liposclerotic skin appears inflamed and

extensive fibrosis is present throughout the skin and subcutaneous tissues in these patients. These events precede ulceration and predispose to tissue breakdown, although the reasons for the increased susceptibility of such to skin ulceration remain unclear.

The pathological processes leading to leg ulceration are still in existence when an active ulcer is present. These can be mitigated by use of compression and surgery to minimize venous hypertension. At least one cause of an ulcer failing to heal will be the continuing damaging effects of these mechanisms.

What evidence is there that a failure of the healing mechanisms is present in leg ulcers? Falanga[2] has proposed that growth factors become bound to the connective tissue proteins and are therefore not available to the healing tissues. He based this assertion on observations from immunohistochemical studies that growth factors including TGF-β1 were located around the capillaries in the perivascular cuff.[3] A possible flaw in this argument is that many of the macrophages which produce the growth factors are also located in the pericapillary region and this may merely represent the site of synthesis and release of these growth factors. In further work, fibroblasts were taken from the skin surrounding leg ulcers and from control subjects. It was found that the responsiveness to stimulation of leg ulcer fibroblasts with TGF-β1 was greatly reduced compared with those taken from normal skin. This was attributable to reduced expression of receptors for this growth factor on the leg ulcer fibroblasts.[4] Further studies have confirmed this observation and suggested that the intracellular signaling mechanisms in ulcer fibroblasts may be impaired.[5]

Lal et al.[6] have shown that, even in non-ulcerated liposclerotic skin, fibroblasts show diminished TGF-β1 responsiveness, despite his earlier publication on the causes of skin fibrosis in lipodermatosclerosis.[6] Similarly, it has been found that PDGF has greatly reduced stimulatory effects on fibroblasts derived from leg ulcers.[7] There has been considerable concentration in much of this work on the effects of the promoters of cellular growth and synthesis of connective tissue components. In most biological systems, such upregulatory mechanisms are balanced by inhibitors. These have been sought in the fluid obtained from venous ulcers and the effects on vascular proliferation have been investigated. It was found that fluid exudate from leg ulcers inhibited vascular proliferation, especially if the fluid came from a slowly healing ulcer.[8] Further study has shown that there are considerable amounts of the cytokine vascular endothelial growth factor (VEGF) in the wound fluid which would normally promote angiogenesis.[9] The inhibitory effect of wound fluid on angiogenesis suggests that undefined inhibitors of angiogenesis are also present in the wound fluid.

I conclude that we far from understand the complex processes that occur in a healing ulcer and therefore, at present, trying to manipulate them to obtain leg ulcer healing will remain an empirical science. The fluid bathing the healing ulcer clearly contains many promoters of cellular growth and synthesis as well as many inhibitors. Whether these are deranged to the extent that ulcer healing is impaired is not clear. Fibroblasts obtained from leg ulcers show lack of response to many of the normal growth factors, but how this could be reversed has not been demonstrated. The complexity of this problem has not prevented clinical trials of individual growth factors being carried out to assess the effect of these on ulcer healing.

CLINICAL TRIALS OF TOPICAL AGENTS TO PROMOTE ULCER HEALING

Stacey et al.[10] have investigated the effect of a topically applied lysate of platelets on the healing of venous leg ulcers. Autologous platelets were used and a lysate prepared which would be expected to contain PDGF and other growth factors. This was applied topically to leg ulcers in a study which included 86 patients. Patients were randomized to receive either platelet lysate or buffer solution to their ulcer combined with conventional compression treatment. Patients were followed up until the ulcer healed or for 9 months. The rate of healing in the two groups was identical. Studies have also been performed in diabetic ulcers with human recombinant PDGF where beneficial effects on healing have been observed.[11] TGF-β2 has been investigated in the promotion of venous ulcer healing.[12] No statistically significant evidence of accelerated wound healing was found. Falanga et al.[13] have investigated the efficacy of a topically applied human recombinant growth factor on the healing of venous ulcers. They applied the EGF twice a day and investigated the influence on ulcer healing over a period of 10 weeks. They could find no evidence of influence of this growth factor on leg ulcer healing.

GM-CSF has been investigated in a number of studies. In a small series (10 patients), recombinant human GM-CSF (rhGM-CSF) was injected adjacent to the leg ulcer. Healing was obtained in eight of the patients within 4 weeks.[14] In a double-blind placebo-controlled study, 60 patients were investigated.[15] Patients were assigned to placebo, 200 μg or 400 μg peri-ulcer injections of rhGM-CSF. After 13 weeks, four out of 21 (19 percent) placebo, 12 out of 21 (57 percent) of the 200 μg rhGM-CSF and 11 out of 18 (61 percent) 400 μg rhGM-CSF patients healed their ulcers. This result reaches statistical significance. A further clinical series involved 38 patients with venous leg ulcers. Topical rhGM-CSF was used in combination with compression treatment. Complete healing was observed in 47 of the 52 ulcers (90 percent). The average healing time was 19 weeks. No recurrent ulcer was observed after 40 months of follow-up.

THE ROLE OF TOPICAL GROWTH FACTORS IN THE MANAGEMENT OF VENOUS ULCERATION

I believe it is fair to say that, in venous ulceration, topical growth factor applications are of little or no use in achieving healing. In the UK, no growth factor is registered with regulatory authorities for this purpose. In patients with diabetic ulcers, a commercial preparation of PDGF, becaplermin (Janssen-Cilag, High Wycombe, UK), is available to promote ulcer healing and is used as a topical application. The data I have presented above show that there is the possibility that GM-CSF may be useful in patients with venous ulceration, but its effects have only been examined in relatively small studies. No data on large-scale clinical trials are available.

A philosophical question arises here as to whether the application of a single growth factor to an ulcer can have any material influence on the complex mechanisms at work. The factors that resulted in the ulcer in the first instance are still present. There is considerable production of growth factors by the patient's own cells. This is opposed by many unknown inhibitors of these growth factors, also produced by the patient's cells. The target tissues of this complex mixture are the fibroblasts, endothelial cells and keratinocytes, which may themselves be impaired in their function by all of these processes. We still are not clear as to whether venous ulcers are perpetuated by the destructive processes which are discussed in detail in Chapter 7 or by faulty healing. My interpretation of the data I have presented above is that faulty healing has not been conclusively demonstrated in venous ulcers. Therefore, it may not be possible to improve it, even if we did understand the complex interaction between the individual processes that have been measured. There is clearly detailed scope for research in this field in order to clarify matters. It may be more profitable to attempt to use pharmacological manipulation of the destructive processes leading to the leg ulcer rather than to promote the healing mechanisms.

REFERENCES

1. Pappas PJ, You R, Rameshwar P et al. Dermal tissue fibrosis in patients with chronic venous insufficiency is associated with increased transforming growth factor-beta1 gene expression and protein production. J Vasc Surg 1999; **30**: 1129–45.
2. Falanga V. Growth factors and chronic wounds: the need to understand the microenvironment. J Dermatol 1992; **19**: 667–72.
3. Higley HR, Ksander GA, Gerhardt CO, Falanga V. Extravasation of macromolecules and possible trapping of transforming growth factor-beta in venous ulceration. Br J Dermatol 1995; **132**: 79–85.
4. Hasan A, Murata H, Falabella A et al. Dermal fibroblasts from venous ulcers are unresponsive to the action of transforming growth factor-beta 1. J Dermatol Sci 1997; **16**: 59–66.
5. Kim BC, Kim HT, Park SH et al. Fibroblasts from chronic wounds show altered TGF-beta-signaling and decreased TGF-beta type II receptor expression. J Cell Physiol 2003; **195**: 331–6.
6. Lal BK, Saito S, Pappas PJ et al. Altered proliferative responses of dermal fibroblasts to TGF-beta1 may contribute to chronic venous stasis ulcer. J Vasc Surg 2003; **37**: 1285–93.
7. Vasquez R, Marien BJ, Gram C et al. Proliferative capacity of venous ulcer wound fibroblasts in the presence of platelet-derived growth factor. Vasc Endovasc Surg 2004; **38**: 355–60.

8. Drinkwater SL, Smith A, Sawyer BM, Burnand KG. Effect of venous ulcer exudates on angiogenesis *in vitro*. *Br J Surg* 2002; **89**: 709–13.

9. Drinkwater SL, Burnand KG, Ding R, Smith A. Increased but ineffectual angiogenic drive in nonhealing venous leg ulcers. *J Vasc Surg* 2003; **38**: 1106–12.

10. Stacey MC, Mata SD, Trengove NJ, Mather CA. Randomised double-blind placebo controlled trial of topical autologous platelet lysate in venous ulcer healing. *Eur J Vasc Endovasc Surg* 2000; **20**: 296–301.

11. Smiel JM, Wieman TJ, Steed DL *et al.* Efficacy and safety of bacaplermin (recombinant human platelet derived growth factor-BB) in patients with non-healing lower extremity diabetic ulcers: a combined analysis of randomised studies. *Wound Repair Regen* 1999; **7**: 335–46.

12. Robson MC, Phillips LG, Cooper DM. The safety and effect of transforming growth factor beta 2 for the treatment of venous stasis ulcers. *Wound Repair Regen* 1995; **3**: 157–67.

13. Falanga V, Eaglstein WH, Bucalo B *et al.* Topical use of human recombinant epidermal growth factor (h-EGF) in venous ulcers. *J Dermatol Surg Oncol* 1992; **18**: 604–6.

14. Borbolla-Escoboza JR, Maria-Aceves R, Lopez-Hernandez MA, Collados-Larumbe MT. Recombinant human granulocyte-macrophage colony-stimulating factor as treatment for chronic leg ulcers. *Rev Invest Clin* 1997; **49**: 449–51.

15. Da Costa RM, Ribeiro Jesus FM, Aniceto C, Mendes M. Randomized, double-blind, placebo-controlled, dose-ranging study of granulocyte-macrophage colony stimulating factor in patients with chronic venous leg ulcers. *Wound Repair Regen* 1999; **7**: 17–25.

Index